Connecting the Quality of Life Theory to Health, Well-Being and Education

Alex C. Michalos

Connecting the Quality of Life Theory to Health, Well-Being and Education

The Selected Works of Alex C. Michalos

Springer

Alex C. Michalos
University of Northern British Columbia
Prince George, BC
Canada

ISBN 978-3-319-51160-3 ISBN 978-3-319-51161-0 (eBook)
DOI 10.1007/978-3-319-51161-0

Library of Congress Control Number: 2017934322

Printed on acid-free paper

This Springer imprint is published by Springer Nature
The registered company is Springer International Publishing AG
The registered company address is: Gewerbestrasse 11, 6330 Cham, Switzerland

Other Books by Alex C. Michalos

North American Social Report, 5 volumes
Global Report on Student Well-Being, 4 volumes
Essays on the Quality of Life
Ancient Views on the Quality of Life
Militarism and the Quality of Life
Foundations of Decision Making
Trade Barriers to the Public Good
Good Taxes
A Pragmatic Approach to Business Ethics
Principles of Logic
Improving Your Reasoning
The Popper-Carnap Controversy

For Deborah, with love

Acknowledgements

Most of the previously published papers in this set of four volumes (and most of my books) appeared in a publication of Springer, Kluwer, Reidel or Nijhoff, a chain of publishers that I have had the opportunity to work with since the 1960s. Since the original source of each paper in the collection is given on its first page in this collection, there is no need to repeat all these sources and express my thanks for permission to reprint them in each occurrence. I am happy to express here my gratitude for the lot and for the many years of our pleasant and productive work together.

In each of the volumes in this set, I have acknowledged permission to reprint each of the previously published papers appearing in scholarly journals, books or newspapers apart from the chain of publishers listed above. In this fourth volume, there are no previously published papers appearing in publications outside the chain.

In the Appendix of each volume, I included some photographs and pictures to provide a somewhat different kind of historical context to my narrative. What I have been able to contribute over the past 50 years or so have been influenced by many more people than I have been able to picture here, but when I reflect on what I have done, most of the people pictured here are very much a part of the story. Most of the photos and pictures are from my family albums, but some have come from friends and a couple newspapers. I would like to express my thanks to the following for allowing me to reprint their items: Wolfgang Glatzer for photographs in How Good Policies and Business Ethics Enhance Good Quality of Life, numbered v2.1 (short for photo #1, volume 2), in Development of the Quality of Life Theory and its Instruments (v3.3, v3.5, and v3.6), and in Connecting the Quality of Life Theory to Health, Well-Being and Education (v4.1); to Ferran Casas for photographs v2.6, 3.1, v3.2 and v3.4; to Filomena Maggino for v4.4, v4.5, and v4.6; to Anna L.D. Lau and Robert A. Cummins for v4.3, v4.8, and v4.9; to Valerie Moller for V3.7 and v3.8; to Joanna Kit-Cun Lam for v3.11; to Daniel T.L. Shek for v4.2; to the Cleveland Plain Dealer for Philosophical Foundations of Quality of Life v1.4, and to the Detroit Free Press for v1.7.

Contents

Overview of the "The Selected Works of Alex C. Michalos"

Philosophical Foundations of Quality of Life

How Good Policies and Business Ethics Enhance Good Quality of Life

Development of Quality of Life Theory and Its Instruments

Introduction to "Selected Works of Alex C. Michalos"

Biographical Notes

The central aim of this set of volumes is to describe and explain the context and connections among a subset of papers and books produced over the past 50 years. Rather than a mere reproduction of work already published, this will be an attempt to disclose the productive processes in their various historic contexts that led to the various research projects and publications. In Michalos (2003), I published a collection called *Essays on the Quality of Life* containing 20 articles focused on the quality of life, 3 of which appear in other volumes of this set because they seemed to be so central to the array of issues in the 70 articles in these volumes. For completeness, I mention articles from the earlier collection and books that are directly relevant to the themes in these volumes.

Some years ago (these days it seems that most things begin with 'some years ago', unfortunately), in a debate about the existence of God, a member of the audience put the question to us 'Why would God want to watch re-runs?'. The question made sense from the point of view of one of the debaters, since God was supposed to know everything that is going to happen before it happens. As the atheist in the debate, I could only say that I have no idea why, although a lot of people seem to enjoy them.

While I also enjoy some re-runs, I would not find much joy in re-binding some old papers for a new audience. I do, however, find the idea of describing the historical context in which similar research questions more or less simultaneously appeared to people in diverse parts of the globe and were addressed first individually and then collectively. Here, the historical context includes some of my own biographical material. This is offered as a kind of second-best effort substituting for an autobiography that I have never had the courage to write, notwithstanding having thought about it many times.

My father ended his formal education in the sixth grade and my mother ended hers in the eighth grade. As far as I have been able to discern, in 1917, when he was about 17, my father, Charles K. Michalos, emigrated from the island of Chios,

Greece, to work in the steel mills of Gary, Indiana. He arrived with a pocket-sized Greek–English dictionary, learned to speak English with a heavy Greek accent, moved from the mills to driving a Nabisco bread and pastry truck for another 17 years, bought a small hamburger joint, then a somewhat bigger one and finally something more like a diner on Euclid Avenue in Cleveland, Ohio. Its claim to fame was the fact that many of the Cleveland Browns ate there, which was quite a big deal in 1947 when the Browns were the All American Football Conference champions and I was one of their biggest junior high school fans. My father died in January 1951, at about 51. We were never sure, because he was never sure, how old he was. I was daddy's boy and his loss was a great loss to me.

My mother, Josephine Pucci, was born in Akron, Ohio, one of eight children of immigrants from Palermo, Sicily. She worked at the May Company department store, sang in the chorus of the Cleveland Opera Company, married my father in 1931, produced my brother in 1932 and me in 1935, and provided the mom part of our mom and pop diner. Unlike my dad, she was not a particularly happy person, but she lived to be 93 years old, dying in June 1998. Like my dad, and the rest of us I guess, she did the best she could with what she had.

I was generally an above average but not outstanding primary and secondary school student. In secondary school and the first half of university, I was more interested in sports and girls than scholarship, though I enjoyed mathematics and history. I went to what was then Western Reserve University (now Case-Western Reserve University) in 1953, majoring in history with minors in philosophy and religion. When I read Plato's *Republic*, I felt as if he was talking directly to me. It had never occurred to me to ask what a good life might be, but the more I thought about it, the more I *had* to think about it.

I grew up in a very mixed religious family. The story my mother told was that her family were Catholics until the local priest did something that led my grandfather to tell him to go to hell and he took the whole gene pool into a more friendly Baptist church. My father seemed to practice the religion of washing his car on Sundays, but he thought his sons had to be baptized Greek Orthodox in order to preserve something or other that was important to him. So, we were. However, because our house was one block away from a small Quaker church, my brother, Chuck Michalos, and I were sent off together as soon as we were old enough to find our way there and back. I have a gold medal showing that I accumulated three years' of Sundays without missing Quaker Sunday school.

Given this background, when I began to think seriously about a good life, I thought I should make my peace with God if there were one. So, besides studying philosophy, I studied the history of religions. Then, I went to graduate school at the University of Chicago. Because I was what one would have called a doubter, I wanted to study religion in a school of believers, assuming that if anyone could convince me that I was wrong, they could. At least, they would be inclined to try. So, in 1957, I enrolled in the Divinity School, which seemed to have the most diverse faculty, including visiting experts in Buddhism, which especially interested me.

I also married in the summer of 1957, a marriage that lasted about 23 years and produced Cyndi (1960), Ted (1961) and Stephanie (1963). In 1985, I married the love of my life, Deborah Poff, a lucky break for both of us at the time and ever since.

While studying the history of religions, I took courses in philosophy and it seemed to me that philosophers had more precise and decisive methods of pursuing the truth than theologians. The University of Chicago had a wonderfully flexible approach to higher education, allowing students to pursue more than one degree at a time. To get a Bachelor of Divinity degree, a student was required to pass 7 comprehensive examinations and have a year internship in some relevant field of practice. I took some courses designed to prepare one to take the exams and some courses in philosophy that I found interesting. At the 1961 convocation, I received a B.D. and an M.A. in philosophy and then proceeded to pursue a Ph.D. in philosophy of science. I completed the latter in 1965 with a dissertation on a dispute between Rudolf Carnap and Karl Popper on the nature and use of probability theory in the assessment of scientific theories (Michalos 1971).

Many of the most salient and important features of the following 50 years of research and other activities may be regarded as relatively natural developments of these earlier initiatives. In a memorable essay on the best teacher he ever had, Keyfitz (2003) said that scholars should replace the metaphor of providing building blocks for a relatively durable corporate body of knowledge with that of providing biodegradable nutrition out of which new knowledge would grow. In a sense, today's nutrient is tomorrow's fertilizer. What I did until 1965 provided the ingredients for what followed, just as the latter will feed what comes afterward. Most importantly, I think my general approach has been informed by a pragmatic and philosophic interest in a holistic, comprehensive understanding of any particular object of investigation. I will try to explain this approach in the next few paragraphs.

Broadly speaking, there are two ways to define '*philosophy*'. From a *functional* point of view, philosophy may be identified as critical thinking about anything at all, from asphalt to zebras. From a *content* point of view, philosophy may be identified as a body of knowledge answering three questions. What is it? What good is it? How do you know?

Answering the question 'What is it?' gives one a discussion of the nature or being of something. In short, it gives one an *ontology*, a word derived from the Greek 'on' meaning nature or being, and logos, meaning discourse (among other things). Descriptions of the nature of things, ontologies, have at least two aspects. Everything has, after all, a form, structure, morphology or anatomy on the one hand, and a function, activity or physiology on the other. A duck, smile or football game, for examples, can be described at a minimum by describing their structural parts and how the parts function. What Isaac Newton might have referred to as natural philosophy and we now would call natural science is close to what philosophers would call ontology.

Answering the question 'What good is it?' gives one a discussion of the value, worth or goodness in some sense of something. In short, it gives one an *axiology*, a word derived from the Greek 'axios' meaning worthy or valuable, and logos. Of the variety of kinds of value that may be described, it is most useful to distinguish intrinsic from instrumental value. *Intrinsic value* refers to the worth or goodness of a thing in itself, its value as an end in itself rather than as a means to something else. *Instrumental value* refers to the worth or goodness of a thing as a means to something else, not as a thing in itself. Standard examples include things such as eating an apple or throwing a ball at a target having instrumental value insofar as the former produces nutrition and the latter scores points, which in this context have intrinsic value.

Since practically anything might be a useful means to something else for someone in some circumstances for some purposes, practically anything can have instrumental value. However, some people believe that all alleged sorts of intrinsic value may be reduced to a single one. For example, they would argue that the nutrition obtained from eating an apple is really only instrumentally valuable as a means to good health, which is itself instrumentally valuable for a life of pleasure, happiness or satisfaction. Those who believe that there is finally only one intrinsically valuable thing such as pleasure, happiness or satisfaction may be called monists with respect to the ultimate nature (ontological status) of value, while those who believe that there are many intrinsically valuable things may be called *pluralists*.

For a monist, then, it may be said that ontologically distinct things such as music, cheese and justice have different degrees of some sort of value such as pleasure, happiness or satisfaction, while for a pluralist, such ontologically distinct things have ontologically distinct values (music value, cheese value and justice value) regardless of how much pleasure, happiness or satisfaction these things produce. From an ontological point of view, then, a monist would have a numerically smaller number of ontologically distinct things in his or her world (e.g., music, cheese, justice and some degree of pleasure, happiness or satisfaction generated by the other three), while a pluralist's world would have music, cheese, justice plus music value, cheese value and justice value.

For a monist, the task of measuring the total value of something, a person, event, object, attitude, belief, proposition, action or life itself, is in principle straightforward. One simply needs to measure the degree of intrinsic value generated by that thing in terms of or operationalized as pleasure, happiness or satisfaction. For pluralists, the task of measuring the total value of something is not at all straightforward because there may be no way to compare ontologically distinct values like the value of music versus the value of cheese or justice. There does not appear to be any common measure, scale or instrument available to answer questions such as 'How much is music worth compared to the value of justice or cheese?' or 'What is the value of this piece of music in terms of the value of justice or cheese?'

Given the severe comparability problems faced by all value pluralists, it is not surprising that the most frequently studied theories of economists and decision theorists, namely preference theory, choice theory, utility theory and game theory, and one of the most popular ethical theories studied by philosophers, utilitarianism, assume value monism of some sort. As we will see in many of the papers in this collection and many more cited in those papers, scholars have invented a great variety of methods for living in and managing a world apparently containing a plurality of values. In particular, I will describe my own efforts over about 50 years, which have been interesting but largely unsuccessful.

Answering the question 'How do you know?' gives a discussion of one's knowledge of something. In short, it gives one an *epistemology*, a word derived from the Greek 'episteme' meaning knowledge and logos, hence, a theory of knowledge. Strictly speaking, one ought, prudentially and morally, to have a fairly clear answer to the epistemological question before one attempts to answer the ontological and axiological questions. Since a philosopher aims to obtain a body of knowledge about the nature and value of things to be used in the practice of living a good life, a patently necessary condition of achieving that aim is clarity with respect to knowledge itself and its production. That is why the earliest essays in these 4 volumes concern epistemological issues.

Comments on the Articles

All of the papers in this set of volumes are arranged partly in chronological order and partly by their logical connections. Each volume has its own major themes and within those themes, articles have been selected and arranged to provide some idea of the time at which they appeared and its relation to my own and others' research agendas around that time.

Following this introduction, Chap. 1 is an early attempt to show that "a rule for the acceptance of scientific hypotheses called the principle of cost-benefit dominance is more effective and efficient than the principle of the maximization of expected (epistemic) utility". Readers who are familiar with my decision-theoretic papers in the first two volumes of this set will recognize some conceptual and logical consequences of those investigations in this study. Here, I tried to blend observations on a classic in the history of medical science with the latest work in the philosophy of science. At the time the paper was written, historians and philosophers of science, technology and medicine worked largely in independent silos. I tried to show that what was going on inside one silo could make important contributions to what was going on inside another. Readers familiar with Michalos (1997 reprinted in Michalos 2003) will notice that I became somewhat more concerned about the limits of our ability to craft comprehensive indexes of acceptability for scientific theories, although the Canadian Index of Well-Being (Michalos et al. 2011b) is formally roughly equivalent to such an index. An overview of the Canadian Index is provided below in Chap. 17.

The aim of Chap. 2 was "to build a bridge between two intersecting areas of research, social indicators research on the one hand and health-related quality of life research on the other". I was not and have not been the only scholar trying to bring these two closely related research traditions together, but none of us have had much success. The main participants in the two traditions seem to have their interests and expertise developed in different subcultures with very little attention paid to each other, in spite of profound similarities in ultimate aims, and conceptual and formal structures of methods of investigation, laws and theories. Based on the analyses of the chapter, the most important recommendation made was for researchers to avoid using the splendid measure of health status, SF-36, as a measure of the quality of life. A decade later, Michalos et al. (2011a, reprinted below in Chap. 9) demonstrated beyond any reasonable doubt that good measures of the overall quality of life (life satisfaction, happiness, contentment with life, overall satisfaction with the quality of life and subjective well-being) had a significantly different set of predictors from good health measured by SF-36. Fifteen years later still, that message does not appear to have changed the behavior of many researchers in the health-related quality of life tradition.

The paper by Mallard, Lance and Michalos (Chap. 3) is placed in this volume because it applies a relatively rarely used statistical analysis to data collected for my *Global Report on Student Well-Being* (Michalos 1991a, b, 1993a, b) to reveal the impact of culture on people’s assessments of their perceived quality of life overall and in 11 domains of life, including health and education in particular. Using data from 32 of the 39 countries involved in the global survey, the authors found that the Bi-Directional model in which causal arrows ran from life satisfaction to domain satisfaction and from the latter to the former had more support than either a Top-Down model or a Bottom-Up model. Regarding the health satisfaction domain, they found that for samples from 10 countries, the Bottom-Up model was best (health satisfaction influenced life satisfaction), for 7 countries the Top-Down model was best (life satisfaction influenced health satisfaction) and for 6 countries the Bi-Directional model worked best. They also found that the 32 country samples were distributed into 7 clusters across 11 domains. The cluster with Cameroon, Canada and the USA had Bi-Directional relationships in 52% of the domain satisfaction-life satisfaction pairs, which was the greatest percentage for this relationship in all 7 clusters.

Chapters 4–7 are reports of 4 research projects undertaken by participants of UNBC’s Institute for Social Research and Evaluation focused on one set of residents of the Bella Coola Valley of British Columbia. From August to November 2001, a number of procedures were used to get as many as possible of the estimated 1736 residents over 17 years of age in the valley to complete our 11-page questionnaire. About 40% of the residents in the valley are of Aboriginal descent, most from the Nuxalt nation, and about 36% of our sample of 687 respondents had Aboriginal or métis backgrounds. The Provincial Health Officer’s designated determinants of health were measured by 31 items in four clusters, biological, social and economic, health behaviors and health services determinants. These included our standard measures of overall quality of life and domain satisfaction, the gold standard self-reported health status measure SF-36, healthy days measures from the U.S. Centers for Disease Control and demographic measures. Most of our measures revealed that the health status and quality of life of Bella Coola Valley respondents were less satisfactory than those of typical Prince George respondents. The four clusters of health determinants accounted for 24% of general self-reported health and life satisfaction, while our standard array of domain satisfaction scores accounted for 12% of general health and 61% of life satisfaction, indicating considerable perceived differences in general health and overall satisfaction with life.

Using matching subsets by age and gender of Aboriginal respondents in the Bella Coola Valley survey who were residential school survivors versus Aboriginal respondents who had not been residential school attendees, Chap. 5 reports that both groups "experience poorer health and quality of life compared to non-Aboriginals, as well as higher rates of diabetes". Of all the health status measures employed in our survey, only the "self-health rating" item revealed statistically significant lower scores for Aboriginal residential school survivors compared to Aboriginal non-residential school attendees.

Based on comprehensive reviews of patient medical charts from the Bella Coola Medical Clinic, which serves the entire population of the Bella Coola Valley, 127 diabetics were identified, their charts were given identification numbers that could be matched with numbers on questionnaires from our survey and examination of data from charts and questionnaires could be made. About 90 diabetics completed our questionnaire. The study reprinted as Chap. 6 reports that "Participants without diabetes tended to rate their health significantly better than participants with diabetes", diabetics "who used insulin rated their current health significantly lower than those who did not use insulin" and diabetics were "no more likely to be unhappy or dissatisfied with their lives as a whole or with the overall quality of their lives compared to people without diabetes".

Chapter 7 is another report based on comparing information from the Medical Clinic patient charts and 674 respondents to our Valley survey. The authors concluded that "the relationship between chart review and self-report health information observed in this rural population is similar to findings from other populations". In particular, they found "excellent agreement between self-report and clinic data for age, sex, height, weight and Aboriginal ancestry" and for "self-reported and clinically recorded diabetes", but "poor agreement for diagnoses of depression, back/neck problems, eye problems, walking problems, stroke, hearing problems and bone/joint problems". Aggregated Body Mass Index scores tended to have greater error margins because individual estimates of their own weight are biased by their ideals of what that weight should be.

In September 1999, we undertook a health and quality of life survey of residents 55 years old or older in the Northern Interior Health Region of British Columbia and published the results in Michalos et al. (2001 reprinted in Michalos 2003). Chapter 8 is a report of a replication of that survey taken in September 2005. Based on mean scores for the 8 dimensions of health measured by SF-36, it was clear that "the overall health status of males and females aged 55 years and older in the region in 2005 was at least as good as that in 1999." As well, we found that mean scores on 28 measures of satisfaction in diverse domains, overall happiness, life satisfaction and quality of life for the 2005 sample were at least as good as those for the 1999 sample. Smaller percentages of the 2005 sample "avoided going out at night, feared for their safety, had crime-related worries, engaged in crime-related defensive behaviors and were actually the victims of any crimes". As I remarked in the introduction to Chap. 6 in Development of the Quality of Life Theory and its Instruments, the reduction of crime in the city was regularly indicated as something to do to improve the quality of life in Prince George. So, considering these crime-concern measures, there had been some significant improvement. Applying the 7 core discrepancy predictors from Multiple Discrepancies Theory (Michalos 1985) to 8 dependent variables, including overall happiness, life satisfaction, satisfaction with the overall quality of life and subjective well-being, we found that the most influential predictors were the gaps between what respondents wanted and had, what they had and thought others the same age and sex had, and the what they had compared to the best they ever had in the past.

In 2009, my wife (Deborah Poff) began a five-year appointment as President and Vice Chancellor of Brandon University in Manitoba. The report published as Chap. 9 is the result of an attempt to get some baseline self-reported information about our new community in the summer of 2010. Besides the standard measures of health and quality of life I had used in Prince George, the Bella Coola Valley and elsewhere, our Brandon team crafted a Good Neighborhood Index, Social Support Index and Community Health Index. After examining all our measures from diverse points of view, it seemed to me that the main message of the investigation was that good health is not the same as a good life. This was something I had reported before, as we have been reminded in the preceding paragraphs of this introduction, but it seemed to me that the point had not received the attention it deserved. So, putting it boldly in the title of our paper was a strategy of emphasizing its importance. So far as I know, there has been no significant reduction in the use of the gold standard measure of health status, SF-36, as a measure of the overall perceived quality of life. Based on our new sample, we also recommended again that quality of life researchers should always use more than one measure for their dependent variable.

Chapters 10–15 have some association with education, the first two involving survey research results and the last four somewhat more philosophical. Chapter 10 contains an analysis of an aggregated collection of 7 yearly samples of students' perceived quality of life and satisfaction with their school experiences at the University of Northern British Columbia in the years from 1998 to 2005. The Institute for Social Research and Evaluation collaborated with the staff of several student services to produce a survey with core items replicated each year along with additional special-focused items. When we combined satisfaction with school-related domains to satisfaction with ordinary life domains in a Bottom-Up model, we found that we could explain 62% of the variance in life satisfaction and 59% of the variance in satisfaction with the overall quality of life. Satisfaction with school-related domains increased the explanatory power of all predictors of life satisfaction by only 1% and added nothing to our explanatory power of satisfaction with the overall quality of life. For both dependent variables, the most influential school-related satisfaction item was satisfaction with UNBC instructors.

The investigation reported in Chap. 11 was based on an aggregated collection of data from 16 surveys of the Prince George community taken in the period from November 1997 to February 2005. The total sample (N = 8800) was large enough to provide reasonably large subsamples of typically under-represented survey respondents, namely youth aged 18–24 (N = 416), unemployed (N = 304) and those with Aboriginal or Métis ethnic backgrounds (N = 416). Regarding satisfaction with the overall quality of life, we found that the unemployed group were least satisfied, followed by the Aboriginal/Métis group, then youth, with the average total population scores superior to all the others. We did not find any signs of a mid-life crisis for our respondents aged 38–44, although Helliwell et al. (2013) did find signs of such for their much larger world survey sample using 40–50-year-old respondents as those in mid-life. The strongest predictor of life satisfaction for the Aboriginal/Métis group was satisfaction with friendships, but it was satisfaction with one's own self-esteem for youth and the unemployed.

Chapter 12 is based on a paper presented at an international conference at the University of Rome in April 2007 sponsored by the Joint Research Centre of the European Commission, OECD, Centre for Economic and International Studies, and the Bank of Italy. The substance of the paper is a bit more philosophical and conceptual than quantitative. The main point I tried to make is that there are more or less narrow and broad conceptual understandings of the ideas of education, happiness and well-being, and what one finds from quantitative research is strongly determined by how one conceptualizes and operationalizes these ideas. Using a conceptual net with relatively broad notions of the basic ideas and multi-leveled quantitative analyses, one can find plenty of evidence of the impact of education on happiness and well-being, and the reverse, as illustrated in the paper. Unfortunately, most studies only notice the direct effects of formal education, neglecting all kinds of indirect effects from all kinds of learning outside of formal education.

In Chap. 13 I explicated four views of liberal education that I called pragmatic, aristocratic, residualist and developmental, and I argued for the superior adequacy of the idea of liberal education as education aimed at self and social development. Among other things, defining liberal education by certain aims avoids the essentialist trap of supposing that each of us has some basic nature awaiting the proper nourishing environment to actualize that nature and it allows us to evaluate educational programs by their relative success at achieving designated aims. Using the proposed definition, any sort of vocational or technical education may also be liberal, and some programs of study in humanities and arts may fail to be liberal. Finally, liberal education thus defined will contribute to the development of character and moral virtue, and students "getting their heads and hearts together" as we sometimes say.

In 2005, there were many conferences, symposia, special editions of journals and ad hoc articles written in celebration of Albert Einstein's remarkable papers on relativity theory published 100 years earlier. Chapter 14 is a contribution to such a symposium presented at a regional meeting of the Royal Society of Canada at the University of Guelph in May 2005. At the time of the symposium, there was some discussion in Canada of the role of so-called public intellectuals in public policy making. Readers of any of the volumes in this set will be aware that I have always tried to find ways to integrate my academic research with public policy making, even more generally to create bridges for people working in diverse fields within the academy and beyond to cross over giving and receiving aid from others. I prefer the phrase ‘citizen scholar’ to ‘public intellectual’ because there seems to me to be something a bit elitist about the term ‘intellectual’, but the substance of the commitments referred to in both phrases may be the same. In my paper, I note that Einstein was probably too willing to use his well-deserved scholarly reputation as a soapbox from which he could utter alleged gems of wisdom quite beyond his range of expertise. He seems to have been some sort of moral consequentialist pursuing the good life for all people along the lines of a robust Aristotelian Eudaimonia. (See Michalos 2015.) While he often expressed the view that science or scientific research could be used to discover means but not ends, I tried to show that “in the sense that good scientific research specifies and demands certain kinds of theorizing or hypothesizing, it creates appropriate ends”.

As a scholarly journal and book series editor for over 40 years, I sometimes had to deal with alleged cases of plagiarism or what we now more often refer to as cases of unacknowledged authorship. Compared to the over 7000 articles published in the seven journals I founded or co-founded over all those years, I had to investigate and adjudicate fewer than two hands full of alleged plagiarism cases, mostly from the *Journal of Business Ethics*. In Chap. 15, I describe some historically early views about unacknowledged authorship to illustrate its relationships with diverse purposes and contexts. At the end of the article, I review two cases I adjudicated concerning such authorship. The first is offered as an illustration of the sort of case study typically published on the Web site of the Committee on Publication Ethics (COPE) and the second as an illustration of procedures following the Springer *Policy on Publishing Integrity*. The policies and adjudication procedures of COPE and Springer vary over time as new cases appear and more nuanced rules are developed.

When I was gathering information to help me decide whether or not I should edit the *Encyclopedia of Quality of Life and Well-Being Research*, I read several introductory chapters of established encyclopedias and talked to friends who had edited other encyclopedias. Since I had consulted many encyclopedias connected to my research over the years and had never read the introduction to any encyclopedia, I wrote the introduction to my encyclopedia as if most, if not all, of the readers of the introduction were potential editors and/or authors of encyclopedia entries. Because the original text that I wrote was longer and had considerably more detail than the publisher’s staff believed would be appropriate for the encyclopedia, it was severely reduced for publication. However, because I think there are many useful insights and bits of historical information, I decided to include the original text here as Chap. 16. I offer it to all future editors, wishing you the very best of luck.

The final Chap. 17 in this volume is a brief history of the development of quality of life research in Canada from the 1960s to 2014. There is certainly much more to be said than I could say in 40 pages, but I hope I have provided at least a running start to anyone interested in writing a more comprehensive history. There are many histories of varying lengths of the social indicators/quality of life movement worldwide, many identified and summarized in Land and Michalos (TBP). Readers interested in the broader story should consult that article.

References

Helliwell, J. F., Layard, R. & Sachs, J. (Eds.). (2013). *World happiness report 2013*. New York: UN Sustainable Development Solutions Network.

Keyfitz, N. (2003). Nathan Keyfitz on Mr. Somerville and others. In A.C. Michalos (Ed.), *The best teacher I ever had: Personal reports from highly productive scholars* (pp. 126–131). London, Ontario: Althouse Press.

Land, K. C. & Michalos, A. C. (2017). TBP. Fifty years after the social indicators movement: Has the promise been fulfilled? An assessment and an agenda for the future. *Social Indicators Research*.

Michalos, A. C. (1971). *The Popper-Carnap controversy*. Hague: Martinus Nijhoff.

Michalos, A. C. (1985). Multiple discrepancies theory (MDT). *Social Indicators Research, 16*, 347–413.

Michalos, A. C. (1991a). *Global report on student well-being, Vol. 1: Life satisfaction and happiness*. Dordrecht: Springer-Verlag.

Michalos, A. C. (1991b). *Global report on student well-being, Vol. 2: Family, friends, living partner and self-esteem*. Dordrecht: Springer-Verlag.

Michalos, A. C. (1993a). *Global report on student well-being, Vol. 3: Employment, finances, housing and transportation*. Dordrecht: Springer-Verlag.

Michalos, A. C. (1993b). *Global report on student well-being, Vol. 4: Religion, education, recreation and health*. Dordrecht: Springer-Verlag.

Michalos, A. C. (1997). Combining social, economic and environmental indicators to measure sustainable human well-being. *Social Indicators Research, 40*, 221–258.

Michalos, A. C. (2003). *Essays on the quality of life*. Dordrecht: Kluwer Academic Publishing.

Michalos, A. C. (2015). *Ancient views on the quality of life*. Dordrecht: Springer.

Michalos, A. C., Hubley, A., Zumbo, B. C., & Hemingway, D. (2001). Health and other aspects of the quality of life of older people. *Social Indicators Research, 54*, 239–274.

Michalos, A. C., Ramsey, D., Eberts, D., & Kahlke, P. M. (2011a). Good health is not the same as a good life: survey results from Brandon, Manitoba. *Social Indicators Research, 107*, 201–234.

Michalos, A. C., Smale, B., Labonté, R., Muhajarine, N., Scott, K., Guhn, M., et al. (2011b). *The Canadian index of well-being: Technical paper 1.0*. Waterloo, Ontario: Canadian Index of Well-Being and the University of Waterloo.

Chapter 1
Cost-Benefit Versus Expected Utility Acceptance Rules

Alex C. Michalos

The Problem

One of the fundamental problems of life in general and the philosophy of science in particular is the specification of reliable criteria for the determination acceptable hypotheses (in the broad sense of ordinary sentences, laws and theories) and courses of action. While no one has been able to provide a set of criteria that could be regarded as necessary and sufficient for all sorts of hypotheses and circumstances, a number of more or less plausible rules specifying sufficient conditions of acceptability *given* certain data, purposes and attitudes have obtained fairly wide acceptance. These include such familiar principles as Gauss's least squares rule of estimation, Fisher's method of maximum likelihood, Wald's minimax loss rule, Savage's minimax regret rule, Bernoulli-Bayes's rule for the maximization of expected utility, and so on.[1] The last rule in this list is of particular importance for this paper.

A number of influential philosophers have recommended the Bernoulli-Bayes rule or some variation of it as a first approximation or step in the right direction toward a solution of the problem of providing a criterion, principle or rule for determining the acceptability of scientific hypotheses (e.g., Carnap 1950; Hempel 1960, 1966; Leach 1968; Levi 1967). But, so far as I know, no one has suggested that some sort of benefits-less-costs rule might be more advantageous, and it is roughly this idea that I wish to explore and ultimately vindicate. More precisely, I

Michalos, A.C.: 1970. Cost-benefit versus expected utility acceptance rules. Theory and Decision, 1, pp. 61–88.

[1]All but the last of these rules are reviewed in Michalos (1969b).

A.C. Michalos (✉)
University of Northern British Columbia, Prince George, BC, Canada
e-mail: michalos@brandonu.ca

A.C. Michalos, *Connecting the Quality of Life Theory to Health, Well-Being and Education*, DOI 10.1007/978-3-319-51161-0_1

shall attempt to prove the *normative* claim that a cost and benefit dominance principle of acceptance ought to be preferred to any sort of Bernoulli-Bayesian principle because right now and for the foreseeable future the former performs better and cannot perform worse than the latter (in a sense of 'perform' that will be elucidated below).[2]

Although most of the paper consists of a detailed analysis and comparison of the two relevant principles, their requirements and applications, I shall begin with a brief outline of the basic elements of each in order to provide a general orientation and more or less common background for our discussion.

Maximization of Expected Utility

Proponents of the rule enjoining the maximization of expected utility, which we shall hereafter abbreviate as MEU, imagine a decision-maker confronted with a set of (practically speaking) mutually exclusive and exhaustive possible courses of action from which one that is optimal must be adopted. The decision-maker knows that the payoff or *utility* (in some sense of this word which will be explained later) that he obtains from his choice will be partially determined by events which are (practically speaking) mutually exclusive, exhaustive and beyond his control. If he has objective probability values (i.e., relative frequencies, propensities, physical range measures, etc.) for the occurrence of these events then he is operating under conditions of risk. If he does not have such values then he is in a situation of uncertainty, but he will transform it into a situation of risk by determining appropriate subjective probability values (i.e., betting quotients, degrees of belief, etc.) for the events. Given all these data he is ready to use MEU, which, as a normative principle, prescribes the acceptance of that course of action whose sum of probability-weighted utilities is larger than that of any of its alternatives. If 'U_i' and 'p_i' represent the utility and probability values, respectively, of the ith of n payoffs obtainable by adopting some hypothesis, then

$$\sum p_i U_i (i = 1, 2, \ldots, n) \tag{1.1}$$

or

$$p_1 U_1 + p_2 U_2 + \cdots + p_n U_n \tag{1.2}$$

represents the expected utility of accepting that hypothesis. Clearly, when there is no risk involved then formulae (1.1) and (1.2) shrink to the single utility value

[2]MacCrimmon (1968) and Pruzan (1966) contain less thorough comparisons of these and similar rules, with respect to different applications. Raiffa (1969) contains a defense of the Bemoulli-Bayes principle for "multi-attribute" problems. Hinrichs and Taylor (1969) and Prest and Turvey (1965) contain excellent surveys of recent work on cost-benefit analysis.

whose procurement is certain (has a probability value of unity) given the acceptance of that hypothesis. Following MEU then, one would simply accept that hypothesis whose expected-utility (or utility in the limiting case) was greater than that of its alternatives. If two or more hypotheses have the same expected-utility and it is higher than those of the alternatives, then each of the former should be regarded as equally acceptable.

For our purposes we may think of the decision-maker described above as a practicing theoretical or applied scientist, and we may assume that his possible courses of action are the adoption of certain hypotheses as bases for further action. Although one *can,* as Isaac Levi has shown us (Levi 1962), imagine a person accepting a hypothesis not as a basis for action but as somehow suitable for admission into his total corpus of knowledge, our concern here is with the provision of hypotheses more or less directly related to action (cf. Chisholm 1968). If we regard a hypothesis as acceptable then, at the very least, it merits the investment of further resources such as research facilities and activity, time, money, energy, and so on. Note, however, that our concern with the acceptability of hypotheses as bases for action does not alter any of the formal or logical aspects of the problem. Only the content of the utility function or the arguments to be included in that function would be different for Levi's decision-makers and mine.

Cost-Benefit Dominance

Our exposition of a variation of a benefits-less-costs rule, which we will call 'the principle of cost-benefit dominance' and abbreviate CBD, may begin with a decision-maker in roughly the same situation we described for MEU. He is confronted with a similar set of (practically speaking) mutually exclusive and exhaustive hypotheses and events. He may be able to assign some sort of probability value to the occurrence of each event and he may not. In any case, such values are not required. Similarly, utility values are not required. Instead of assigning a utility value to the payoffs he will receive as a result of this or that combination of accepted hypothesis and turn of events, he merely determines the "raw forms" of the benefits and costs attached to each combination. For example, instead of noting that a hypothesis adequately accounts for a certain phenomenon provided that certain events take place rather than some others, coheres with a well-established theory in another domain given those events and has a Reichenbachian weight of 0.7, *and* that all of this gives it a utility value of 0.8, he merely lists its benefits in their "raw form" (i.e., it coheres provided that such and such is the case, etc.). Similarly, he lists its costs and the benefits and costs for its alternatives given the various contingencies. It must be assumed, of course, that he is able to weakly order the "raw form" data *within* each attribute and the corresponding preferences. For example, he must be able to determine whether two hypotheses are equally explanatory or one explains more than the other; he must be able to rank order any three distinct levels of explanatory power transitively; and he must recognize that his preferences ought to be perfectly positively correlated with the "raw form" data, e.g., he ought to prefer a hypothesis that explains more phenomena to one that explains less (if all other things are equal). It does not have to be assumed that he is able to weakly order the "raw form" data across attributes, e.g., he never has to be able to rank order different levels of explanatory power, coherence, testability, etc. on a single scale of some sort. In other words, he is obliged to make intra-attribute comparisons but not interattribute comparisons.

The net result of this analysis is a battery of matrices (i.e., a different matrix for each attribute) which constitute a comparative "profile" of each hypothesis with respect to its alternatives. Schematically, the matrices in such a battery for the attributes of, say, simplicity, explanatory power, precision, coherence, testability, etc. would each look like this.

$$\begin{array}{llcccc}
 & & \multicolumn{4}{c}{\textit{Possible Events} \text{ (States of Nature)}} \\
 & & E_1 & E_2, & \ldots, & E_n \\
 & H_1 & p_1B_1^1, & p_2B_2^1, & \ldots, & p_nB_n^1, \\
 & H_2 & p_1B_1^2, & p_2B_2^2, & \ldots, & p_nB_n^2, \\
 & \cdot & \cdot & \cdot & & \cdot \\
\textit{Hypotheses} & \cdot & \cdot & \cdot & & \cdot \\
 & \cdot & \cdot & \cdot & & \cdot \\
 & H_n & p_1B_1^n, & p_2B_2^n, & \ldots, & p_nB_n^n,
\end{array}$$

The entry for row H_1 column E_2, for example, would tell us that if the hypothesis represented by 'H_1' is accepted and the event(s) represented by 'E_2' occur, then we will obtain a benefit represented by 'B_2^1' with a probability represented by 'p_2'. Since 'p_2' and 'B_2^1' need not represent numerical values of any sort, the juxtaposition of these two signs must not be taken to mean multiplication [as in formulae (1.1) and (1.2)]. The superscript on 'B_2^1' indicates the hypothesis 'H_1' and the subscript indicates the event(s) 'E_2'. The 'B' is short for 'benefits'. They might be a high degree of explanatory power, simplicity, coherence with other theories, precision, etc. While various philosophers and scientists (e.g., Ackermann 1961; Buchdahl 1969; Bunge 1959, 1961; Good 1968; Goodman 1959; Hempel 1960, 1962, 1966; Hertz 1956; Jeffreys 1957; Laudan 1968; Levi 1967; Margenau 1950; McLaughlin 1970; Michalos 1965a, 1969a, d; Popper 1959; Schlesinger 1963; Williams 1969) have made recommendations as to which attributes ought to be included in an optimal set, all that is assumed here is that such a set would contain, say, more than a couple and less than a couple dozen members, none of which would have to be entirely independent (in any sense) of the others. In matrices for such costs as required set-up time, computational effort, special facilities, technical assistance, money, operationalization, etc. the 'B' would be replaced by a 'C' for costs'.[3]

---

[3] A fairly thorough analysis of decision-making costs may be found in Michalos (to be published).

As with formulae (1.1) and (1.2), when there is no risk involved then such matrices shrink to a single item, namely, a column indicating the various benefits (costs) that will be obtained (borne) with certainty given the acceptance of a particular hypothesis.

If for every possible contingency and for every attribute, the benefits and costs of accepting one hypothesis are preferable (i.e., ought to be preferred) to those of accepting another then the former *strongly dominates* the latter. If for some contingency and for some attribute, the benefits and costs of accepting one hypothesis are preferable to those of another *and* for all of the remaining contingencies and attributes the benefits and costs of accepting the latter are not preferable to those of the former (i.e., some are exactly alike and others are less preferable), then the former dominates the latter.[4] Hence, if one hypothesis strongly dominates another then the former also dominates the latter, but the converse is not true. According to CBD then, the hypothesis that ought to be accepted is the one which dominates all of its alternatives. If two or more hypotheses have the same benefits and costs but dominate all others then they should be regarded as equally acceptable. In general, depending on the particular benefits and costs involved, research in a given problem-area should continue until some hypothesis emerges as dominant over all of its alternatives.

Preferability and Superior Performance

I am assuming that one principle of acceptance is *preferable* to another provided that the former may perform better and cannot perform worse than the latter. Moreover, one principle *performs better* than another if and only if it is more effective and more efficient than the other. An acceptance principle is *effective* exactly insofar as it is possible in every sense of this term to isolate, identify or select acceptable hypotheses by applying it. If it were impossible in any sense to apply a principle then it could not be applied and, consequently, could not identify anything. So it would be completely ineffective. The *efficiency* of an acceptance principle may be defined and measured by the ratio of its effectiveness to the number of assumptions and the degree of sophistication of the kinds of information required for its application.[5] The *degree of sophistication* of a particular piece of information may be determined by the sorts of scales (nominal, ordinal, interval or ratio) or concepts (qualitative, comparative or quantitative) required to accurately express that information, e.g., 'this is hot' may be regarded as a less sophisticated piece of information than 'this is hotter than that' which is less sophisticated than 'this has a temperature of 90 °F'. Hence, if it could be shown that CBD and MEU

[4]These two definitions, of course, are merely special applications of the famous Pareto Principle that has been used widely by economists since Vilfredo Pareto's *Cours d'tconomie politique*, 1877, e.g., Arrow (1951), Harsanyi (1955), Hildreth (1953), Luce and Raiffa (1964), Newman (1965), Rothenberg (1961), Tullock and Buchanan (1962).

[5]'Effectiveness' and 'efficiency' are analyzed in greater detail in Michalos (1970b).

are equally effective or that CBD is more effective than MEU *but* that CBD requires fewer assumptions and/or less sophisticated information than MEU, then the superior efficiency of CBD would be established. That, of course, would establish its superiority of performance and, therefore, its preferability over MEU, which is my central thesis. In the next two sections I shall attempt to establish this thesis roughly as follows. In section "MEU Versus CBD: Comparison of Requirements" it will be shown that MEU requires information of a more sophisticated sort and, consequently, more assumptions than CBD. Some of this information is not now nor will it be in the foreseeable future available. It follows then, that MEU is now and will be for some time to come *completely ineffective.* In section "Harvey's Implicit Use of CBD" we review Harvey's defense of his theory of the motion of the heart and blood against that of Galen as a paradigm case study of an undoubtedly successful defense of a scientific hypothesis *and* of an implicit application of CBD. Any adequate acceptance rule would have to disclose the superiority of Harvey's view over Galen's and, as a matter of fact, it is fairly apparent that something like CBD was behind Harvey's presentation of the evidence for his view. By means of this historical example then, the *effectiveness* of CBD is established. Thus, because CBD is more effective and must have a higher efficiency ratio than MEU, the former performs better and cannot perform worse than MEU for the present and foreseeable future. Hence, the superiority and preferability of CBD over MEU is established.

MEU Versus CBD: Comparison of Requirements

The requirements and general prospects of our two principles may be thoroughly compared in five respects.

5.1. In the first place it is apparent that MEU does but CBD does not require numerical probability values. With MEU it is not enough to be able to determine that a certain event and concomitant attribute value is probable, very probable, improbable, more probable than some other, as probable as some other, etc. Such frequently useful qualitative and comparative probabilistic judgments are worthless for MEU, because the latter can only "process" quantitative judgments; e.g., judgments of the form 'The degree of probability of obtaining a value of x for attribute A in the event that E is r'. Thus, one who uses MEU must assume that all of the notoriously difficult philosophic problems involved in obtaining initial numerical probability values (for the particular procedures employed) have been satisfactorily solved. (See, for example, Barker 1957; Hintikka and Suppes 1966; Keynes 1957; Lakatos 1968; Michalos 1965b, 1966, 1967, 1969b, to be published; Popper 1959; Salmon 1966). Moreover, granted that a given position is philosophically unobjectionable in itself, it must still be assumed that every contingency that might be relevant to the acceptance of any hypothesis can be meaningfully assigned a numerical value by that procedure, i.e., that in one way or another it is always meaningful to transform conditions of uncertainty into conditions of risk. As

Ellsberg has shown (Ellsberg 1961), however, proponents of minimax, maximin and maximax decision rules cannot and would not accept this assumption. (See also Burks 1968; Keynes 1957; Milner 1960.) On the other hand, both the assumption and its denial are irrelevant to CBD, for the latter does not require probability values of any sort but it can always use them when they are available.

5.2. Just as CBD can but MEU cannot get along without numerical probability values, the former can and the latter cannot proceed without numerical utility values. There seem to be two *prima facie* possible ways to produce these values, the first of which will be shown to be abortive and the second of which is largely wishful thinking. The former will be considered in this subsection and the latter in the next.

To begin, it should be noted that the numerical utility values required are cardinal and not merely ordinal. The former are necessary because they are the only ones that can be meaningfully added or multiplied, and both of these operations must be performed on the utility values used by MEU. So, some means of obtaining at least an interval scale of numerical utility values must be found.[6]

One way to tackle the problem of securing an interval scale of utility values is to try to generate them from a simple rank ordering of attribute values. The most popular and manageable means to this end is the standard-gamble technique of von Neumann and Morgenstern (1947). Unfortunately (for defenders of MEU), while this technique can [in principle though not always in fact (Michalos 1967)] be used to produce an interval scale of utility, the utility involved is not the sort that is of interest to philosophers of science. The latter are concerned with "epistemic utilities". In Hempel's words,

> *epistemic utilities* ... represent "gains" and "losses" as judged by reference to the objectives of "pure" or "basic" scientific research; in contradistinction to ...*pragmatic utilities,* which would represent gains or losses in income, prestige, intellectual or moral satisfaction ... (Hempel 1962, p. 156).

And Levi writes

> when an investigator declares himself to be engaged in an effort to replace agnosticism by true belief ... there is no need to ascertain his "true feelings" ... (Levi 1967, p. 76).

Presumably the fundamental logical distinction between a scale of "epistemic utility" and "pragmatic (including psychological) utility" is that only the former could have some normative force for a scientist *as* a scientist.[7] Moreover, it might be thought that by making certain adjustments in the von Neumann-Morgenstern technique, a scale with normative force could be constructed. Indeed, this idea

[6]On the problem of scales and their transformations see Ackoff (1962), Fishbum (1964), Luce and Raiffa (1964) and Rothenberg (1961).

[7]A vast amount of literature has been produced by proponents and opponents of "pragmatic utility", and it is doubtful that I could contribute anything novel to the discussion here. Interested readers may find critiques of the concept in Arrow (1951), Ellsberg (1961), Kuhn (1963), MacCrimmon (1968), Manheim and Hall (1968), Michalos (1965a, 1966, 1967), Rothenberg (1961) and Stedry and Chames (1966).

seems to be behind Levi's efforts in *Gambling With Truth* (p. 50). It is easy to demonstrate, however, that the von Neumann-Morgenstern technique cannot yield the required scale. According to that technique,[8] a decision-maker begins by rank ordering attribute values. To keep things simple, suppose he has a single attribute, say, explanatory power, and can distinguish in a publically observable or inter-subjectively testable fashion, three ranks, low, average and high. The latter may be represented by '*L*', '*M*' and '*H*', respectively. Clearly, he prefers

$$H \text{ to } M \text{ to } L.$$

He then assigns a value of 0 to the lowest rank and 1 to the highest rank. To determine the numerical value of the remaining rank, he considers various choices (gambles) that might be put to him having the form

$$M \text{ versus } pL + (1 - p)H,$$

where '*pL*' is short for 'obtaining a low ranking hypothesis with a probability value of *p*' Clearly, if $p = 0$ then the right side of the gamble would be preferred (because the choice is then between *M* and *H,* and *H* is preferred to *M*), and if $p = 1$ then the left side is preferred (because *M* is preferred to *L*). By varying the value of*p* appropriately, the decisionmaker can (often if not always) reach a point where both sides seem equally attractive. At that point he merely computes the numerical value of the right side and that tells him the value of the left side, i.e., the value of the remaining rank.

Now, in order to put this whole procedure to work *normatively,* one would have to have some criterion, rule or principle that prescribes the appropriate probability values. For the case before us, it might have the form: Given a gamble between '*M*' and '*p*L + (1 − *p*) *H*' a decision-maker (with his eye on the "gains" and "losses" to "pure" science) ought to reach a state of indifference when and only when $p = r$. The only way to justify such a prescription, however, is to show that *M* must have a certain "epistemic utility" value, and that can only be shown *after* the interval scale of "epistemic utility" values for explanatory power has been constructed. That, of course, is much too late for anyone who thought the standard-gamble technique would be useful. It is *not* useful, because one must already possess the very information it is supposed to, but can only redundantly provide. Hence, it is impossible to use this technique to construct a scale of "epistemic utility" values which would have normative force for a scientist *as* a scientist. Therefore, the first *prima facie* possible way of producing the scale required by MEU has been shown to be abortive (cf. Raiffa 1969, p. 5).

5.3. The other *prima facie* plausible way to obtain the required scale is to construct interval scales of measurement for *every* relevant attribute and then transform the attribute values into utility values. Mathematically, at least, the

[8] A more thorough analysis of the technique may be found in Miller and Starr (1960).

transformations would be relatively straightforward. As a matter of fact, both Hempel and Levi have begun their constructions of "epistemic utility" measures from approximately this point. (See Hempel 1962, p. 154; Levi 1967, p. 71.) Both of them have worked primarily *from* a "content measure" which yields values unique up to a linear transformation *to* a measure of "epistemic utility" which yields similar values. While there is nothing objectionable about this procedure in itself, it must be emphasized that it is at best a first step on a very long journey. Even if we had an acceptable measure of content, we would still almost certainly need measures of simplicity, explanatory power, precision of predictions, coherence with theories in other domains, probability, etc. in order to apply MEU. Needless to say, such measures are not available now and, judging from the history and present status of the unresolved issues surrounding the measurement of probability, they will not be available in the foreseeable future either. Again, however, such measures (interval scales) are not necessary for CBD, which may be applied as soon as one is able to construct a simple rank ordering of attribute values.

5.4. As has been suggested, the transformation of one interval scale into another is mathematically straightforward. If 'u' and 'a' represent the "epistemic utility" and attribute values, respectively, of accepting a certain hypothesis then

$$u = f(a),$$

where 'f' represents any transformation function up to and including the linear one

$$u = ma + n,$$

where 'm' and 'n' represent constants and $m \neq 0$. The extremely difficult problems before proponents of MEU with respect to these transformations are not, therefore, mathematical or merely technological. They are plainly philosophical. In particular, they involve the appropriate selection of 'f', or, in the linear case, the values of the constants 'm' and 'n'. In the latter case, for example, given interval scales of measurement for every relevant attribute, in order to apply MEU one must be able to systematically choose the appropriate constants and to present a plausible justification of his choices. The burden of proof then, that such and such a value for a certain attribute is worth this or that much 'epistemic utility' falls squarely upon MEU's adherents, and it is a burden which can hardly fail to create interminable haggling. After all, what principles could one invoke to show that, say, a hypothesis with a degree of simplicity of 0.8 ought to be assigned an "epistemic utility" of 0.8 or 0.6 or anything else? What principles could be used to prove that, say, a coherence value of 0.8 ought to be worth more or less than a simplicity value of 0.8? What could we use as a basis of comparing the significance of various attributes in order to transform their values into "epistemic utility" values? Clearly some sort of interattribute comparisons will be required to justify the transformation functions, but there is no basis for such comparisons. Of course, if we already knew the "epistemic utility" values corresponding to every attribute value for all attributes, then such comparisons would be self-evident. But that is beside the point. It is precisely those utility values that we are unable to obtain, because the required principles and bases for comparison do not exist. Indeed, even the idea that they (not to mention their justifications) might be forthcoming in the near future seems farfetched to say the least. Thus, we have another good reason for expecting perennial ineffectiveness from MEU and for turning to CBD instead.

5.5. Supposing, for the sake of argument, that all of the aforementioned problems were satisfactorily solved, proponents of MEU would still be faced with an amalgamation problem, i.e., with a problem of combining all of the individual "epistemic utility" values into a single most representative or appropriate value. Since they were forced beyond ordinal to cardinal values from the very beginning, they need not be troubled by Arrow's paradox (Arrow 1951; Michalos unpublished manuscript), Nevertheless, some rule of combination must be constructed and its plausibility defended, and this just creates more unnecessary work in view of the availability of CBD. Because a number of amalgamation rules have already been developed, however, this final step may be the least troublesome of all. (See, e.g., Harsanyi 1955; Hildreth 1953; Rescher 1969; Rothenberg 1961.) But it is still a piece of excess baggage.

To summarize the arguments in this section, I have been attempting to establish the ineffectiveness of MEU on the ground that it requires a more sophisticated sort of information than is now or will be in the foreseeable future available. To obtain this information, a number of problematic assumptions have yet to be made and substantiated. CBD, on the other hand, does not require such sophisticated information or, consequently, its attendant assumptions. Thus, a *prima facie* case for CBD over MEU has been established. But this is not enough. It is one thing to show that CBD does not have the infelicities of MEU and another to show that CBD is effective. It is to the latter task that we shall now turn. If it can be shown that CBD is at all effective now or can be expected to be effective in the foreseeable future, then both its superior effectiveness and efficiency over MEU will be established.

Harvey's Implicit Use of CBD

In Chap. 14 of his classic *Anatomical Disquisition on the Motion of the Heart and Blood in Animals* (Harvey 1889), Harvey summarizes his position as follows.

> Since *all things,* both argument and ocular demonstration, show that the blood passes through the lungs, and heart by the force of the ventricles, and is sent for distribution to all parts of the body, where it makes its way into the veins and porosities of the flesh, and then flows by the veins from the circumference on every side to the centre, from the lesser to the greater veins, and is by them finally discharged into the vena cava and right auricle of the heart, and this in such a quantity or in such a flux and reflux thither by the arteries, hither by the veins, *as cannot possibly be supplied by the ingesta* and *is much greater than can be required for mere purposes of nutrition*; it is absolutely necessary to conclude that the blood in the animal body is impelled in a circle, and is in a state of ceaseless motion; that this is the act or function which the heart performs by means of its pulse; and that it is the sole and only end of the motion and contraction of the heart (p. 93, italics added).

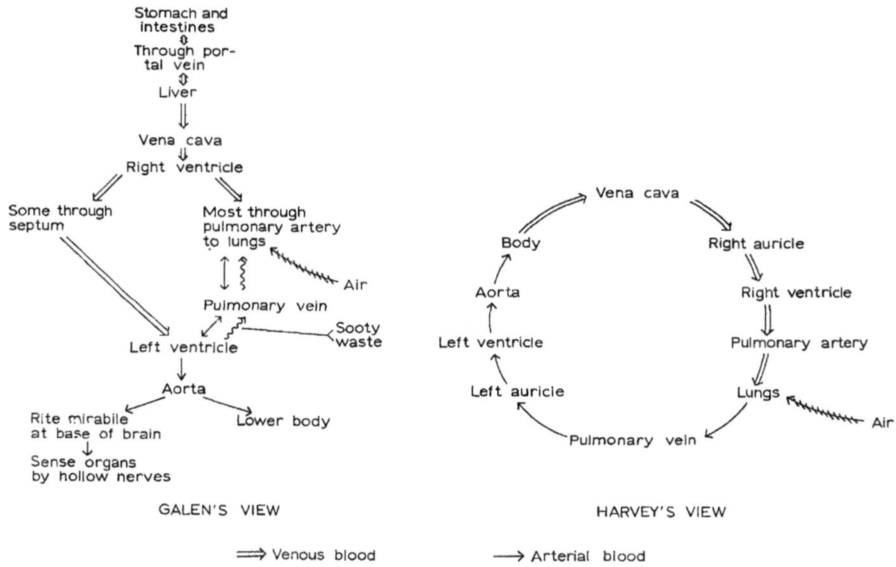

Fig. 1.1 Galen vs. Harvey on Motion of Blood

This famous paragraph is instructive in a number of ways, four of which are relevant to our discussion.

First, the fact that Harvey insists that "all things" show that his position is sound reveals an implicit acceptance of the methodological rule we have been adocating, namely, CBD. He obviously assumes that the sort of complete dominance that his hypothesis (theory) has over its rivals is a sufficient reason for accepting it. Some of the details of that dominance will be described below.

Second, the long conjunction from "show" to the italicized phrases outlines the circular path taken by the blood through a body. This is illustrated in Fig. 1.1 beside its most widely held alternative which was developed by Galen.[9] We shall have more to say about these diagrams below, but for now it is enough to notice that beginning with the vena cava, the arrows indicating the direction of flow in Harvey's view form a circle while those in Galen's view proceed along two straight paths with some "back-up". This illustrates the fundamental discrepancy between the view that Harvey is advocating and the alternative that he is rejecting.

Third, the italicized phrases refer to Galen's theory that the blood is produced from ingesta and dispersed outward continuously from the liver to the rest of the body for nutrition. Although Cesalpino (Crombie 1959, II, pp. 226–227) had somewhat vaguely and inconsistently advocated the theory that there was a daily ebbing and flowing (like the tides) between the heart and the veins and arteries, and

[9]The path outlined here for Galen's view has been put together from excerpts from *On the Functions of Parts of the Human Body* in Crombie (1959), Fleming (1955), Graubard (1964) and Singer (1957) and from the remarks of the historians themselves.

although there was some two way movement in Galen's view certainly in the pulmonary and portal veins and possibly throughout the system as a result of his theory of "attractive" and "expulsive faculties" (explained below), Harvey's primary target is the idea that the blood flows more or less continuously from the liver. It is this hypothesis especially that his continuous circulation theory is to replace.

Fourth, the remarks following the italicized phrases emphasize the main aspects of his theory, namely, that the blood in animals (not just men) is moved continuously in a circle by the contraction of the heart.

A careful examination of Harvey's text suggests that Harvey considered the following attributes as especially relevant to the comparison of his theory with Galen's: explanatory power, analogies with accepted theories in other domains, simplicity and logical (internal) consistency. A priori this set of attributes has no more to recommend it than a number of others one might suggest. But for our purposes it is not necessary to reach an agreement on the optimal set of appraising attributes. All that is required here is a generally satisfactory set, or as Herbert Simon would say, a 'satisficing' set (Simon and March 1958). Our primary goal is to show that with respect to each of these attributes, Harvey's theory is superior to Galen's.

Explanatory Power

Although Galen's theory could not account for any observable phenomena for which Harvey's theory had no explanation, the latter could but the former could not account for the facts that: (1) The amount of blood that passed into the aorta in an hour weighed much more than the total amount found in an animal (Harvey 1889, pp. 74–78, 87), (2) This amount of blood did not drain all the veins or rupture the arteries (Harvey 1889, p. 94). (3) It could not be produced from the juices of ingested aliment or absorbed as nutriment (Harvey 1889, pp. 75–78, 80, 87), (4) When the vena cava is closed the heart becomes pale and smaller, and when the aorta is closed the heart becomes deep purple and larger (Harvey 1889, pp. 46–47, 79), (5) A middling ligature closing a vein can cause a limb to swell and a tight ligature closing an artery can cause it to turn pale (Harvey 1889, pp. 81, 83), (6) Dissected bodies have much more blood in their veins than in their arteries and much more in the right ventricle than the left (Harvey 1889, pp. 76, 111). (7) The valves are situated in order to prevent the passage of blood from the large to the small veins which would cause swelling and rupture (Harvey 1889, pp. 89–90), (8) Tumefaction follows a blow to the temple (Harvey 1889, p. 85). (9) In phlebotomy a ligature must be applied above the puncture (Harvey 1889, p. 85). (10) When a patient undergoing a phlebotomy becomes weaker the blood drains more slowly (Harvey 1889, p. 87), (11) A whole system may become contaminated although the originally infected part is apparently sound (Harvey 1889, p. 96). (12) Medicine applied externally influences internal organs (Harvey 1889, p. 97),

As if all of this were not enough, Harvey includes the following general remark near the end of his penultimate chapter.

> Finally, reflecting on every part of medicine, physiology, pathology, semeiotics and therapeutics, when I see how many questions can be answered, how many doubts resolved, how much obscurity illustrated by the truth we have declared, … I see a field of such vast extent in which I might proceed so far, and expatiate so widely, that this my tractate would not only swell out into a volume, … but my whole life, perchance, would not suffice for its completion (Harvey 1889, pp. 99–100).

External Analogies

While the sort of movement envisaged by Galen's theory suggested little more than a perpetually flowing stream, the cyclic motion of Harvey's theory was analogous to and fit together admirably with a number of ideas and theories that he accepted in other domains. Indeed, immediately following his description of the path followed by the blood, he cites four analogies that would have been familiar to most of his readers.

> This motion we may be allowed to call circular, in the same way as Aristotle says that the air and the rain emulate [a] the circular motion of the superior bodies; [b] for the moist earth, warmed by the sun, evaporates; the vapours drawn upwards are condensed, and descending in the form of rain, moisten the earth again, [c] By this arrangement are generations of living things produced; [d] and in like manner are tempests and meteors engendered by the circular motion, and by the approach and recession of the sun (Harvey 1889, p. 71).[10]

Seven chapters later we find him again arguing in peripatetic fashion that since "under all circumstances" motion generates and preserves "heat and spirits" which are necessary for life, a body must have its "particular seat and fountain, a kind of home and hearth, where … the original of the native fire, is stored and preserved". This "original" in animals was none other than their pulsating hearts (Harvey 1889, p. 94; Pagel 1961, p. 181).

Simplicity

Harvey's theory was simpler than Galen's in the sense that the former required fewer basic assumptions and ad hoc hypotheses than the latter. In the first place, Galen regarded the liver as the center of the venous system and the heart as the center of the arterial system, with anastomosis between the two systems and

[10]Both Crombie (1959, II, pp. 235–237) and Pagel (1961, pp. 177–182) regard these analogies as highly influential on Harvey's thinking.

"communication between the cavities of the heart" through "the tiny pores which appear above all toward the middle of the partition between the cavities…" (Harvey 1889, pp. 34, 38–39; Galen 1916, p. 321). Harvey's theory of course had a single center, the heart, and as for "the tiny pores" in the septum, he exclaimed "By Hercules! no such pores can be demonstrated, nor in fact do any such exist" (Harvey 1889, p. 42). Furthermore, the ad hoc assumption of anything passing through the septum raised more questions than it answered.

> … how could one of the ventricles extract anything from the other… when we see that both ventricles contract and dilate simultaneously? Why should we not rather believe that the right took spirits from the left, than that the left obtained blood from the right ventricle…? But it is certainly mysterious and incongruous that blood should be supposed to be most commodiously drawn through a set of obscure and invisible ducts, and air through perfectly open passages, at one and the same moment. And why… is recourse had to secret and invisible porosities, to uncertain and obscure channels, to explain the passage of the blood to the left ventricle, when there is so open a way through the pulmonary veins (Harvey 1889, p. 42).

It is perhaps worthwhile to notice here that although the capillaries required by Harvey's theory to permit blood to pass from arteries to veins were as "obscure and invisible" as the "uncertain and obscure channels" through the septum required by Galen's theory,[11] the assumption of the existence of the former did not create more problems than it solved. Indeed, it seems to be primarily this aspect of the hypothesis of invisible capillaries which makes it decidedly not ad hoc.

Second, Galen's view of the *causes* of the movement of "material" to and from the heart was enormously more complicated than Harvey's. The latter's view was mentioned in the fourth point that was cited above following his summary of Chap. 14. In Galen's view "almost all parts of the animal" possessed an "attractive faculty" by means of which they obtained their "proper juice", a "retentive faculty", which was responsible for the retention of whatever was of "some benefit", an "alterative faculty", which accounted for the conversion of attracted material into "nourishment", and an "expulsive faculty" that explained the elimination of whatever was not of "some benefit" (Galen 1916, pp. 223–225, 247–249, 307). For example, with respect to the stomach he explains:

> … the attractive faculty in connection with swallowing, the retentive with digestion, the expulsive with vomiting and with the descent of digested food into the small intestine – and digestion itself we have shown to be a process of alteration (Galen 1916, p. 275).

He also distinguishes *"two kinds of attraction,* that by which a vacuum becomes refilled and that caused by appropriateness of quality" (Galen 1916, p. 319). All "hollow organs" such as the heart and arteries display both kinds of attraction during diastole, with the former "always attracting lighter matter first" and perhaps from some distance, while the latter "acts frequently… on what is heavier" and usually nearby (Galen 1916, pp. 317–319, 325),

[11]The flow of blood through capillaries was not observed until 1661 by Marcello Malpighi (Crombie 1959, II).

> The arteries draw into themselves on every side; those arteries which reach the skin draw in the outer air… those which pass up from the heart into the neck, and that which lies along the spine… draw mostly from the heart itself; and those which are further from the heart and skin necessarily draw the lightest part of the blood out of the veins (Galen 1916, p. 317).

This should be enough for our purposes. Rather than providing a general causal explanation of the movement of "material" to and from the heart as described in his *On the Functions of Parts of the Human Body* and outlined in Fig. 1.1, Galen has given us reasons to expect *not* that but another kind of movement. For with this explanatory scheme "almost all" of the single arrows in Fig. 1.1 should be replaced by double arrows.[12]

Furthermore, considering the fact that he only uses the term 'faculty' "so long as we are ignorant of the true essence of the cause which is operating" (Galen 1916, p. 17), even if his view were internally consistent, it would not be very informative. And finally, to return to our original point, even if the scheme worked, it was much more complicated and contained many more loose ends than Harvey's.

Internal Consistency

Galen was fully aware that the uncoordinated activity of the "attractive" and "expulsive faculties" could lead to paralysis or chaos. But he thought that the whole system could run smoothly if the faculties operated "consecutively" like inhaling and exhaling (Galen 1916, pp. 303–307). Harvey knew that explanation was inadequate. If, as noted above, the "ventricles contract and dilate simultaneously" and if they only attract with dilation and repel with contraction, then they could not be exchanging anything "consecutively" (Harvey 1889, p. 42). So either there was no exchange or the "faculty" scheme was faulty, or, as Harvey claimed, both. Similarly, Harvey claimed that on Galen's view the "spirits"[13] in the aorta (which were necessary to the life of the heart as well as every other organ) should have been drawn into the left ventricle as a result of its "attractive faculty", but somehow they always escaped (Harvey 1889, p. 40). This is merely a special case of the

[12]Crombie (1959, I, pp. 164–165) and Fleming (1955) completely missed this point, and criticized historians who had referred to a general ebbing and flowing in the whole venous system. See also section "Internal Consistency" below.

[13]Galen imagined that the vital functions were produced by the activity of three kinds of "spirits", namely, the "vital spirit" of the heart, the "natural spirit" of the liver and the "animal spirit" of the brain. The first "accounted for" the "vital faculty" or "principle of animal life", the second for the "vegetative faculty" or "principle of nutrition and growth" and the third for the "psychic faculty" or "spiritual principle of life" (Crombie 1959; Ackermann 1961, pp. 163–167).

general point made above, namely, that "almost all" of the arrows on Galen's view in Fig. 1.1 turn out to be both double and single at the same time, which is impossible. Again, Harvey saw that the idea that the mitral valve[14] should allow the "spirituous blood" to pass from the left ventricle to the lungs while at the same time it prevented the "thinner" air from retrogressing through the same channel was plainly inconsistent (Harvey 1889, p. 40). And finally, he noted a similar infelicity in the alleged "cooling and cleaning system" operating between the left ventricle and lungs by means of the pulmonary vein. If the mitral valve prevented the "cooling" air from escaping once it arrived in the left ventricle then it could not fail to prevent the "fuliginous vapours" from escaping also, in which case there would be no "cleansing" activity (Harvey 1889, p. 40).

This completes my review of Harvey's comparison of his theory with that of Galen's on the movement of the blood and the function of the heart with respect to the four attributes of explanatory power, analogies with other theories, simplicity and internal consistency. The implicit application of CBD with these attributes was *effective.* It produced a decision in favor of Harvey's view over Galen's. Harvey was certainly not "all right", especially in his selection of acceptable scientific theories in other domains, which is quite understandable.[15] But his errors are only relevant to the content of his argument, not to its logical form. From the logical or methodological point of view, his argument was perfectly non-demonstratively valid. His theory dominated its alternatives and was, therefore, more acceptable. Fortunately (for Harvey at least), unlike most theories, his theory has continued to dominate its alternatives. In fact, by the time he and his contemporaries had passed away, serious alternatives were no longer put forward (Graubard 1964, pp. 172–176). Hence, today it is appropriate to describe his theory not merely as more acceptable than its alternatives, but as acceptable.

Considering the results of sections "MEU Versus CBD: Comparison of Requirements" and "Harvey's Implicit Use of CBD" together now, I take it that the effectiveness and efficiency, and therefore, the superiority and preferability of CBD over MEU has been established. Before closing this investigation, however, two more general topics merit our attention. The first pertains to a certain infelicity shared by both MEU and CBD, and will be discussed in the next section. The second concerns various strategies that could be used to increase the effectiveness of CBD and, therefore, strengthen our case for it. These issues are taken up in section "Increasing the Effectiveness of CBD".

---

[14]The mitral valves are located between the auricles and ventricles in the mitral orifices on both sides of the heart. The one referred to here is on the left side and known as the 'bicuspid valve' because it has two flaps or doors.

[15]According to the first quotation in section "External Analogies" above, he evidently accepted a geocentric theory of the planetary system.

An Infelicity of MEU and CBD

The major drawback of both of these principles is that they do not provide any built-in evaluation for the variety of evidence for or against a hypothesis. If, for example, one hypothesis has a utility of 0.2 on the basis of a single attribute and a probability of 0.6 of obtaining its full value, while another hypothesis has a utility value of 0.2 for each of three attributes (two plus the one on which the other hypothesis is superior) with probabilities of 0.2 each, then the expected utility of each hypothesis is the same 0.12. Similarly, neither hypothesis dominates the other. However, the hypothesis with a greater variety of support might plausibly be regarded as warranting a higher assessment. What can be said about this discrepancy?

It seems to me that this problem of assessing variety may be treated in much the same way that voting theorists treat the problem of "no election". That is, we may introduce the attribute of 'variety' into our analysis just as voting theorists introduce the option 'no election' along with the list of candidates. (See, e.g., Dodgson 1963.) Then, just as a voter is allowed to judge the merits of each candidate in the presence of the option to have the whole election rescinded, our decision-makers are allowed to judge the variety of support for or against a hypothesis and assign it some appropriate value. Whether or not this strategy would work as well for our decision-makers as its analogue works for voters, a priori it certainly seems that it would.

Increasing the Effectiveness of CBD

There are a number of ways to increase the effectiveness of CBD, some of which put more severe demands on the number of assumptions and kinds of information required than proponents of CBD would be willing to satisfy. In the remaining paragraphs of this section I shall introduce five general tactics and indicate their peculiar costs.

8.1. You recall that one hypothesis was said to dominate another if *for all* attributes and contingencies the benefits and costs associated with the latter are not preferable to those of the former and for some attribute and contingency the benefits and costs associated with the former are preferable to those of the latter. The italicized phrase 'for all' may be regarded as an abbreviation of the longer locution 'for all n ($n \geq 1$) relevant attributes and m ($m \geq 1$) contingencies'. As long as n is sufficiently large, we may weaken the notion of dominance by degrees, by replacing 'for all n' by 'for all $n - 1$', 'for all $n - 2$', and so on up to 'for all $n(n - 1)$'. Thus while strong dominance and dominance place certain requirements on all attributes, $(n - 1)$-dominance puts requirements on all but one attribute, $(n - 2)$-dominance on all but two, etc. For example, a hypothesis whose benefits and costs were preferable to those of another with a single exception in which the latter's benefits (or costs) were preferable to the former might be said to $(n-1)$-dominate the latter, although it could not dominate the latter. Clearly, the chances of obtaining a single acceptable hypothesis with CBD increase as the degrees of dominance decrease from n. Moreover, no new information is required. On the other hand, it must be assumed that the data from some *prima facie* relevant attribute(s) may be safely ignored. That, of course, may be difficult to justify, especially in the completely general fashion proposed. For notice that, say, $(n-1)$-dominance does not specify any particular attribute to be ignored. It merely permits a reversal in any attribute whatsoever, and one may be reluctant to grant such sweeping permission.[16]

Just as one can reduce n to $n-1$, etc. one can reduce m to $m-1$, etc. when there are a sufficient number of contingencies. This would produce the same advantages and disadvantages as reductions in n.

Finally, it should be mentioned that one could again use the analogy between this investigation and voting theory, and consider such familiar notions of dominance as simple majority dominance, absolute majority dominance, $\frac{2}{3}$ dominance, and so on.[17] For specific n's and m's, all of these phrases could be translated into the 'n minus something' terminology.

8.2. Having considered the apriori elimination of attributes and contingencies, there are two fairly natural tacks to take. One may consider the elimination of specially selected contingencies or of specially selected attributes. I shall discuss the former in this subsection and the latter in the next.

It is a familiar fact that the decision rules known as 'minimax loss', 'minimax regret', 'maximin gain', 'maximax gain' and 'Hurwicz's rule' focus a decision-maker's attention on only some of the contingencies before him. For example, minimax loss tells one to merely review the maximum losses (costs) possible as a result of accepting any hypothesis given each contingency, and to act so as to guarantee the smallest of the maximum losses possible. Similarly, one might eliminate all of the data on benefits from one's analysis and define a concept of minimax-dominance. To determine which hypothesis minimax-dominated which, one would review the maximum costs attached to each hypothesis for every contingency and regard that one as minimax-dominant which insured the smallest maximum possible cost. Concepts of minimax regret-dominance, maximax-dominance, etc. could be constructed analogously.

All of these qualified types of dominance would be easier to obtain than unqualified dominance. So their use would increase the effectiveness of CBD. Furthermore, they do not require any more information. Indeed, some of them require less information, because they completely disregard either benefits or costs.

---

[16]Most of the case histories cited in Bunge (1961) seem to have admitted some reversals, although a more careful analysis might reveal a different picture.

[17]From a formal or logico-mathematical point of view, voting theory and the theory of multi-attribute decision-making are virtually indistinguishable. See, for example, Mackenzie (1967), Michalos (1969c, 1970a, to be published, unpublished manuscript).

However, this demands the rather bold assumption that such data *and more* can be safely ignored, and a priori there seems to be no justification for this assumption.

8.3. As Miller and others have shown (Archer et al. 1955; Hayes 1962; Miller 1956; Osgood et al. 1957; Shepard 1964), there is a general tendency for decision-makers to unwittingly let one or two of many relevant attributes determine their final judgment. Moreover, as MacCrimmon (1968) and Raiffa (1969) have recently emphasized, for one reason or another, a decision-maker may *choose* to regard one attribute as more important than all of the others together. In the latter case then, concepts of specific attribute dominance might be defined such as 'probability-dominance', 'explanatory power-dominance', etc. to be used with CBD. While such an approach presupposes interattribute comparisons of importance and, therefore, additional evaluative criteria, "weighing" devices, assumptions and justifications, it is still less demanding than MEU. Hence, with this modification, CBD would probably (depending primarily on the number of vitally important attributes selected) still be more effective than MEU.

8.4. If the total expulsion of some attributes and/or contingencies from the set of relevant evidence seems unjustifiable, a less drastic procedure may seem attractive. It has already been noted that evaluative criteria and "weighing" devices would have to be developed in order to select the one or two supremely important attributes mentioned in the previous paragraph. *If* every attribute could be assigned a numerical value indicating its weight of importance *and* all attribute values could also be expressed numerically, then each hypothesis could be assigned a numerical value equal to the sum of its weighted attribute values and the hypothesis with the largest sum could be regarded as the most acceptable. By requiring all weights of importance to be real numbers greater than zero, one could be certain that every relevant attribute had *some* influence on the total evaluation sum for each hypothesis. Neat as it sounds, such a procedure could not be practicable, because it demands even more information and assumptions, and could not be more effective than MEU.

8.5. As Simon and March (1958) and Ellsberg (1961) have insisted, it is sometimes easier to determine that something is unsatisfactory than it is to determine just how satisfactory something is. It is usually easier to decide which shirts, suits, socks, or ties "just won't do" than it is to decide which of a couple fairly decent ones one should buy. Following Simon, we may say that an attribute value is satisficing if and only if hypotheses with such a value could in every sense of this term be acceptable. It follows then, that any hypothesis with a non-satisficing value for some attribute in some contingency cannot be acceptable. Hence, such hypotheses may be immediately eliminated from consideration, with CBD applied to the remainder. By providing a good reason for rejecting some hypotheses that might otherwise remain in the set of live options, a review of attribute values from a satisficing point of view could increase the a priori chance of obtaining a single acceptable hypothesis with CBD. The apparent additional information required is the minimum satisficing attribute value for every attribute. Even if such comprehensive data was not available, however, it might still be worthwhile (i.e., increase the effectiveness of CBD) to know *some* minimum satisficing values. Naturally the identification of such values presupposes assumptions and justifications for the evaluative criteria employed.

8.6. Finally, it should be noted that one could combine some of the tactics described in 8.1–8.5.[18] For examples, one could use a satisficing review of attribute values (8.5) along with a weaker concept of dominance (8.1); a contingency eliminating rule (8.2) with a weaker concept of dominance; (8.1), (8.2) and (8.5) together; and so on. What must always be remembered, of course, is that increases in the number of tactics employed create corresponding increases in the number of assumptions and justifications required. Furthermore, the very reason CBD has been recommended here in the first place is that it is supposed to reduce the latter without excessive costs.

Conclusion

Since I have summarized the argument for my central thesis at the end of section "Preferability and Superior Performance", it is not necessary to repeat it here. All that remains to be said now is that what is required at this point is a strong defense of a particular set of relevant attributes or, in Bunge's words (1961), "assaying criteria" for the evaluation of all hypotheses. Perhaps no single set will do for all kinds of hypotheses. What we require of acceptable laws may be different from what we require of acceptable theories. Attributes that are relevant for the determination of the acceptability of ordinary sentences (rather than laws or theories) may well be something else again. At any rate, if my case for CBD over MEU has been argued persuasively, then it is clearly the relevant attributes or "assaying criteria" that should be the focus of our attention now.

Acknowledgements The number of friends who have kindly given me suggestions and encouragement is almost embarrassingly large, but I would like to express my gratitude to Myles Brand, Cliff Hooker, David Hull, Scott Kleiner, Hugh Lehman, Werner Leinfellner, Andrew McLaughlin and Tom W. Settle.

References

Ackermann, R. (1961). Inductive simplicity. *Philosophy of Science, 28,* 152–161.
Ackoff, R. L. (1962). *Scientific method.* New York.
Archer, E. J., Bourne, L. E., & Brown, F. G. (1955). Concept identification as a function of irrelevant information and instructions. *Journal of Experimental Psychology, 49,* 153–164.
Arrow, K. J. (1951). *Social choice and individual values.* New York.
Barker, S. F. (1957). *Induction and hypothesis.* Ithaca.
Buchdahl, G. (1969). *Metaphysics and the philosophy of science.*

[18]This is also suggested by MacCrimmon (1968).

Bunge, M. (1959). *Metascientific queries*. Springfield.
Bunge, M. (1961). The weight of simplicity in the construction and assaying of scientific theories. *Philosophy of Science, 28,* 120–149.
Bunge, M. (1967). *Scientific research* (Vol. II). Berlin.
Burks, A. W. (1968). The pragmatic-Humean theory of probability and Lewis' theory. In P. A. Schilpp (Eds.), *The philosophy of C. I. Lewis* (pp. 415–464). LaSalle.
Carnap, R. (1950). *Logical foundations of probability.* Chicago.
Chisholm, R. M. (1968). Lewis' ethics of belief. In P. A. Schilpp (Eds.), *The philosophy of C. I. Lewis* (pp. 223–242). LaSalle
Crombie, A. C. (1959). *Medieval and early modem science* (Vol. I and II). Garden City.
Dodgson, C. L. (Lewis Carroll). (1963). *A discussion of the various methods of procedure in conducting elections* (reprinted in D. Black. *The theory of committees and elections* (pp. 214–222). Cambridge.).
Ellsberg, D. (1961). *Risk, ambiguity, and the savage axioms, P-2173.* Santa Monica: The RAND Corporation.
Fishbum, P. C. (1964). *Decision and value theory.* New York.
Fleming, D. (1955). Galen on the motions of the blood in the heart and lungs. *Isis, 46,* 14–21.
Galen. (1916). *On the natural faculties* (A. J. Brock Trans.). London.
Good, I. J. (1968). Corroboration, explanation, evolving probability, simplicity and a sharpened razor. *British Journal for the Philosophy of Science, 19,* 123–143.
Goodman, N. (1959). Recent developments in the theory of simplicity. *Philosophy and Phenomenological Research, 19,* 429–446.
Graubard, M. (1964). *Circulation and respiration.* New York.
Harsanyi, J. C. (1955). Cardinal welfare, individualistic ethics and interpersonal comparisons of utility. *Journal of Political Economy, 63,* 309–321.
Harvey, W. (1889). *An anatomical disquisition on the motion of the heart and blood in animals* (Willis's translation revised and edited by A. Bowie, London, 1889 and reprinted in C. M. B. Camac (Ed.). (1959). *Classics of medicine and surgery.* New York).
Hayes, J. R. (1962). Human data processing limits in decision making. *Electronics System Division Report,* ESD-TDR-62-48.
Hempel, C. G. (1960). Inductive inconsistencies. *Synthese, 12,* 439–469.
Hempel, C. G. (1962). Deductive-nomological versus statistical explanation. In H. Feigl & G. Maxwell (Eds.), *Minnesota studies in the philosophy of science* (Vol. III, pp. 98–169). Minneapolis.
Hempel, C. G. (1966). Recent problems of induction. In R. G. Colodny (Ed.), *Mind and cosmos* (pp. 112–134). Pittsburgh.
Hertz, H. (1956). *The principles of mechanics.* New York.
Hildreth, C. (1953). Alternative conditions for social orderings. *Econometrica, 21,* 81–91.
Hinrichs, H. H., & Taylor, G. M. (Eds.). (1969). *Program budgeting and benefit-cost analysis.* Pacific Palisades, CA.
Hintikka, J., & Suppes, P. (1966). *Aspects of inductive logic.* Amsterdam.
Jeffreys, H. (1957). *Scientific inference.* Cambridge.
Keynes, J. M. (1957). *A treatise on probability.* London.
Kuhn, A. (1963). *The study of society* (p. 111). Homewood.
Lakatos, I. (1968). Changes in the problem of inductive logic. In I. Lakatos (Ed.), *The problem of inductive logic.* Amsterdam.
Laudan, L. (1968). Theories of scientific method from Plato to Mach. *History of Science, 6,* 1–63.
Leach, J. (1968). Explanation and value neutrality. *British Journal for the Philosophy of Science, 19,* 93–108.
Leinfellner, W. (1968). Generalization of classical decision theory. In L. Borch & J. Mossin (Eds.), *Risk and uncertainty* (pp. 196–210). London.
Levi, I. (1962). On the seriousness of mistakes. *Philosophy of Science, 29,* 47–65.
Levi, I. (1967). *Gambling with truth.* New York.
Little, I. M. D. (1950). *A critique of welfare economics.* Oxford.

Luce, R. D., & Raiffa, H. (1964). *Games and decisions.* New York.
MacCrimmon, K. R. (1968). *Decisionmaking among multiple-attribute alternatives: A survey and consolidated approach, memorandum RM-4823-ARPA.* Santa Monica: The RAND Corporation.
Mackenzie, W. J. M. (1967). *Free elections.* London.
Manheim, M. L., & Hall, F. L. (1968). *Abstract representation of goals, P-67–24.* Department of Civil Engineering, M.I.T.
Margenau, H. (1950). *The nature of physical reality.* New York.
McLaughlin, A. (1970). Science, reason and value. *Theory and Decision, 2* (to be published).
Michalos, A. C. (1965a). *Probability and degree of confirmation: A study of the disagreement between Karl Popper and Rudolf Carnap from 1934 to 1964.* Doctoral dissertation, University of Chicago.
Michalos, A. C. (1965b). Two theorems of degree of confirmation. *Ratio, 7,* 196–198.
Michalos, A. C. (1966). Estimated utility and corroboration. *British Journal for the Philosophy of Science, 16,* 327–331.
Michalos, A. C. (1967a). Postulates of rational preference. *Philosophy of Science, 34,* 18–22.
Michalos, A. C. (1967b). Descriptive completeness and linguistic variance. *Dialogue, 6,* 224–228.
Michalos, A. C. (1969a). An alleged condition of evidential support. *Mind, 78,* 440–441.
Michalos, A. C. (1969b). *Principles of logic.* Englewood Cliffs.
Michalos, A. C. (1969c). A theory of decision-making evaluation. Paper read at the Annual Meeting of the Eastern Division of the American Philosophical Association.
Michalos, A. C. (1969d). Positivism versus the elermeneutic-dialectic school. *Theoria, 35*(Part 3), 267–278.
Michalos, A. C. Analytic and other "dumb" guides of life. *Analysis* (to be published).
Michalos, A. C. (1970a). Decision-making in committees. *American Philosophical Quarterly, 7,* 91–106.
Michalos, A. C. (1970b). *Efficiency and morality.* Paper read at the Annual Meeting of the Western Division of the American Philosophical Association.
Michalos, A. C. The costs of decision-making. *Public Choice* (to be published).
Michalos, A. C. *The impossibility of an ordinal measure of acceptability* (unpublished manuscript).
Miller, G. A. (1956). The magical number seven, plus or minus two. *Psychological Review, 63,* 81–97.
Miller, D. W., & Starr, M. K. (1960). *Executive decisions and operations research.* Englewood Cliffs.
Milner, J. (1960). Games against nature. In R. M. Thrall, C. H. Coombs, & R. L. Davis (Eds.), *Decision processes* (pp. 49–60). New York.
von Neumann, J., & Morgenstem, O. (1947). *The theory of games and economic behavior.* Princeton.
Newman, P. (1965). *The theory of exchange.* Englewood Cliffs.
Osgood, C. S., Suci, G. J., & Tannenbaum, P. H. (1957). *The measurement of meaning.* Urbana.
Pagel, W. (1961). The position of Harvey and van Helmont in the history of European thought. In R. M. Palter (Ed.), *Toward modern science* (Vol. II, pp. 175–191). New York.
Popper, K. R. (1959). *The logic of scientific discovery.* New York.
Prest, A. R., & Turvey, R. (1965). Cost-benefit analysis: A survey. *The Economic Journal, 75,* 683–735.
Pruzan, P. M. (1966). Is cost-benefit analysis consistent with the maximization of expected utility? In J. R. Lawrence (Ed.), *Operational research and the social sciences* (pp. 319–336). London.
Raiffa, H. (1969). *Preferences for multi-attributed alternatives, memorandum RM-5868-DOT/RC.* Santa Monica: The RAND Corporation.
Rescher, N. (1969). *Introduction to value theory.* Englewood Cliffs.
Rothenberg, J. (1961). *The measurement of social welfare.* Englewood Cliffs.
Salmon, W. C. (1966). *The foundations of scientific inference.* Pittsburgh.
Schlesinger, G. (1963). *Method in the physical sciences.* London.

Shepard, R. N. (1964). On subjectively optimum selection among multi-attribute alternatives. In M. W. Shelly & G. L. Bryan (Eds.), *Human judgments and optimality* (pp. 257–281). New York.

Simon, H. A., & March, J. G. (1958). *Organizations.* New York.

Singer, C. (1957). *A short history of anatomy and physiology from the Greeks to Harvey.* New York.

Stedry, A. C., & Chames, A. (1966). The attainment of organization goals through appropriate selection of subunit goals. In J. R. Lawrence (Eds.), *Operational research and the social sciences* (pp. 147–164). London.

Tullock, G., & Buchanan, J. M. (1962). *The calculus of consent.* Ann Arbor.

Wilkie, J. S. (1965). Harvey's immediate debt to Aristotle and to Galen. *History of Science, 4,* 103–124.

Williams, P. M. (1969). The structure of acceptance and its evidential basis. *British Journal for the Philosophy of Science, 19,* 325–344.

Wilson, C. Z., & Alexis, M. (1962). Basic frameworks for decisions. *Journal of the Academy of Management, 5,* 151–164.

Chapter 2
Social Indicators Research and Health-Related Quality of Life Research

Alex C. Michalos

Introduction

Research related to quality-of-life ought to benefit from efforts of researchers trained in diverse disciplines, addressing more or less similar problems, with more or less similar aims. One of the early, great philosophers of science of the twentieth century, Rudolf Carnap, said that what surprised and distressed him most about his work in philosophy of physics was that while he thought his research bridging two disciplines would be welcomed by both sides, in fact it was unwelcomed (Schilpp 1963). Both sides thought his work was neither fish nor fowl, and it was only when the field of philosophy of science reached something like disciplinary status, with its own journals, recognized authorities, classic texts, paradigms, standard courses and so on, that his work received the attention and approbation it deserved.

I do not think social indicators research and health-related quality of life research constitute distinct disciplines, but there are relatively independent research groups devoted to the range of issues in each field. In this paper I try to build something like a modest footbridge between the two fields in order to make it easier for researchers in both fields to draw on the body of knowledge accumulated in each field. I hope I have more success than Carnap, but whether or not I do, I am happy

---

This essay was written for presentation at an invited plenary session of the annual meeting of the International Society for Quality of Life Research held in Amsterdam, 7–10 November 2001. The original plan was to give special attention to research on happiness, but the focus became broader as the story unfolded.

Michalos, A.C.: 2004. Social indicators research and health-related quality of life research. Social Indicators Research, 65, pp. 27–72.

A.C. Michalos (✉)
University of Northern British Columbia, Prince George, BC, Canada
e-mail: michalos@brandonu.ca

A.C. Michalos, *Connecting the Quality of Life Theory to Health, Well-Being and Education*, DOI 10.1007/978-3-319-51161-0_2

to report that my own understanding of the research undertaken on each side of the bridge has been immensely enriched by this investigation. So, I am grateful to the organizers of this conference for the invitation to write this paper.

The structure of the essay is as follows. In the next section "Social Indicators of the Quality of Life: Basic Definitions" I briefly review some basic definitions concerning social indicators of the quality of life. After that, there is a section "Historical Origins and Motives" reviewing some of the historical origins and motives behind social indicators research. I assume, with some evidence, that measures of happiness provide at least one important way to operationalize the variety of ideas referred to by the phrase 'quality of life'. In section "Explaining Happiness with Life as a Whole from Selected Domain Satisfaction Items" I review results of eleven surveys undertaken to explain happiness on the basis of the personal satisfaction respondents got from a dozen specific domains of their lives, e.g., satisfaction with their jobs, their living partners, their financial security and their health. Following that, in section "Explaining Happiness with Life as a Whole from Health and Other Variables" I review results of three surveys undertaken to explain happiness on the basis of respondents' health measured by such things as SF-36, chronic illnesses and Body Mass Index scores. Then there are two sections in which I review studies designed to explain satisfaction with one's health on the basis of measured health status (section "Explaining Satisfaction with One's Own Health") and on the basis of Multiple Discrepancies Theory (MDT, section "Multiple Discrepancies Theory (MDT)"). While the material in the sixth section is based on a single study, that in the seventh section is based on 58 studies of undergraduate student samples taken from 83 universities in 39 countries, involving over 18000 students. In section "Health-Related Quality of Life" I review nearly two dozen studies in the tradition of health-related quality of life in order to illustrate the serious confounding and question-begging that one encounters with explained and explanatory variables in this tradition. Finally, there is a short overview and concluding section "Conclusion".

Social Indicators of the Quality of Life: Basic Definitions

Since the middle of the 1960s there have been people working all over the world in what many of us used to call the "social indicators research movement". The term "social indicator" is used to denote a social statistic that is supposed to have some significance for the quality of life, and the term "social report" designates an organized collection of social indicators. From a linguistic point of view, social indicators usually consist of a term denoting a subject class and a term denoting what I call an "indicator property". For example, the second term of the phrase "infant mortality" denotes the indicator property mortality and the first term denotes a particular class of things, namely, infants that may possess that property. By replacing the subject term "infant" by "one year old", "two year old", etc., we can routinely generate (social) mortality indicators for as many age groups as we like.

Similarly, by replacing the subject term by "male", "Indian", etc., we can routinely generate mortality indicators for as many kinds of groups as we like.

Social indicator *phrases* are like variable *names* in logic and mathematics, and social indicators are like the variables themselves. Furthermore, just as we speak of the values of variables in logic and math, we may speak of the indicator-values of social indicators. For example, human body weight is a (social) health indicator which may have an indicator-value of 120 lb. Finally, and most importantly, strictly speaking it is the indicator-value of a social indicator which indicates whatever it is that a particular indicator is supposed to indicate. For example, if the indicator-value of one's body weight is 600 lb then this indicates that one is probably obese (or very, very tall), eats more carbohydrates, starches and fats than most people, shops at special clothing stores, suffers fatigue and shortness of breath from little exertion, cannot sit comfortably in a theatre seat, and may have difficulty finding a suitable mate. Usually, the relationship between an indicator-value and what it indicates is a one-many relationship, as my example indicates.

Social indicators that refer to personal feelings, attitudes, preferences, opinions, judgments or beliefs of some sort are called *subjective indicators,* e.g., satisfaction with one's health, attitudes toward exercise, beliefs about the benefits of some therapy. Social indicators that refer to things that are relatively easily observable and measurable are called *objective indicators*, e.g., the height and weight of people, numbers of people admitted to hospital, numbers of people dying per year.

Positive indicators are such that most people will assume that if their indicator-values increase, some facet of the quality of life is improving, e.g., elderly citizens incomes and minority-group educational attainment. *Negative indicators* are such that most people will assume that if their indicator-values increase, some facet of the quality of life is deteriorating, e.g., infant mortality rates and murder rates. (Notice that an indicator is here regarded as positive or negative not in virtue of whether or not its values in fact increase or decrease, but only in virtue of whether or not most people would like its values to increase or decrease, i.e., not in virtue of the *fact* but in virtue of the *desirability* of an increase or decrease in its values.) *Unclear indicators* are such that either (a) most people will not be willing or able to say whether bigger indicator-values indicate a better or worse state of affairs, e.g., welfare payments, or (b) there is serious disagreement about whether bigger indicator-values indicate a better or worse state of affairs, e.g., divorce rates. In the case of welfare payments, we do not know what to say because as the values increase there may be an increase of people in need of such assistance, which is bad; while, at the same time, there is an increase in the amount of assistance given, which is good. In the case of divorce rates, on the other hand, many people know exactly what they want to say, and they happen to disagree with what some other people want to say.

Input indicators indicate some sort of inputs into a process or product, e.g., daily exercise time. *Output indicators* indicate some sort of output of a process or product, e.g., Body Mass Index. Unlike the previous classifications of indicators, what counts as an input or output indicator depends on the purposes of the classification. For example, from the point of view of a therapist or coach, a person's daily exercise time could be regarded as the output resulting from advice, admonitions

Table 2.1 Types of social indicators for health domain

Positive (P)			Negative (N)	
Input (I)				
Objective (O)	IOP	(e.g., daily exercise time)	ION	(e.g., cigarettes smoked per day)
Subjective (S)	ISP	(e.g., positive attitude toward exercise)	ISN	(e.g., positive attitude toward smoking)
Output (U)				
Objective (O)	UOP	(e.g., normal BMI score)	UON	(e.g., stained fingers and teeth)
Subjective (S)	USP	(e.g., satisfaction with weight)	USN	(e.g., dissatisfaction with staines)

and threats given to a patient or student. Similarly, a person's BMI could be regarded as an input indicator for a therapist or coach trying to decide what sort of exercise to prescribe.

All of these kinds of indicators are summarized in Table 2.1, with examples of each. (Michalos 1988 shows how these distinctions could be used to systematically expand UNESCO's annual international reports.)

When people use the phrase 'quality of life', they sometimes intend to contrast it with *quantities* or *numbers* of something. There are, then, two quite different sorts of things that one might want to refer to when using the phrase 'quality of life'. In the first place, one might want to refer to sorts, types or kinds of things rather than to mere numbers of things. For example, one might want to know not merely how many people were admitted to a hospital last year and for how long, but also what sorts of people they were, male or female, young or old, rich or poor, and so on. When the term quality in the phrase 'quality of life' is used in this sense, one may say that it and the phrase in which it occurs is intended to be primarily *descriptive*.

In the second place, however, one might want to refer to the *value* or *worth* of things by using the term 'quality' in the phrase 'quality of life'. For example, one frequently hears of people making a trade-off between, say, a high salary on the one hand and better working conditions on the other. Presumably the exchange here involves monetary and some other value. That is, one exchanges the value of a certain amount of money for the value of a certain set of working conditions. When the term 'quality' in the phrase quality of life is used in this sense, one may say that it and the phrase in which it occurs is intended to be primarily *evaluative*. (Different theories about values are reviewed in Michalos (1980, 1981), and aggregation problems are reviewed in Michalos (1970a, b, c, d, 1997, 2001).)

Both senses of the phrase 'quality of life' are important. It is important to be able to describe human existence in a fairly reliable and valid fashion, and it is important to be able to evaluate human existence in the same way. In philosophic jargon, one would say that a complete account of the quality of life requires a thorough examination of its nature or being as well as an examination of its value or good, i.e., an ontological account answering the question 'What is its nature?' and an axiological account answering the question 'What is its value?'. I suppose it is trivially true (tautological) that the improvement of one's relatively objective and subjective conditions implies an improvement in the quality of one's life in an evaluative sense. From a consequentialist moral point of view, our aim should be to improve or increase the value or worth of the lives of all people (Michalos 1995). Thus, the general line of my approach is in the naturalistic subjectivist tradition of the American pragmatists, especially James (1909), Perry (1926, 1954), Dewey (1939) and Lewis (1946). Since the tradition has been around for a long time, there is no need to review its strengths and weaknesses. From this point of view, the quality of a person's or community's life, in an evaluative sense, is directly proportionate to the net levels of satisfaction generated by that life for everyone affected by it. As James put it in an essay first published in 1891,

> That act must be the best act ... which makes for the *best whole,* in the sense of awakening the least sum of dissatisfactions. In the casuistic scale, therefore, those ideals must be written highest which prevail at the least cost, or by whose realization the least possible number of other ideals are destroyed.... The course of history is nothing but the story of men's struggles from generation to generation to find the more and more inclusive order (James 1977, p. 623).

When researchers measure a person's overall quality of life in terms of his or her reported happiness or satisfaction, they are most likely assuming that people are the best judges of the value or worth of their own lives and that as their reported levels of happiness or satisfaction increase or decrease, the quality of their lives (its value or worth) is increasing or decreasing. If all other things are equal, it is reasonable and morally right to give personal reports some privileged status in assessing the quality of a person's life (e.g., Nord et al. 2001). Nevertheless, one hardly needs scientific research to realize that all other things are often not equal, although there is plenty of research to prove it (Michalos 1990, 1991a). Thus, giving people the first word to assess the overall quality of their own lives does not imply that each person's word is always the only, best or final word, or that such first words are in principle incorrigible (Lewis 1946; Braybrooke 1967). It is quite possible that some external observers might assess the value or worth of some person's life with different results based on different and even more reasonable and morally acceptable methods, all things considered. Essentially, that is why loyal agency to a patient or any sort of client cannot bear the weight of serving as a supreme moral principle (Michalos 1979; Brunk 1987; Poff 1987). In his broad approach to quality of life measurement, Hornquist (1989) explicitly, systematically and I think quite properly allows for such circumstances. Apriori one cannot say for all people and for all time what is the single best method for assessing the overall quality of everyone's life, all things considered. As I explained in Michalos (1978, 1992, 1995), one can not even give a rigorous account of what it would mean to consider all things. Thus, the best one can do is try to assemble a reasonable profile of the objective and subjective features of people's lives, and to evaluate the profile in a reasonable and morally acceptable way. In short, in the end, we muddle our way through to something we think is worthy of being called a good or bad quality of life (Michalos 2001).

Historical Origins and Motives

Since good histories of the recent origins of the social indicators movement have been published by Michalos (1980, 1999), Land (1983), MacRae (1985), Ferris (1990), Noll and Zapf (1994), Vogel (1994) and Sirgy (in press), there is no need for an extensive review here. By the middle 1950s and 1960s there was a flurry of activity in all industrialized countries and in international organizations. It was a period in which governments were committed to activism. Government sponsored social programs blossomed across the globe, bringing with them the need to monitor results in order to evaluate the programs. It was reminiscent of the 1930s when everyone struggled to pull the world out of recession and planning associations sprung up at all levels of government (Karl 1974; President's Research Committee on Social Trends 1933; League for Social Reconstruction Research Committee 1935).

The longer historical tradition of social indicators researchers may be traced back fairly directly to Jeremy Bentham's ideas about a 'felicific calculus' that would allow decision makers to calculate the net pleasure or pain connected to every action for everyone affected by that action, with public policy choices made to get the greatest net pleasure or least net pain for the greatest number of people (Bentham 1789). For economists, utility theory is the apparent heir of Bentham's calculus (Mitchell 1918). Utility theory is formally elegant and has been an enormously fruitful source of research programs in individual and group decision making related to commercial markets, social and political relations, bargaining, conflict resolution, gaming and scarce resource allocation in practically all areas, including health (Nussbaum and Sen 1993; Torrance 1986). It is the heart of micro economics. Unfortunately, utility theory (as many other theories) is much better on paper and in classroom exercises than it is in practice, especially in public policy making. What is worse, utility theory begins with revealed preferences which are the mere tips of socially, psychologically and pragmatically constructed icebergs of more or less coherent systems of knowledge, opinions, attitudes, desires and needs (Michalos 1967, 1978, 1985; Schwarz and Strack 1999) While economists and other utility theorists see the iceberg tips and ask 'How can we use them?', psychologists and sociologists see them and ask 'What is their source?' and 'Is it reasonable to use them?'. More often than not, social indicators researchers have been on the side of psychologists and sociologists.

At least since the mid 1930s, statistics from National Income and Product Accounts have been routinely used for public policy making in total disregard of any microeconomic utility analysis. Thus, many of us (social indicators researchers) thought that what was required for public policy making was a set of social and later environmental indicators that could be combined with the National Accounts to create a System of Social, Economic and Environmental Accounts. In most industrialized countries today, government funded research on this project is continuing. I believe one of the motivating forces that most social indicators researchers have in common is this vision of a grand accounting system with a place for everything important and everything important in its place (Juster and Land 1981; Fox 1985). A Task Force of the International Society for Quality of Life Studies recently published a long paper in which some adequacy criteria for such a grand system were presented, along with some analyses of some contemporary constructions (Hagerty et al. 2001). Needless to say, we are far from any generally accepted system. Some researchers in the health-related quality of life tradition seem to envision comprehensive systems that are similar to those envisioned by social indicators researchers, e.g., Hörnquist (1989), Renwick and Brown (1996).

Given most social indicators researchers' shared vision of a grand accounting scheme, it will come as no surprise that most of us also share a love for crunching numbers. While most of us grant the importance of qualitative speculative and empirical work, we are primarily interested in attaching numbers to things and to the value of things, and using quantitative information to solve public policy problems. It will also come as no surprise that most social indicators researchers are males and that, silly as it is, many of us seem to have the attitude that our numbers can beat their numbers. 'Our' numbers are the numbers produced by sociologists, psychologists and environmentalists, while 'their' numbers are the ones produced by economists. Admitting some oversimplification, most social indicators researchers think that it is a mistake for people interested in the quality of life to limit their focus of attention to commercial market activities and to evaluate everything countable by the single measure of money. We would judge it equally mistaken to limit one's attention to human health. Put positively, we think the quality of people's lives can be measured and compared directly using indicators of such things as life expectancy free of disability, educational attainment, crime rates, literacy rates, resource depletion rates, air pollution rates, stress at work, satisfaction with family relations, self-esteem and so on. Most likely, we suppose that if a grand accounting scheme is ever designed, it will involve some sort of an input-output matrix of a profile of social, economic and environmental indicators that collectively capture the quality of human existence in descriptive and evaluative senses. Although in much of this paper it is assumed that, from the point of view of a person's personal experience or feelings, the quality of a person's life may be measured by reported happiness, there is in fact much more to life and its varied qualities than happiness. While happiness may be one of the best global indicators of the quality of life, it is certainly not the only one (Veenhoven and Ouweneel 1995; Diener and Lucas 1999, 2000).

Several researchers working in the area of health-related quality of life regard health as an aspect or domain of the broader field of overall quality of life. For example, members of the Quality of Life Research Unit at the Centre for Health Promotion (CHP) of the University of Toronto regard the quality of peoples' lives as multidimensional, touching on their "being, belonging and becoming" (Renwick and Brown 1996) in ways that are reminiscent of Allardt's (1975) "having, loving and being". Fletcher et al. (1987, p. 557) were clear that "The concept of quality of life encompasses many components: cultural and political values as well as more tangible measures such as living and educational standards and freedom from disease." But they limit their explorations to "those dimensions of quality of life which are affected by a disease and its treatment, and which have the potential to be changed by the therapeutic situation". Najman and Levine (1981) took a similar line in their review of the impact of medical technologies on the quality of patients' lives.

Explaining Happiness with Life as a Whole from Selected Domain Satisfaction Items

I suppose the ideas designated by the term 'happiness' or their various synonyms in different languages are the oldest candidates as global indicators of an overall good quality of life. It is necessary to use the plural 'ideas' because different people have had very different ideas about the nature of happiness or of an overall good quality of life (Tatarkiewicz 1976). Virtually all research has shown that happiness and life satisfaction share some common meaning, e.g., see Tatarkiewicz (1976), Veenhoven (1984), Argyle (1987), Michalos (1991a), Michalos and Zumbo (1999, 2001). When people talk about satisfaction or happiness with their whole lives, they are typically referring to a relatively lasting, justified, good feeling and attitude about their lives. So, a theory of life satisfaction could be interpreted as a theory of happiness, and in general such theories would be theories of subjective well-being. However, because measures of happiness and life satisfaction do not have identical connotations or denotations, it is worthwhile to analyze their components and correlates separately.

Table 2.2 provides some comparative figures from eleven surveys taken over 20 years resulting from regressing mean happiness scores on mean scores for satisfaction with various domains of life. The simple linear model used to obtain these figures was one of the first models applied by social indicators researchers and it is still one of the most frequently used models (Michalos 1991a). It is based on the idea that people's overall or global levels of happiness are the result of some sort of combination of the satisfaction that they get from different aspects of their lives. The model allows one to precisely measure the impact of satisfaction with, for examples, people's family relations, health, housing and jobs on their perceived overall happiness with life. Although there are plenty of indexes of happiness and subjective well-being generally, in most of my work I use variants of the single item, 7-point measures that were thoroughly investigated by Andrews and Withey (1976), and especially by Andrews (1984). In the latter paper, Andrews showed that "a typical survey item [e.g., 7-point measures], when administered by a respected survey organization to a general population sample, can be expected to yield 50–83% valid variance, 0–7% method effects variance, and 14–48% residual variance … over two-thirds of the variation in measurement quality could be explained by 13 survey design characteristics" (p. 409). Although McDowell and Praught (1982, pp. 949, 958) recommended the Bradburn Affect Balance Scale (Bradburn and Caplovitz 1965) as a general measure of "well-being or happiness" in population

Table 2.2 Comparison of happiness regressions from 11 surveys

	1979	1981	1982	1984	1985/86	1997	1997	1999n	1999s	2000	2000
	A[a]	B	C	D	E	F	G	H	I	J	K
Percent of variance explained in happiness	45	32	36	39	28	38	27	45	47	35	46
Predictors											
Satisfaction with:	Standardized regression coefficients										
Health	0.12	0.12	0.18	0.17	0.09	b	b	0.10	b	b	b
Financial security	0.09	0.06	0.21	b	0.13	0.14	0.19	0.09	b	0.19	0.06
Family relations	0.38	−0.03	0.09	0.14	0.06	0.14	b	b	b	0.14	b
Job	0.03	c	0.09	0.18	b	b	b	0.14	0.20	b	0.16
Friendships	0.23	0.23	0.01	0.21	0.10	0.09	b	b	0.21	b	b
Housing	0.01	−0.01	0.10	b	0.07	b	b	b	b	b	b
Area lived in	b	0.01	0.05	b	c	b	b	c	c	b	b
Recreation activity	0.03	0.04	0.05	b	0.07	b	b	b	b	0.14	b
Religion	c	0.01	0.03	b	b	b	b	b	b	0.15	b
Self-esteem	0.07	0.09	0.14	0.26	0.13	0.27	0.25	0.38	0.29	0.23	0.32
Transportation 0.05	0.05	b	b	b	b	c	c	c	c	c	
Gov. services	c	0.08	0.03	c	c	0.09	b	c	c	b	c
Living partner[c]	0.30	c	c	0.18	0.22	0.22	0.13	0.17	b	0.24	
Education	−0.3	c	c	b	0.10	c	c	c	c	b	b
Fed. Gov. Off.	c	c	c	c	c	c	c	0.10	b	b	b
Personal safety	c	c	c	c	c	c	c	0.08	0.16	b	b

$P < 0.01$

[a] *A* Clerical staff (N = 312), *B* Rural seniors (N = 273), *C* Cochrane residents (N = 328), *D* Guelph students (N = 296), *E* World students (N = 5036), *F* Prince George residents (N = 466). *G* Jasper residents (N = 210), *H* B.C. northerners (N = 713), *I* B.C. southerners (N = 348). *J* Quesnel (N = 370), *K* Prince George residents Nov. 2000

[b] Significance level too low to enter equation

[c] Not in questionnaire. Sources of the surveys are identified in the References using the letters heading each column; e.g., A = Michalos (1980)

surveys, their examination of that scale and a single item happiness measure revealed that "The latter performed remarkably well on many of [their] … analyses and probably provides the best single approach to measuring well-being". Unfortunately, other researchers have gone along with the recommendation instead of with the most likely "best single approach", e.g., Diabetes Control and Complications Trial (1988). Serious problems with the Bradburn scale were reported in Sandvik et al. (1993). Good cases for self-reported, single-item, global indicators of health status were made by Idler and Benyamini (1997), and Verbrugge et al. (1999).

On average, for the eleven samples represented in Table 2.5, we were able to explain 38% of the variance in reported happiness from some subset of the 16 predictor variables listed in the exhibit. Our best success came from the sample of southern British Columbians in 1999 (column I), at 47%. A dozen of the 16 domain variables were drawn from Andrews's (1974) extensive research. When all variables are standardized to have means of zero and standard deviations of one, the standardized regression coefficients (Betas) measure the percent of movement in the dependent variable when a predictor variable moves one full unit and every other predictor in the set is held constant. For example, under column A one finds that the Beta value for satisfaction with one's family relations is $\beta = 0.38$, which means that for every full standard deviation increase in satisfaction with one's family relations, one's happiness increases about 38% of a standard deviation. Figuratively speaking, this means that for every full step increase in how good one feels about one's family relations, one's overall happiness goes up about 38% of a step. Inspection of the other figures in that column reveals that satisfaction in no other domain had as great an impact on overall happiness for the 312 members of the sampled clerical staff.

For our purposes, it is most important to notice that satisfaction with one's own health was *never* the strongest predictor of happiness in any sample. In five of the eleven samples, satisfaction with one's own health failed to enter the final explanatory regression equation for lack of statistical significance. In another three samples, it failed to appear as one of the top three predictors, it ran third in two of the three samples in which it did appear in the top three and in the remaining sample it ran only second. Clearly, the old adage about having everything when you have your health is false for the people in these eleven samples.

Reading across the row to the right from 0.38 in column A, one sees that satisfaction with one's family relations was not the strongest predictor of happiness for any other sample. Satisfaction with one's own self-esteem was the strongest predictor in seven samples, and by that fact alone a good candidate for the most important domain in the set of 16. More often than not, the better one feels about one's own self, the happier one will be.

The figures just reviewed clearly illustrate the fact that different groups of people with different life circumstances, resources and constraints use different mixtures of ingredients to determine their happiness. The explanatory model used here allowed the groups represented in Table 2.2 to draw satisfaction from roughly the same set of domains. Analytically speaking, some groups used more and some used fewer of these domains to build their happiness. The Jasper group used only 3 of the 12 possibilities open to them while the rural seniors used all 12 of 12 open to them. There is no evidence that people consciously selected more or fewer domains to craft their happiness, but different people did in fact use different building blocks. Supplementing these findings, in several provocative studies Schwarz and colleagues have demonstrated that the order in which domain and global items are presented in questionnaires, as well as the number of competing domains presented can have profound effects on the measured relationships among all the variables; e.g., Schwarz and Strack (1991, 1999), Schwarz and Bless (1992). Concluding a fine review article, Schwarz and Strack (1999, p. 79) wrote,

> … reports of well-being are subject to a number of transient influences. Like other social judgments, they are best considered constructions in response to particular questions posed at a particular time. Although the information that respondents draw on reflects the reality in which they live, which aspects of this reality they consider and how they use these aspects in forming a judgment is profoundly influenced by features of the research instruments.

Explaining Happiness with Life as a Whole from Health and Other Variables

An astute observer would say that while *satisfaction with one's health* may be a weak predictor of overall happiness, *health itself* should be a strong predictor. Tables 2.3, 2.4 and 2.5 show the results of our examination of this suggestion using three different samples and different sets of potential predictors. In each case, self-reported health was measured by the near-gold standard eight dimensions of the Medical Outcomes Study Short Form (SF-36) (Ware et al. 1993), although in the third case additional health measures were also used. I will discuss each case in turn.

Table 2.3 summarizes results of a survey of 875 adults aged 55 to 95 living in the Northern Interior Health Region of British Columbia in September 1999 (Michalos et al. 2001). Our interests lie in the first and last numerical columns. The first numerical column shows that 2 of the 8 SF-36 health dimensions explained 34% of the variation in happiness scores. The dimension of Mental Health ($\beta = 0.49$) was over three times as influential as that of Social Functioning ($\beta = 0.14$), and the other 6 dimensions of SF-36 were not statistically significantly associated with happiness. As one moves across the columns from left to right, results of regressing happiness scores on other things are listed. Other things include, for examples, a 4-item index of social support, worries about crime, satisfaction with what one is accomplishing in life now, satisfaction with family relations, and so on. The last column gives the results of regressing happiness scores on all the significant predictors from the previous columns. It shows, first, that in the context of that set of potential predictors, only the Mental Health dimension of SF-36 remained significant and its influence was reduced

Table 2.3 Regressions of happiness on health, worries, social support and domain satisfaction

	Health dimensions[a]	Crime worries, soc. supp.[b]	Other worries, age identity[c]	Domain satisfaction[d]	All pred.[e]
% of variance explained	34	21	21	40	44
	N = 623	N = 807	N = 411	N = 584	N = 431
Predictors	Betas	Betas	Betas	Betas	Betas
Mental health	0.49	[f]	[f]	[f]	0.24
Social functioning	0.14	[f]	[f]	[f]	[g]
Social support index	[f]	0.34	[f]	[f]	0.1
Fair treatment index	[f]	0.16	[f]	[f]	[g]
Physical age identity	[f]	[f]	−0.17	[f]	[g]
Difficulties with housing costs	[f]	[f]	−0.22	[f]	[g]
Personal worries (Factor 1)	[f]	[f]	−0.18	[f]	[g]
Living area (Factor 5)	[f]	[f]	−0.15	[f]	−0.09
Retail store access (Factor 3)	[f]	[f]	−0.12	[f]	[g]
Ideal age preference	[f]	[f]	0.13	[f]	[g]
Friendships	[f]	[f]	[f]	0.11	0.13
Present age	[f]	[f]	[f]	0.17	0.15
Self-esteem	[f]	[f]	[f]	0.19	0.12
Accomplishing in life now	[f]	[f]	[f]	0.17	0.14
Local government officials	[f]	[f]	[f]	0.09	[g]
Family relations	[f]	[f]	[f]	0.09	[g]
Opportunities to socialize	[f]	[f]	[f]	0.09	[g]

[a]8 dimensions from SF-36
[b]Index of crime-related worries, personal fair treatment index, social support index
[c]Five factors from preferences and problems items, 5 age-identity items, difficulties and % of income spent on housing
[d]24 domain satisfaction scores
[e]a + b + c + d
[f]Variable not in equation
[g]Significance level too low for variable to enter equation

Table 2.4 Regressions of happiness on health, leisure benefits and activities, domain satisfaction and social support

	Health dimensions[a]	Leisure benefits[b]	Domain satisfaction[c]	Dom. sat. + Health[d]	All pred.[e]
% of variance explained	22	16	42	42	42
	N = 390	N = 418	N = 323	N = 306	N = 296
Predictors	Beta	Beta	Beta	Bela	Beta
Mental health	0.47	f	f	0.12	g
Psych. benefits	f	0.4	f	g	g
Social support	f	f	f	f	0.15
Self-esteem	f	f	0.3	0.28	0.32
Job	f	f	0.19	0.18	0.19
Family relations	f	f	0.12	0.12	g
Living partner	f	f	0.17	0.19	0.22
Present age	f	f	0.11	g	g

[a]8 dimensions from SF-36
[b]6 indexes of perceived leisure benefits + 7 indexes of *Catalogue* benefits + 4 indexes of active and sedentary recreation
[c]15 domain satisfaction scores
[d]a + c
[e]a + b + c + social support index
[f]Not in equation
[g]Significance level too low to enter equation

Table 2.5 Regression of happiness scores on health and domain satisfaction scores

Explanatory variables	Beta values	Beta values	Beta values
General health	0.1	a	a
Mental health	0.24	a	0.14
CES-D	−0.32	a	−0.26
Stress index	−0.16	a	−0.1
Role physical	a	a	0.06
Vitality	a	a	−0.04
Role emotional	a	a	0.07
Chronic cond.	a	a	0.04
Family rel. sat.	a	0.17	0.1
Living partner sat.	a	0.16	a
Financial sec. sat.	a	0.15	a
Self-esteem sat.	a	0.33	0.17
Prov. Gov. sat.	a	0.13	a
Fed. Gov. sat	a	a	0.07
Present age sat.	a	a	0.14
Variance explained (%)	45	40	53

[a]Variable not in equation

considerably ($\beta = 0.24$). Second, although Mental Health was the most influential of the seven significant predictors, it had much less influence than the other six predictors combined. Third, the addition of Mental Health to the seven significant domain satisfaction predictors from the fourth column increased our total explanatory power by only four percentage points, i.e., from 40 to 44% explained variance in happiness scores. From this point of view, self-rated health had very little indeed to offer toward respondents' happiness. Fourth, it shows clearly that the measured importance of health to happiness varies with the total number and kinds of potential predictors employed. If one were to judge that importance merely on the basis of the information in the first column, one's judgment would be severely distorted. This is an excellent example of the sort of balanced view that social indicators research can provide of the importance of health to one's overall quality of life (here operationalized merely as happiness).

Table 2.4 summarizes the results of a survey of a random sample of 440 adults aged 18 years and older living in Prince George in November 1999 (Michalos and Zumbo 2003). The primary focus of the survey was to examine relationships between self-rated health measured by the 8 dimensions of SF-36 and leisure activities measured in a variety of ways. As in the previous paragraph, our interests lie mainly in the first and last numerical columns of the exhibit. The first numerical column of Table 2.4 shows that only one of the 8 SF-36 health dimensions explained 22% of the variation in happiness scores. Mental Health did all the work, with $\beta = 0.47$. The last numerical column shows that of the 8 potential predictors in the regression equation, only four had any statistically significant influence and together these four explained 42% of the variance in happiness scores. What is more important for our purposes, however, is the fact that while the set of predictors varied in the last three columns, the percent of variance explained was always only 42%. A set of five domain satisfaction variables alone, or four domain satisfaction variables plus Mental Health, or three domain satisfaction variables plus a 4-item index of social support provided equally efficient explanations of respondents' reported happiness.

Table 2.5 summarizes the results of a survey of a random sample of 723 adults aged 18 years and older living in Prince George in November 1998 (Michalos et al. 2000). The main aim of the survey was to gather some baseline data related to health and health care, and to assess its impact on the quality of people's lives measured in different ways. Besides SF-36, our questionnaire included the 20—item Center for Epidemiologic Studies Depression (CES-D) scale (Radloff 1977), 12 items measuring general life stress, 11 items measuring stress at work, 5 items on smoking and drinking behaviour, Body Mass Index scores, a list of chronic health conditions and 10 items on health care services in our area. The first column in the exhibit shows the results of regressing happiness scores on all of our health-related potential predictors. 45% of the variation in these happiness scores was explained. From SF-36, only two dimensions had statistically significant influence, namely, General Health ($\beta = 0.10$) and Mental Health ($\beta = 0.24$). As one would have expected, CES-D weighed in negatively ($\beta = -0.32$), as did the general stress index ($\beta = -0.16$). The second column shows that a set of five domain satisfaction scores accounted for 40% of the variation in happiness scores, and the third column shows that the two sets together accounted for 53% of the variation in happiness scores, with CES-D scores having the greatest influence ($\beta = -0.26$). Altogether, the seven health-related predictors accounted for 60% of the total variance explained and the four domain satisfaction predictors accounted for the remaining 40%. This again shows us that depending on the number and kinds of potential predictors employed, self-rated health appears to be more or less important to happiness.

In all these explanations, good mental health makes a substantial contribution to happiness. While that is not surprising or troubling in itself, it has an implication that is both. I will not dwell on the problem, but the following remarks from an intriguing review essay by Taylor and Brown (1988, pp. 204–205) are worth repeating here.

> The mentally healthy person appears to have the enviable capacity to distort reality in a direction that enhances self-esteem, maintains beliefs in personal efficacy, and promotes an optimistic view of the future. These three illusions, as we have called them, appear to foster traditional criteria of mental health, including the ability to care about the self and others, the ability to be happy or contented, and the ability to engage in productive and creative work. ... The individual who responds to negative, ambiguous, or unsupportive feedback with a positive sense of self, a belief in personal efficacy, and an optimistic sense of the future will, we maintain, be happier, more caring, and more productive than the individual who perceives the same information accurately and integrates it into his or her view of the self, the world, and the future. In this sense, the capacity to develop and maintain positive illusions may be thought of as a valuable human resource to be nurtured and promoted, rather than an error-prone processing system to be corrected. In any case, these illusions help make each individual's world a warmer and more active and beneficent place in which to live.

Explaining Satisfaction with One's Own Health

Having discovered that one's self-rated health and one's reported satisfaction with it each have some independent influence on one's happiness, a researcher naturally wonders how much influence *selfrated health* has on one's reported *satisfaction with one's health.* Table 2.6, from Michalos et al. (2000), answers this question. Using the same set of health-related potential predictors described two paragraphs

Table 2.6 Regression of health satisfaction scores on health scores

Explanatory variables	Beta values
General health	0.51
Vitality	0.17
Body mass index	−0.06
Health worries	−0.14
Stress index	−0.09
Explained variance	56%

above, we were able to explain 56% of the variance in respondents' satisfaction with their own health. The General Health dimension from SF-36 clearly dominated the set of significant predictors, with a Beta value of $\beta = 0.51$. The Vitality dimension had a relatively small impact, $\beta = 0.17$, and scores for Body Mass, Health Worries and Stress were appropriately negative at $\beta = -0.06$, $\beta = -0.14$ and $\beta = -0.09$, respectively. Using the Pratt measure (Thomas et al. 1998), we found that the General Health dimension accounted for 65% of all the variance explained by our variables.

Multiple Discrepancies Theory (MDT)

In Michalos (1985), I proposed and tested a theory of subjective well-being called Multiple Discrepancies Theory (MDT). Operationally, 'subjective well-being' was measured by single-item, seven-point scales of reported happiness and satisfaction. MDT was supposed to explain why people are happy or satisfied with their whole lives as well as with their jobs, living partners, finances, housing, friendships and so on. It was also supposed to explain people's revealed preferences or actual choices in terms of their levels of reported satisfaction, which would make it a deeper theory (Bunge 1961) as well as an empirical alternative to utility theory. Most importantly for present purposes, it was supposed to explain satisfaction with one's own health. In fact it performed this function very well, as I will now show.

The basic postulates of MDT are as follows.

H1: Reported net satisfaction (happiness or subjective well-being) is a positive linear function of perceived discrepancies between what one has and wants, relevant others have, the best one has had in the past, expected to have 3 years ago, expects to have after 5 years, deserves and needs.

H2: All perceived discrepancies, except that between what one has and wants, are positive linear functions of objectively measurable discrepancies, which also have direct effects on satisfaction and actions.

H3: The perceived discrepancy between what one has and wants is a mediating variable between all other perceived discrepancies and reported net satisfaction, i.e., besides the direct effects posited in H1, six discrepancies have indirect effects.

H4: The pursuit and maintenance of net satisfaction motivates human action in direct proportion to the perceived expected levels of net satisfaction.

H5: All discrepancies, satisfaction and actions are directly and indirectly affected by age, sex, education, ethnicity, income, self-esteem and social support.

H6: Objectively measurable discrepancies are linear functions of human action and conditioners.

Figures 2.1 and 2.2 illustrate the relations specified in the six postulates. More detailed explanations of the postulates and their sources may be found in Michalos (1985, 1991a). It is perhaps worth mentioning here that although MDT is deeper

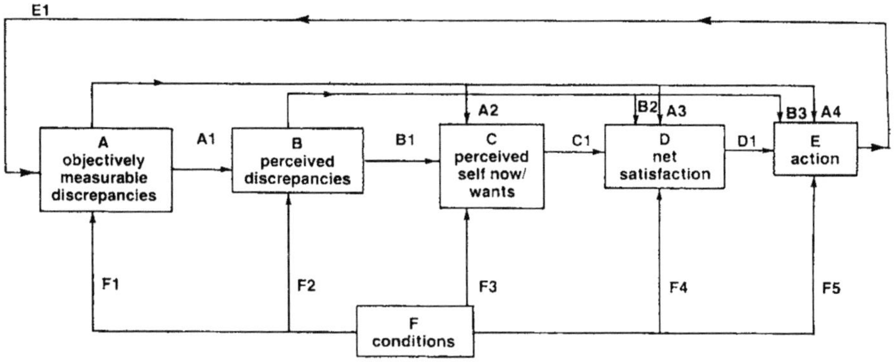

Fig. 2.1 Multiple discrepancies theory

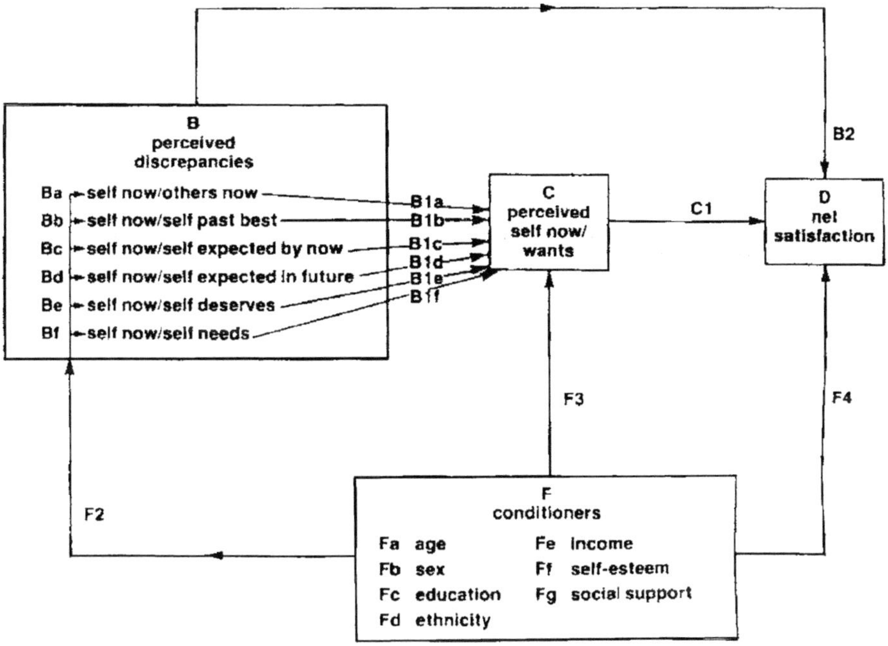

Fig. 2.2 Perceptual core of MDT

than utility theory, it suffers from some circularity roughly similar to that suffered by utility theory. After all, judgments about the best one has had in the past, what one deserves and needs (H1) are essentially evaluations. So, although my view of the nature of value is in the naturalistic subjectivist tradition, insofar as MDT is supposed to provide an explanation of satisfaction, my view is both less naturalistic and more circular than the classic naturalists or I would have liked.

Applying MDT to convenience samples of undergraduates from the University of Guelph, I was able to explain 46% of the variation in men's (N = 296) and 53% of the variation in women's (N = 341) satisfaction with their own health (Michalos 1985). For men and women, the most influential predictors of all those postulated were the gaps between the levels of health wanted and the levels actually obtained. Encouraged by this success, I went after bigger fish.

With the help of 68 colleagues around the world, in the 1984–86 period, data were collected from over 18000 undergraduates in 39 countries, using 19 different languages. The complete results of the investigation were given in Michalos (1991a, b, 1993a, b). Table 2.7 gives the results of using MDT to explain satisfaction with one's own health. In the column under S (for "satisfaction with one's own health") we find a total sample of N = 8076 students, including 4,116 males and 3960 females. MDT explained 51% of the variance in reported health satisfaction scores for the whole group, 52% for males and 51% for females.

Regarding discrepancies for the whole group, the self/wants gap (SW = 0.46) had the greatest impact on health satisfaction, followed by self/others (SO = 0.37). Note that the impact of the self/wants variable on satisfaction is measured by its beta value, which equals its *direct effect,* while the impact of every other gap variable is measured by the product of the various betas involved in its *direct and indirect effects* on satisfaction.

From the column under SW one finds that the MDT set of predictors explains 42% of the variance in scores indicating the perceived gap between the sort of health students have and the sort they want. In the TESW column, one finds that it is social comparison scores (SO = 0.34) that dominate the lot of predictors. The next most influential predictor is self/needs (SN = 0.19).

Considering perceived discrepancies relative to health satisfaction, the rank ordering of the three most influential predictors for females is exactly the same as the ordering for the group as a whole. For females, we have self/wants (SW = 0.45), self/others (SO = 0.35) and self/needs (SN = 0.15). For males, we have self/wants (SW = 0.46) and self/others (SO = 0.39), followed by self/deserved (SD = 0.13).

Regarding the relative impacts of self/needs versus self/deserved for males and females in the domain of health, considerations of equity are more influential than considerations of need for males, while considerations of need are more influential than considerations of equity for females.

Considering the relative impacts of my predictors on the gaps between what one has and wants regarding one's own health, the rank orderings of the two most influential variables for males and females are the same. The self/others gap has the greatest impact for males (SO = 0.35) and females (SO = 0.33), followed by self/needs for males (SN = 0.17) and females (SN = 0.21).

Since different samples were used to measure the relationships among scores for health status, health satisfaction and MDT predictors, we have no way of knowing the relative strength of the relationships in general. Lest anyone concludes too rapidly from the numbers we have just seen that self-rated health status predictors are always superior to MDT predictors of reported health satisfaction, the following

Table 2.7 Satisfaction with one's health regressed on MDT predictors (decimal points omitted)

	S*	SW	SO	SD	SN	SP	SF	SB	TES	TESW
N	8076	8107	0	8562	8762	8705	8624	0	–	–
R^2	51	42	0	1	1	1	1	0	–	–
Predictor	[a]	[a]	[a]	[a]	[a]	[a]	[a]	[a]	–	–
Sex	−3	5	0	3	0	4	−3	0	0	6
Age	−3	0	0	−4	−6	−3	0	0	−4	−2
WS	5	0	0	4	5	4	−3	0	6	2
LED	2	0	0	0	0	0	3	0	2	0
ETH	−2	3	0	5	4	7	−7	0	1	5
SO	21	34							37	34
SD	6	12							12	12
SN	4	19							13	19
SP	6	12							12	12
SB	6	9							10	9
SW	46								46	
Males										
N	4116	4132	0	4375	4494	4456	4415	4482	–	–
R^2	52	42	0	1	1	1	I	1	–	–
Age	−2	0	0	−3	−6	−3	0	−4	−4	−2
WS	5	0	0	5	5	4	−5	−4	6	2
LED	0	0	0	0	0	0	5	0	0	0
ETH	0	5	0	7	7	9	−9	5	5	9
SO	23	35							39	35
SD	7	13							13	13
SN	0	17							8	17
SP	4	13							10	13
SB	9	7							12	7
SW	46								46	
Females										
N	3960	3975	0	0	0	0	0	0	–	–
R^2	51	42	0	0	0	0	0	0	–	–
WS	6	0	0	0	0	0	0	0	6	0
ETH	−3	0	0	0	0	0	0	0	−3	0
SO	20	33							35	33
SD	6	10							11	10
SN	5	21							15	21
SP	8	11							13	11
SB	3	11							8	11
SW	45								45	

*Abbreviations are as follows. *S* Satisfaction with one's health, *WS* Work status, *LED* Level of education, *ETH* Country of birth, *SO* Self/other gap, *SD* Self/deserved gap, *SN* Self/needs gap, *SP* Self/progress gap, *SB* Self/best gap, *SW* Self/wants gap, *SF* Self/future gap, *TES* Total effects (=sum of direct and indirect effects) on satisfaction, *TESW* Total effects on self/wants variable remarks are worth considering. For the 38 countries in my global survey, on average MDT explained 48% of the variance in health satisfaction scores for the whole group and males, and 49% for females. For the whole group, percents of variance explained in scores indicating satisfaction with one's health ranged from a high of 73% in Finland to a low of 24% in Jordan. There was one other country with a figure in the 70s, Korea = 71%, and there were 4 countries with figures in the 60s, Belgium = 69%, Austria = 64%, and Germany and Switzerland = 60%. Altogether, there were 10 (26%) countries in which at least 55% of the variance in health satisfaction scores for the whole group was explained. For males, percents of variance explained in health satisfaction scores ranged from a high of 72% for Korea to a low of 21% for Greece. There were 4 countries with figures in the 60 s, namely, Finland = 69%, Austria and Portugal = 64%, and Switzerland = 61%. Altogether, there were 8 (24%) countries with at least 55% of the variance explained in health satisfaction scores. For females, percents of variance explained in health satisfaction scores ranged from a high of 76% for Finland to a low of 25% for Chile. There were 5 countries with figures in the 60 s, namely, Austria = 65%, Sweden = 64%, Germany and the Netherlands = 62%, and Switzerland = 60%. Altogether, there were 11 (38%) countries with at least 55% of the variance explained in health satisfaction scores (Michalos 1993b, pp. 77–80).

Clearly, in certain circumstances, the potential predictors assembled in MDT can provide considerable power to explain people's reported satisfaction with their own health, occasionally perhaps *even more power* than a reasonably broad set of measures of self-reported health. Of course the only way to measure the relative explanatory power of actual health status predictors versus MDT predictors is by undertaking surveys in which all relevant predictors are included. I have never done that, but someone probably will do it some day. It would also be worthwhile for someone to employ MDT in an examination of the impact of response-shift bias related to pre-, post- and then-test scores (Sprangers and Schwartz 1999; Sprangers 1996). Given the rich array of judgment standards in MDT, a wide variety of response-shifts might occur across the period of time from a patient's initial diagnosis, through and beyond therapy.

Regarding overall happiness with life, MDT explained 42% of the variance in happiness scores for the whole student group, 41% for males and 44% for females. The most influential predictors for all three groups were the gaps for self/best, self/others and self/wants, in that order (Michalos 1991, pp. 115–125).

Health-Related Quality of Life

Broadly speaking, there are two types of measures of health-related quality of life, namely, those that are specific to diseases, conditions, functions and/or populations and those that are not (Guyatt et al. 1989; Patrick and Deyo 1989). Disease-specific quality of life measures are designed to measure the quality of diseased life (QDL) and as such they are not likely to be confused with general measures of the quality of life of ordinary, normal or non-diseased people. For example, the Functional Living Index-Cancer (FLIC) measures cancer patients' functioning and feelings about the impact of their disease on their lives (Schipper et al. 1984). No-one could reasonably mistake a FLIC score as a general measure of the overall quality of a normal, non-diseased person's life. The Oswestry Low Back Pain Disability Questionnaire measures the degree to which the quality of a person's life is constrained or impaired by a specific condition, low back or leg pain (Fairbank et al. 1980). The FACT-general (FACT-G) cancer quality-of-life scale is a straightforward measure of the quality of a cancer-diseased life. It is noteworthy that "Most of the concepts measured by the FACT-G are not specific to oncology and therefore lend themselves to evaluation in other diseases" (Cella et al. 1993, p. 577). The Illness Behavior Questionnaire measures the degree to which the quality of a sick person's life is compromised by that person's perception and management of his or her illness (Pilowsky et al. 1983). Again, the scale would be an unlikely candidate as a measure of the general quality of life of normal people.

Andresen et al. (1999) briefly reviewed some of the differences, strengths and weaknesses of using condition-specific versus generic measures of health-related quality of life. For present purposes, perhaps their most important remark was that "condition-specific measures prohibit comparisons of persons with SCI [spinal cord injuries] to the general population or to other groups with impairments" (p. 977). This is important because it highlights two of the most important differences between the aims of social indicators researchers and health-related quality of life researchers. From the beginning, social indicators researchers have been focused on measuring the quality of life of average people living in diverse circumstances, and they have been interested in measuring people's health primarily as a determinant of the quality of their lives. Certainly more than social indicators researchers, health-related quality of life researchers have been primarily interested in measuring the health of people as something good in itself and, secondarily as a cause, effect, component, or all three, of the quality of their lives. Also more than social indicators researchers, health-related quality of life researchers have been interested in developing measuring instruments that are useful for a great variety of health care workers and purposes, from clinicians with relatively few subjects with extraordinary problems to population health managers with relatively many subjects with ordinary problems.

Unlike disease-specific quality of life measures, so-called generic or general health-related quality of life measures are very problematic, primarily because they are so confounded. Recognizing the importance of distinguishing validation of measures or instruments from validation of interpretations of such measures or instruments (McDowell and Newell 1996), it is probably more accurate to say that measures and interpretations are each confounded. I grant immediately that if one accepts the World Health Organization's broad definition of health as "complete physical, mental and social well-being", there may not be confounding. Depending on what one loads into the notions of physical, mental and social well-being, if one has complete physical, mental and social well-being, then the quality of one's life may well be excellent. Again, depending on what one loads into those notions, a reasonable measure of excellent health might be an equally reasonable measure of an excellent quality of life.

The trouble is, there is no rule book to tell us exactly what should be loaded into the notions of physical, mental and social well-being. For example, if one interpreted ‘physical’ well-being broadly enough to include people’s physical environment (e.g., their housing, neighbourhood, area air, water and land quality) and then insisted on including measures of these sorts of things in a profile of human health, then that profile would probably capture more of the broad sense of quality of life understood as happiness. The same game could be played with the notions of mental and social wellbeing, with similar results. I would not recommend it because I think it would expand our ordinary ideas of human health far beyond reasonable recognition. In fact, the game being played would be nothing less than that of expanding ordinary ideas of health to make them equivalent to the broader ideas of quality of life or happiness. Insofar as the game was successfully played, ‘health’ would become synonymous with ‘quality of life’ (or perhaps ‘happiness’) and the phrase ‘health-related quality of life’ would be equivalent to the hopelessly redundant ‘health-related health’ or ‘quality of life- related quality of life’. So, broad as the WHO definition of ‘health’ is, it is still not as broad as the idea of quality of life understood as happiness and it would be a mistake to try to make the ideas equivalent. As long as some distinction is consistently maintained between the two notions, remarks such as the following are both meaningful and important.

> The objective [of quality of life research in the area of nursing science] must be to acquire knowledge of the influence of various degrees of health failure upon quality of life throughout the life cycle and to establish what constitutes a good life in the context of treatment and care (Hanestad 1990, p. 30).

Epistemologically, I go a long way with constructionists (Michalos 1991a) and I think the ideas of health and quality of life are socially constructed, but I believe that they are ordinarily constructed as different notions with some overlapping sense (strictly, overlapping connotation and denotation as logicians would say) and I believe that this is appropriate. I am not convinced, as Nord et al. (2001) apparently are that “To most people, ‘quality of life’ refers to … [only a] … subjective, overall feeling” and I would not support their recommendation to use the term ‘quality of life data’ “only in connection with data about people’s subjective feelings about life”. As a matter of fact, a similar proposal was made by Solomon (1980) at UNESCO and it seemed to attract some adherents in Europe, but it never quite caught on in North America. Birnbacher (1999, p. 30) took that line almost exactly when he wrote,

> Quality of life judgements… are judgements from the subject’s own perspective. To bring this *internal* perspective to bear on medical decision-making was the central point of introducing the concept, in opposition to a medical paternalism that takes its cue exclusively from such external criteria as normal functioning, role fulfilment and social worth. This point is lost unless the concept is understood in a strictly descriptive and psychological way.

During the cold war years, some Eastern European researchers preferred to talk about 'way of life' rather than 'quality of life', with the former term applying only to observable behaviour, especially the use of one's time for daily activities (Andorka and Harcsa 1990). As will become clear shortly, I do think the idea of health-related quality of life is very troublesome and we would probably be better off without it. But maybe if researchers would be more careful in their usage, a lot of the problems would disappear. If we all agreed that, say, 'health-related quality of life' means 'the overall nature and value of life in relation to health', and if all of us were much more careful than we usually are, maybe most of the problems would disappear. Maybe not. In any case, if Birnbacher (1999, pp. 28–29) is right (as I believe he is) in his judgment that some researchers just want to abandon the concept of *quality of life* altogether because it is "too multi-faceted and too controversial", some think "the multiplicity of concepts of quality of life is more or less inevitable", some "welcome the pluralism of interpretations as potentially productive" and some think there are "good reasons to postulate a unitary concept at least for the medical context", it is unlikely that we are going to get general agreement on the best strategy for managing our problems with the idea of *health-related quality of life.*

We have already seen in section "Explaining Happiness with Life as a Whole from Health and Other Variables" that if 'quality of life' is interpreted as 'happiness' then good measures of health explain anywhere from almost a half to only a fifth of the quality of people's lives, when the explanatory models include no other domains of life. When salient other domains are included in one's model, then good health measures have relatively little influence on the quality of life understood as happiness. This strongly suggests that even if one's measures are designed to capture the broad, WHO sense of 'health', they fail to capture the sense of 'quality of life' understood as 'happiness'.

Another way to see the limitations of thinking about quality of life and health as co-extensive notions is to try to explain General Health from the set of domain satisfaction items employed in the simple linear model explaining happiness. Using the data-set from Michalos et al. (2000), I correlated eleven domain satisfaction items with the SF-36 General Health Index and then regressed the latter on the former, with and without the domain of health satisfaction. Table 2.8 shows that each domain satisfaction item was positively and significantly (0.01 or better, two tailed test) correlated with the General Health Index. Table 2.9 shows that without health satisfaction in the model, only 15% of the variance in General Health Index scores could be explained by three domain satisfaction scores, with the other seven potential predictors failing to reach significance. The three predictors were satisfaction with one's self-esteem ($\beta = 0.22$), recreation activities ($\beta = 0.18$) and family relations ($\beta = 0.09$). When health satisfaction was entered into the equation, 44% of the variance in General Health Index scores could be explained and a single predictor, health satisfaction, did all the work ($\beta = 0.66$).

Suppose, then, that we accept the concepts of health and quality of life as different but overlapping notions. What are we to make of ideas of health-related quality of life? If one thinks of the quality of a person's life as divisible into several

Table 2.8 Correlations of general health index scores and domain satisfaction scores

Satisfaction with:	Correlation with general health (N)	Satisfaction with:	Correlation with general health (N)
Your house	0.18 (N = 707)	Your neighbourhood	0.13 (N = 703)
Your family relations	0.20 (N = 698)	Your living partner	0.14 (N = 595)
Your job	0.19 (N = 602)	Your friendships	0.27 (N = 699)
Your health	0.69 (N = 700)	Your spiritual fulfilment	0.20 (N = 656)
Your financial security	0.28 (N = 695)	Your recreation activity	0.36 (N = 693)
Your self-esteem	0.36 (N = 696)		

Table 2.9 Regressions of general health index on domain on domain satisfaction items

Explanatory variables = Satisfaction with:	Without health satisfaction, betas	With health satisfaction, betas
Your self-esteem	0.22	[a]
Your recreation activity	0.18	[a]
Your family relationships	0.09	[a]
Your health	–	0.66
Variance explained (%)	15	44
N	498	496

[a]Significance level too low to enter equation

different domains along the lines of the simple linear model (e.g., family life, job, health, recreation activities), then health-related quality of life may be regarded as a particular species of the genus *domain-related quality of life.* Other species would include, for example, job-related quality of life and marriage-related quality of life. Just as researchers construct descriptive and evaluative measures of people's health and then try to explain people's overall quality of life on the basis of health, researchers construct descriptive and evaluative measures of people's jobs and marriages and try to explain their overall quality of life on the basis of their jobs and marriages. However, so far as I know, only health researchers have dared to confound ideas of the quality of life by joining them in a hyphenated way to specific domains. A perfect example of the confusion that can arise may be found in an otherwise very good review article by Guyatt et al. (1989, p. 1443). Here is what they say in a section on utility measures. "Quality of life is measured as a single number along a continuum, death being 0.0 and full health 1.0." The logical implication is that full health equals excellent quality of life. This is exactly like saying 'Quality of life is measured as a single number along a continuum, terrible job (or terrible marriage) being 0.0 and excellent job (or excellent marriage) 1.0.'

The implication would then be that an excellent job or an excellent marriage equals excellent quality of life. That is clearly false, just as it is false to suppose that good health equals good quality of life. Torrance (1986) and Churchill et al. (1984) make precisely this supposition when they assume that quality of life is measured by a utility score ranging from healthy to dead, as Guyatt et al. assert.

McDowell and Newell (1996, p. 13) recognized that such mis-identification occurs in the literature, but did not identify it as a problem. They wrote,

> Health measurements may also be classified descriptively according to their scope or the range of topics they cover. The spectrum of measures ranges from those that focus on a particular organ system (vision, hearing), to methods concerned with a diagnosis (anxiety or depression scales), to those that measure broader syndromes (emotional well-being), to measurements of overall health, and, broadest of all, to measures of overall quality of life.

This sort of mistake is often made in the health-related quality of life research literature. For example, Eiser and Tooke (1993, p. 86) claimed that

> Two broad approaches can be identified in measurement of quality of life. In the first, it is assumed that quality of life is synonymous with health status. … In the second approach, individual differences in how people perceive and appraise situations are stressed; the individual's perceptions of, and satisfaction with, his or her level of functioning is considered central to any assessment of quality of life.

In my terms, these authors are saying that 'quality of life' is synonymous with 'health measured by objective indicators' or with 'health measured by subjective indicators-satisfaction with health'. So, the question of the impact of one's health on one's overall quality of life is reduced to the question of the impact of objectively measured on subjectively measured health or vice versa, or the question of the impact of objectively measured quality of life on subjectively measured quality of life or vice versa. The reduced questions are all important, but so is the question that is begged, namely, the question of the impact of health (objectively or subjectively measured) *among all other aspects of people's lives* on their overall quality of life (objectively or subjectively measured). More precisely, if the question at issue is 'What is the relative impact of health compared to all other aspects or domains of people's lives on their overall quality of life?', then the logical fallacy of begging the question occurs when a researcher employs definitions of key words or methodological procedures that presuppose the question at issue has already been answered (Michalos 1969).

Bardsley et al. (1993, p. 619) wrote,

> Both the late complications of diabetes and the means used to prevent them have a significant impact on the lives of people with the condition. Measuring quality of life is therefore important in assessing clinical need and evaluating the success of management. Three approaches to measuring health status were therefore compared. … The measures used were the Nottingham Health Profile (NHP), four categories of an anglicized version of the Sickness Impact Profile (the Functional Limitations Profile (FLP)), and a scale of Positive Well-Being (PWB).

For these authors, then, because the quality of people's lives is important, they measured people's *health status,* assuming that validated measures of the latter are equivalent to measures of the former, effectively begging the question of the measurable impact of health on the overall quality of people's lives.

Finding that total stable glycosylated hemoglobin (HbA_1) levels were uncorrelated with young diabetics' scores on the Diabetes Quality of Life Instrument (DQOL) but correlated with their selfperceived health status, Ingersoll and Marrero (1991, p. 118) concluded,

> Practitioners have a tendency to equate good metabolic control with quality of life. While the value of good metabolic control should not be understated, these data suggest that phenomenologic or self-perceived quality of life holds a very different meaning to adolescents with IDDM [insulin-dependent diabetes mellitus]…. Psychosocial quality of life may constitute a qualitatively different, but also important, outcome in conjunction with physiological quality of life, reflected in good metabolic control. … While diabetes practitioners should not lose sight of the centrality of metabolic control, neither should they dismiss or deemphasize quality of life issues.

Thus, for these authors, 'physiological quality of life' is synonymous with 'self-perceived health status' while 'psychosocial quality of life' is synonymous with 'quality of life', although they recognize that 'practitioners have a tendency to equate good metabolic control (=physiological quality of life) with quality of life (=psychosocial quality of life).

People often use SF-36 as a measure of health-related quality of life, when in fact it was designed and validated as a generic measure of health. Thus, Jacobson et al. (1994, p. 267) wrote,

> Consecutive outpatients (n = 240) from a large multispecialty diabetes clinic were studied on a single occasion using two measures of quality of life - Diabetes Quality of Life Measure (DQOL) and the Medical Outcome Study Health Survey 36-Item Short Form (SF-36). … The two measures examine quality of life from different but complimentary perspectives. The DQOL seems more sensitive to lifestyle issues and contains special questions and worry scales oriented toward younger patients, whereas the SF-36 provides more information about functional health status.

When researchers use the SF-36 as a measure of health-related quality of life, they are begging the question about the relationship of *good health* to *good quality of life* because they are assuming SF-36 measures both equivalently. What's worse, by confounding these notions, they are preventing themselves from actually measuring the impact of the former on the latter and they are making it more difficult for others to even recognize this important issue.

Nerenz et al. (1992, pp. MS121–MS122) apparently made that mistake when they wrote,

> The measurement of quality of life for diabetic patients is practical in an ambulatory clinic setting using either mail or in-person methods. … the quantitative approach to assessing health status may allow more explicit agreement between patient and physician on acceptable trade-offs between current quality of life and risk of future diabetes complications. When used routinely, the SF-36 measure could provide a common vocabulary for patient and physician to use in discussing those trade-offs, if both physicians and patients can become comfortable with discussing health status in terms of scores on the SF-36 dimensions.

As illustrated above with the quotation from Bardsley et al. (1993), people often use the Sickness Impact Profile as if it were a measure of the overall quality of life, although it was designed as "a behaviourally based measure of health-related dysfunction" intended "to provide a measure of health status that would be useful in the assessment of individuals or populations with chronic as well as acute illness" (Bergner 1993, p. 95). It was originally validated on hyperthyroid patients, rheumatoid arthritic patients and patients who had total hip replacement, and the published report of those validation investigations does not contain a single occurrence of the phrase 'quality of life' (Bergner et al. 1981). In Bruin et al. (1992) review of the SIP's reliability and validity, it's largest correlation ($r = 0.87$) was with the Arthritis Impact Measurement Scale. For our purposes, it must be noted that "Respondents check only the items that describe them on a given day *and are related to their health,* although the actual medical condition is not an issue" (McDowell and Newell 1996, pp. 431–432, emphasis added). Since only health-related items are in the SIP and respondents are instructed to check only items related to their health, if SIP scores are regarded as measures of the overall quality of people's lives then the question of how health is related to the overall quality of people's lives is clearly begged in favour of a strong positive relation. The following quotation from Prigatano et al. (1984, p. 1619) illustrates precisely such circular reasoning.

> It is of some interest that in this investigation, recent life changes in patients with COPD [chronic obstructive pulmonary disease] were not greater than those found in control subjects except on the health dimension. This suggests that changes in work, home life, marriage, personal and social life, and finances cannot account for the enhanced quality of life differences in patients with COPD and mild hypoxemia. Rather, it appears that it is the changes in health that seem to be most important for quality of life.

On the contrary, given their dependent variable, it only appears that *changes in health* are most important for the behaviourally-measured *health status* of sick people, as one would have expected.

The Diabetes Control and Complications Trial (DCCT) (1988, pp. 275–276) wrote that "Many measures have been developed to assess quality of life … measures such as the Sickness Impact Profile … have been developed to study the general population". Similarly, Guyatt et al. (1987, p. 52) wrote that "McSweeny et al. (1982) applying the Sickness Impact Profile, a quality of life instrument designed for the general population …". It appears as if the authors of both papers identified 'behaviorally-measured health status' with 'quality of life', effectively begging the question of the how health might be related to the overall quality of anyone's life. A similar argument could be made about the use of the Quality of Well-Being Scale by Andresen et al. (1998).

The recently released report from the U.S. Department of Health and Human Services, Centers for Disease Control and Prevention (November 2000) has some stunning examples of confounding. Here are some. "The concept of health-related quality of life (HRQOL) and its determinants have evolved since the 1980s to encompass those aspects of overall quality of life that can be clearly shown to affect health—either physical or mental" (p. 6). So "health-related quality of life" is a dependent variable with "its determinants", but "overall quality of life" is also a predictor because it has "aspects" that "affect" "health", which is now a dependent variable apparently driven by something that encompasses it, namely, "quality of life". Again, "Further, the CDC Chronic Disease, Disability, and Women's Health Programs have evolved to target quality of life as an important health outcome" (p. 7). So, now "health" is the predictor and "quality of life" is the dependent variable. Nevertheless, "Specifying HRQOL represents a unique effort on the part of national policy makers to formally recognize quality of life as an important component of health" (p. 15). That is to say, "quality of life" is an aspect of "health", rather than being determined by or determining "health". In sum, in these three sentences we are told that "health" is a component of a broader notion of "quality of life", that "quality of life" is a component of a broader notion of "health", and that each is driven by and drives the other, as well as some other things. It would be difficult to find more confusion in any three sentences and I suspect its source is the confounded "concept of health-related quality of life".

Conclusion

The aim of this essay was to build a bridge between two intersecting areas of research, social indicators research on the one hand and health-related quality of life research on the other. If researchers on either side of the bridge are enabled to find something of value on both sides, I will have succeeded in my task. The first substantive section of the paper introduced key concepts and definitions in the social indicators research tradition, e.g., social indicators, positive, negative, input and output indicators, social reports and quality of life. After that, there was a section reviewing some historical origins and motives of social indicators researchers, beginning roughly with Jeremy Bentham's 'felicific calculus' and ending with the search for a comprehensive accounting scheme capable of measuring the quality of human existence with social, economic and environmental indicators.

Ideas about human happiness are historically and logically closer to Bentham's views than they are to contemporary views about comprehensive accounting schemes for the quality of people's lives, but research around ideas of happiness continues to provide important insights for social indicators researchers and for health- related quality of life researchers. In the interest of illustrating the usefulness of happiness research to health-related quality of life research, I reviewed results of eleven surveys undertaken to explain happiness on the basis of levels of satisfaction that respondents got from a dozen specific domains of their lives, e.g., satisfaction with their jobs, family relations and health. On average, for the eleven samples, we were able to explain 38% of the variance in reported happiness from some subset of the predictor variables. Our best success came from a sample of southern British Columbians at 47%. Satisfaction with one's own health was *never* the strongest predictor of happiness in any sample. In five of the eleven samples, satisfaction with one's own health failed to enter the final explanatory regression equation for lack of statistical significance. In another three samples, it failed to appear as one of the top three predictors, it ran third in two of the three samples in which it did appear in the top three and in the remaining sample it ran only second. Satisfaction with one's own self-esteem was the strongest predictor in seven samples, i.e., usually, the better one feels about one's own self, the happier one will be. The results in this section of the essay show that different groups of people with different life circumstances, resources and constraints use different mixtures of ingredients to determine their happiness.

After examining some research revealing the relative importance of people's *satisfaction with their health* to their overall happiness, I considered some studies revealing the importance of people's *selfreported health* to their overall happiness. Self-reported health was measured primarily by the eight dimensions of SF-36. In a survey of 875 older Canadians, two dimensions of SF-36 had statistically significant effects on reported happiness when the only potential predictors entered into the regression equation were scores on the eight dimensions. The dimensions of Mental Health and Social Functioning explained 34% of the variation in happiness scores. Most importantly for our purposes, when a variety of other potential predictors were entered into the equation, the total explained variance in happiness scores rose to 44% but only one of the eight dimensions of SF-36 remained, namely, Mental Health. The latter accounted for a mere four percentage point increase in the explanatory power of all the significant predictors. Thus, self-reported health had relatively little to contribute toward respondents' reported happiness, and its measured contribution was significantly affected by the number and kinds of potential predictors employed. This result was replicated with two different samples and sets of potential predictors.

After reviewing studies explaining the variation in reported happiness scores on the basis of health-related potential predictors, I reviewed a couple approaches to explaining people's *satisfaction with their own health*. First, using the same set of health-related potential predictors of overall happiness, we were able to explain 56% of the variance in respondents' satisfaction with their own health. Then, using Multiple Discrepancies Theory, we were able to explain about 51% of the variation in satisfaction with one's own health scores for 8,076 undergraduates, with highs of 76% for a sample of Finnish females and 72% for Korean males. Accordingly, it was reasonable to conclude that if one's aim is to explain people's satisfaction with their own health, the potential predictors assembled in MDT can provide quite a bit and sometimes even more explanatory power than a reasonably broad set of measures of selfreported health. From the point of view of making public policy related to health, this is an extraordinary conclusion. It implies, for example, that insofar as policy makers are primarily interested in voters' satisfaction with their own health rather than with voters' health itself (because net satisfaction may drive voting behaviour more than health drives voting behaviour), they might reap greater benefits by manipulating voters' perceived discrepancies rather than improving their health. The ghost of Machiavelli rises and smiles.

In the penultimate section of the essay a couple dozen publications on health-related quality of life were examined in order to show that some serious confounding and question-begging has accompanied use of the phrase. In particular, it was argued that there are good reasons for carefully distinguishing ideas of health and quality of life, and for not interpreting SF-36 and SIP scores as measures of the quality of life. It was suggested that we might all be better off if the term 'health-related quality of life' was simply abandoned. However, since this is unlikely to happen, it was and is strongly recommended that researchers be much more careful with their usage of the phrase and their interpretation of purported measures of whatever the phrase is supposed to designate.

References

Allardt, E. (1975). *Att ha, alska, attvara. Om valfard i Norden [Having, Loving, Being. On Welfare in the Nordic Countries]*. Borgholm: Argos.

Andorka, R., & Harcsa, I. (1990). Modernization in Hungary in the long and short run measured by social indicators. *Social Indicators Research, 23,* 1–153.

Andresen, E. M., Fouts, B. S., Romeis, J. C., & Brownson, C. A. (1999). Performance of health-related quality-of-life instruments in a spinal cord injured population. *Archives of Physical Medicine and Rehabilitation, 80,* 877–884.

Andresen, E. M., Rothenberg, B. M., & Kaplan, R. M. (1998). Performance of a self-administered mailed version of the Quality of Well-Being (QWB-SA) questionnaire among older adults. *Medical Care, 36*(9), 1349–1360.

Andrews, F. M. (1974). Social indicators of perceived life quality. *Social Indicators Research, 1,* 279–299.

Andrews, F.M. (1984). Construct validity and error components of survey measures: A structural modeling approach. *Public Opinion Quarterly, 48*, 409–442.

Andrews, F. M., & Withey, S. B. (1976). *Social indicators of well-being*. New York: Plenum Press.

Argyle, M. (1987). *The psychology of happiness*. London: Routledge.

Bardsley, M. J., Astell, S., McCallum, A., & Home, P. D. (1993). The performance of three measures of health status in an outpatient diabetes population. *Diabetic Medicine, 10,* 619–626.

Bentham, J. (1789). An Introduction to the Principles of Morals and Legislation. London.

Bergner, M. (1993). Development, testing and use of the sickness impact profile. In S. R. Walker & R. M. Rosser (Eds.), *Quality of life assessment: Key issues in the 1990s* (pp. 95–110). Dordrecht: Kluwer Academic Publishers.

Bergner, M., Bobbitt, R. A., Carter, W. B., & Gilson, B. S. (1981). The sickness impact profile: Development and final revision of a health status measure. *Medical Care, 19*(8), 787–805.

Birnbacher, D. (1999). Quality of life—Evaluation or description. *Ethical Theory and Moral Practice, 2*(1), 25–36.

Bradburn, N. M., & Caplovitz, D. (1965). *Reports of happiness*. Chicago: Aldine.

Braybrooke, D. (1967). Skepticism of wants, and certain subversive effects of corporations on American values. In S. Hook (Ed.), *Human values and economic policy* (pp. 224–239). New York: New York University Press.

Brunk, C. (1987). Professionalism and responsibility in the technological society. In D. C. Poff & W. J. Waluchow (Eds.), *Business ethics in canada* (pp. 60–75). Toronto: Prentice-Hall Canada.

Bunge, M. (1961). The weight of simplicity in the construction and assaying of scientific theories. *Philosophy of Science, 28,* 120–149.

Cella, D. F., et al. (1993). The functional assessment of cancer therapy scale: Development and validation of the general measure. *Journal of Clinical Oncology, 11*(3), 570–579.

Churchill, D. N., Morgan, J., & Torrance, G. W. (1984). Quality of life in end-state renal disease. *Peritoneal Dialysis Bulletin, 4,* 20–23.

de Bruin, A. F., de Witte, L. P., Stevens, F., & Diederiks, J. P. M. (1992). Sickness impact profile: The state of the art of a generic functional status measure. *Social Science and Medicine, 35*(8), 1003–1014.

Dewey, J. (1939). *Theory of valuation.* Chicago: University of Chicago Press.

Diabetes Control and Complications Trial. (1988). Reliability and validity of a diabetes quality-of-life measure for the diabetes control and complications trial. *Diabetes Care, 11*(9), 725–732.

Diener, E., & Lucas, R. E. (1999). Personality and subjective well-being. In D. Kahneman, E. Diener, & N. Schwarz (Eds.), *Well-being: The foundations of hedonic psychology* (pp. 213–229). New York: Russell Sage Foundation.

Diener, E., & Lucas, R. E. (2000). Explaining differences in societal levels of happiness: Relative standards, need fulfillment, culture and evaluation theory. *Journal of Happiness Studies, 1,* 41–78.

Eiser, C., & Tooke, J. E. (1993). Quality-of-life evaluation in diabetes. *PharmacoEconomics, 4*(2), 85–91.

Fairbank, J. C. T., et al. (1980). The Oswestry low back pain disability questionnaire. *Physiotherapy, 66,* 271–273.

Ferriss, A. (1990). Whatever happened, indeed! *Journal of Public Policy, 9,* 401–405.

Fletcher, A. E., Hunt, B. M., & Bulpitt, C. J. (1987). Evaluation of quality of life in clinical trials of cardiovascular disease. *Journal of Chronic Diseases, 40*(6), 557–566.

Fox, K. A. (1985). *Social system accounts: Linking social and economic indicators through tangible behavior settings.* Dordrecht: D. Reidel.

Guyatt, G. H., Townsend, M., Berman, L. B., & Pugsley, S. O. (1987). Quality of life in patients with chronic airflow limitation. *British Journal of Diseases of the Chest, 81,* 45–54.

Guyatt, G. H., Veldhuyzen Van Zanten, S. J. O., Feeny, D. H., & Patrick, D. L. (1989). Measuring quality of life in clinical trials: A taxonomy and review. *Canadian Medical Association Journal, 140,* 1441–1448.

Hagerty, M. R., et al. (2001). Quality of life indexes for national policy: Review and agenda for research. *Social Indicators Research, 55,* 1–96.

Hanestad, B. R. (1990). Errors of measurement affecting the reliability and validity of data acquired from self-assessed quality of life. *Scandanavian Journal of Caring Sciences, 4*(1), 29–34.

Hornquist, J. O. (1989). Quality of life: Concept and assessment. *Scandanavian Journal of Social Medicine, 18,* 69–79.

Idler, E. L., & Benyamini, Y. (1997). Self-rated health and mortality: A review of twenty-seven community studies. *Journal of Health and Social Behavior, 38,* 21–37.

Ingersoll, G. M., & Marrero, D. G. (1991). A modified quality-of-life measure for youths: Psychometric properties. *The Diabetes Educator, 17*(2), 114–118.

Jacobson, A. M., de Groot, M., & Samson, J. A. (1994). The evaluation of two measures of quality oflife in patients with type I and type II diabetes. *Diabetes Care, 17*(4), 267–274.

James, W. (1909). *The meaning of truth: A sequel to pragmatism.* New York: Longmans Green and Co.

James, W. (1977). (originally published 1891), The moral philosopher and the moral life. In J. J. McDermott (Ed.), *The writings of William James: A comprehensive edition* (pp. 610–629). Chicago: University of Chicago Press.

Juster, F. T., & Land, K. C. (1981). *Social accounting systems: Essays on the state of the art.* New York: Academic Press.

Karl, B. D., & Charles, E. (1974). *Merriam and the study of politics.* Chicago: University of Chicago Press.

Land, K. (1983). Social indicators. *Annual Review of Sociology, 9,* 1–26.

League For Social Reconstruction Research Committee. (1935). *Social planning for Canada*. Toronto: Thomas Nelson.

Lewis, C. I. (1946). *Analysis of knowledge and valuation*. LaSalle: Open Court.

MacRae, D. (1985). *Policy indicators: Links between social science and public debate*. Chapel Hill: University of North Carolina Press.

McDowell, I., & Newell, C. (1996). *Measuring health: A guide to rating scales and questionnaires*. New York: Oxford University Press.

McDowell, I., & Praught, E. (1982). On the measurement of happiness: An examination of the Bradburn scale in the Canada health survey. *American Journal of Epidemiology, 116*(6), 949–958.

McSweeny, A. J., et al. (1982). Life quality of patients with chronic obstructive pulmonary disease. *Archives of Internal Medicine, 142,* 473–478.

Michalos, A. C. (1967). Postulates of rational preference. *Philosophy of Science, 34,* 18–22.

Michalos, A. C. (1969). *Principles of Logic*. Englewood Cliffs: Prentice-Hall.

Michalos, A. C. (1970a). Decision making in committees. *American Philosophical Quarterly, 7,* 91–106.

Michalos, A. C. (1970b). Cost-benefit versus expected utility acceptance rules. *Theory and Decision, 1,* 61–88.

Michalos, A. C. (1970c). The impossibility of an ordinal measure of acceptability. *Philosophical Forum, 2,* 103–106.

Michalos, A. C. (1970d). The costs of decision making. *Public Choice, 9,* 39–51.

Michalos, A. C. (1978). *Foundations of decision-making*. Ottawa: Canadian Library of Philosophy.

Michalos, A. C. (1979). The loyal agent's argument. In T. Beauchamp & N. Bowie (Eds.), *Ethical theory and business* (pp. 247–253). Prentice-Hall: Englewood Cliffs. (Reprinted in Michalos 1995).

Michalos, A. C. (1980). *North American social report, Vol. 1: Foundations, population and health*. Dordrecht: D. Reidel.

Michalos, A. C. (1981). Technology assessment, facts and values. In P.T. Durbin (Ed.), *Research in Philosophy and Technology* (Vol.4, pp. 59–81). Dordrecht: JAI press.

Michalos, A. C. (1985). Multiple discrepancies theory (MDT). *Social Indicators Research, 16,* 347–413.

Michalos, A. C. (1988). Integrated development planning using socio-economic and quality of life indicators. In *Innovative approaches to development planning* (pp. 113–216). Paris: UNESCO.

Michalos, A. C. (1990). The impact of trust on business, international security and the quality of life. *Journal of Business Ethics, 9*, 619–638. (Reprinted in Michalos 1995).

Michalos, A. C. (1991a). *Global report on student well-being, Vol. 1: Life satisfaction and happiness*. New York: Springer.

Michalos, A. C. (1991b). *Global report on student well-being, Vol. 2: Family, friends, living partner and self-esteem*. New York: Springer.

Michalos, A. C. (1992). Ethical considerations in evaluation. *Canadian Journal of Program Evaluation, 7*, 61–75. (Reprinted in Michalos 1995).

Michalos, A. C. (1993a). *Global Report on Student Well-Being, Vol. 3: Employment, Finances, Housing and Transportation*. New York: Springer.

Michalos, A. C. (1993b). *Global Report on Student Well-Being, Vol. 4: Religion, Education, Recreation and Health*. New York: Springer.

Michalos, A. C. (1995). *A pragmatic approach to business ethics*. Thousand Oaks: SAGE Publications.

Michalos, A. C. (1997). Combining social, economic and environmental indicators to measure sustainable human well-being. *Social Indicators Research, 40,* 221–258.

Michalos, A. C. (1999). Reflections on twenty-five years of quality-of-life research. *Feminist Economics, 5*(2), 119–123.

Michalos, A. C. (2001). Ethics counselors as a new priesthood. *Journal of Business Ethics, 29,* 3–17.

Michalos, A. C., A. Hubley, B., Zumbo, D., & Hemingway, D. (2001). Health and other aspects of the quality of life of older people. *Social Indicators Research*, 54(1), xxx.
Michalos, A. C., & Zumbo, B. D. (1999). Public services and the quality of life. *Social Indicators Research, 48,* 125–156.
Michalos, A. C., & Zumbo, B. D. (2001). Ethnicity, modern prejudice and the quality of life. *Social Indicators Research, 53,* 189–222.
Michalos, A. C., & Zumbo, B. D. (2003). Leisure activities, health and the quality of life. In A.C. Michalos (Ed.) *Essays on the Quality of Life* (pp. 217–238). Dordrecht: Kluwer Academic Publishing.
Michalos, A. C., Zumbo, B. D., & Hubley, A. (2000). Health and the quality of life. *Social Indicators Research, 51,* 245–286.
Mitchell, W. C. (1918). Bentham's felicific calculus. *Political Science Quarterly, 33,* 161–183.
Najman, J. M., & Levine, S. (1981). Evaluating the impact of medical care and technologies on the quality of life: A review and critique. *Social Science and Medicine, 15F,* 107–115.
Nerenz, D. R., Repasky, D. P., Whitehouse, F. W., & Kahkonen, D. M. (1992). Ongoing assessment of health status in patients with diabetes mellitus. *Medical Care, 30*(5), MS112–MS124. (Supplement).
Noll, H.-H., & Zapf, W. (1994). Social indicators research: Societal monitoring and social reporting. In I. Borg & P. P. Mohler (Eds.), *Trends and perspectives in empirical social research.* Berlin: Walter de Gruyter.
Nord, E., Arnesen, T., Menzel, P., & Pinto, Jose-Luis. (2001). Towards a more restricted use of the term "quality of life". *Quality of Life Newsletter, 26,* 3–4.
Nussbaum, M. C., & Sen, A. (Eds.). (1993). *The quality of life.* Oxford: Clarendon Press.
Patrick, D. L., & Deyo, R. A. (1989). Generic and disease-specific measures in assessing health status and quality oflife. *Medical Care, 27*(3), s217–s232.
Perry, R. B. (1926). *General theory of value.* Cambridge: Harvard University Press.
Perry, R. B. (1954). *Realms of value.* Cambridge: Harvard University Press.
Pilowsky, I., et al. (1983). The illness behavior assessment schedule: Reliability and validity. *International Journal of Psychiatry and Medicine, 13,* 11–28.
Poff, D. C. (1987). The loyal agent's argument revisited. In D. C. Poff & W. J. Waluchow (Eds.), *Business ethics in Canada* (pp. 142–144). Toronto: Prentice-Hall Canada.
President's Research Committee on Social Trends. (1933). *Recent social trends in the United States* (Vols. 1, 2). New York: McGraw-Hill.
Prigatano, G. P., Wright, E. C., & Levin, D. (1984). Quality of life and its predictors in patients with mild hypoxemia and chronic obstructive pulmonary disease. *Archives of Internal Medicine, 144,* 1613–1619.
Radloff, L. S. (1977). The CES-D scale: A self-report deporession scale for research in the general population. *Applied Psychological Measurement, 1,* 385–401.
Renwick, R., & Brown, I. (1996). The centre for health promotion's conceptual approach to quality of life. In R. Renwick, I. Brown, & M. Nagler (Eds.), *Quality of life in health promotion and rehabilitation: Conceptual approaches, issues and applications* (pp. 75–86). Thousand Oaks: SAGE Publications.
Sandvik, E., Diener, E., & Seidlitz, L. (1993). Subjective well-being: The convergence and stability of self-report and non-self-report measures. *Journal of Personality, 61,* 317–342.
Schilpp, P. A. (Ed.). (1963). The philosophy of Rudolf Carnap. LaSalle: Open Court.
Schipper, H., et al. (1984). Measuring the quality of life of cancer patients: The functional living index—Cancer: Development and validation. *Journal of Clinical Oncology, 2,* 472–483.
Schwarz, N., & Bless, H. (1992). Constructing reality and its alternatives: Assimilation and contrast effects. In L. L. Marting & A. Tesser (Eds.), The construction of social judgment (pp. 217–245). Erlbaum: Hillsdale, N.J.
Schwarz, N., & Strack, F. (1991). Evaluating one's life: A judgment model of subjective well-being. In F. Strack, M. Argyle, & N. Schwarz (Eds.), *Subjective well-being: An interdisciplinary perspective* (pp. 27–47). Oxford: Pergamon.

Schwarz, N., & Strack, F. (1999). Reports of subjective well-being: Judgmental processes and their methodological implications. In D. Kahneman, E. Diener, & N. Schwarz (Eds.), *Well-being: The foundations of hedonic psychology* (pp. 61–84). New York: Russell Sage Foundation.

Sirgy, J. (in press). *Handbook of quality-of-life research: An ethical marketing perspective*. Dordrecht: Kluwer Academic Publishers.

Solomon, E. (1980). *Consultation of research network on the quality of life, Division for socio-economic analysis*. UNESCO, Paris, 3–5 December.

Sprangers, M. A. G. (1996). Response-shift bias: A challenge to the assessment of patients' quality of life in cancer clinical trials. *Cancer Treatment Reviews, 22*(Supplement A), 55–62.

Sprangers, M. A. G., & Schwartz, C. E. (1999). Integrating response shift into health-related quality of life research: A theoretical model. *Social Science and Medicine, 48,* 1507–1515.

Tatarkiewicz, W. (1976). *Analysis of happiness*. Hague: M. Nijhoff.

Taylor, S. E., & Brown, J. D. (1988). Illusion and well-being: A social psychological perspective on mental health. *Psychological Bulletin, 103,* 193–210.

Thomas, D.R., Hughes, E., & Zumbo, B.D. (1998). On variable importance in linear regression. *Social Indicators Research, 45*, 253–275.

Torrance, G. W. (1986). Measurement of health state utilities for economic appraisal. *Journal of Health Economics, 5,* 1–30.

Veenhoven, R. (1984). *Conditions of happiness*. Dordrecht: D. Reidel.

Veenhoven, R., & Ouweneel, P. (1995). Livability of the welfare-state, appreciation-of-life and length-of-life in nations varying in state-welfare-effort. *Social Indicators Research, 36*, 1–49.

Verbrugge, L. M., Merrill, S. S., & Liu, X. (1999). Measuring disability with parsimony. *Disability and Rehabilitation, 21*(5/6), 295–306.

Vogel, J. (1994). Social indicators and social reporting. *Statistical Journal of the United Nations ECE, 11,* 241–260.

Ware, J. E., Snow, K. K., Kosinski, M., & Gandek, B. (1993). *SF-36 health survey: Manual and interpretation guide*. Boston: The Health Institute, New England Medical Center.

Chapter 3
Culture as a Moderator of Overall Life Satisfaction—Life Facet Satisfaction Relationships

Alison G.C. Mallard, Charles E. Lance and Alex C. Michalos

Introduction

In 1985, Michalos presented a comprehensive theory of satisfaction which took into account important perceived discrepancies believed to lead to satisfaction or dissatisfaction (what one has versus what others have, what one has versus what one has had in the past, etc.). Known as Multiple Discrepancies Theory (MDT), aspects of this theory have been tested successfully in many populations including senior citizens (Michalos 1986), college students around the world (Michalos 1991; Stassen and Staats 1988), and rehabilitation clients (Gauthier 1987). Several different satisfaction domains have been researched within the MDT framework including satisfaction with work (Harwood and Rice 1992; Rice et al. 1989), health (Wright 1985), and life overall (Michalos 1985). Although some adjustments to MDT have been suggested (Neapolitan 1988), the MDT framework remains perhaps the most widely tested and accepted theory of individual satisfaction judgments (Harwood and Rice 1992; Andrews 1991; Rice et al. 1989).

MDT is based on the following assumptions (for further elaboration, see Michalos 1985):

Mallard, A.C.G., Lance, C.E., & Michalos, A.C.: 1997. Culture as a moderator of overall life satisfaction—life facet satisfaction relationships. Social Indicators Research, 40, pp. 259–284.

A.G.C. Mallard · C.E. Lance (✉)
Departmentof Psychology, The University of Georgia,
Athens, GA 30602-3013, USA
e-mail: clance@uga.cc.uga.edu

A.C. Michalos
University of Northern British Columbia, Prince George, BC, Canada
e-mail: michalos@brandonu.ca

A.C. Michalos, *Connecting the Quality of Life Theory to Health, Well-Being and Education*, DOI 10.1007/978-3-319-51161-0_3

(a) Net satisfaction is a positive linear function of the perceived differences between what one has versus (1) what one wants, (2) what others have, (3) the best one has had in the past, (4) what one expected to have 3 years ago, (5) what one expects to have in 5 years, (6) what one deserves, and (7) what one needs.
(b) Apart from the Have-Want discrepancy, all discrepancies are the result of objectively measurable differences. That is, objective discrepancies lead to perceived discrepancies, which lead to satisfaction or dissatisfaction.
(c) The Have-Want discrepancy serves as a mediator between the other discrepancies and net satisfaction. Combined with (a), it follows that perceived discrepancies have both direct and indirect effects on reported net satisfaction.
(d) The desire for satisfaction motivates people to act. The amount of action taken is in direct proportion to the satisfaction expected from the action.
(e) Discrepancies, satisfaction, and action are influenced by age, sex, education, ethnicity, income, self-esteem, and social support.
(f) The actions and conditions of people lead to their objective discrepancies.

In sum, objective discrepancies lead to perceptions of discrepancy. The influences of these perceptions on net satisfaction are both direct and mediated by the Have-Want discrepancy. This applies to satisfaction with income, health, education, and other life facets, as well as with satisfaction with life as a whole.

What MDT does *not* explain, however, is *how* satisfaction associated with distinct life domains relates to overall life satisfaction and vice versa: Is overall life satisfaction the result of some subjectively weighted aggregate of satisfaction in relevant life domains? Does satisfaction in various life domains arise from the influence of overall life satisfaction? Or, do the two influence each other? Three competing views have been offered to explain the relationship between overall life satisfaction (OLS) and life facet satisfaction (LFS).

Models of the OLS-LFS Relationship

Bottom-up model. The first perspective is a *bottom-up* (BU) or aggregate approach to explaining the relationship between OLS and LFS. Here it is maintained that satisfaction in life facets *leads to* overall life satisfaction (Campbell et al. 1976). In other words, OLS results from the cumulative satisfaction found in relevant life facets. That is, "some mental calculation is used to sum the momentary pleasures and pains" (Diener 1984, p. 565). The BU model is illustrated in Fig. 3.1.

A great deal of research on satisfaction, well-being, and quality of life has taken the BU perspective. For example, Bharadwaj and Wilkening (1977) concluded that "Most life satisfaction is derived from satisfaction domains … which are personal, broader in scope, and central to the individual" (p. 436). Headey et al. (1985) concluded that marriage and sex, friends and leisure, job, standard of living, and health were direct determinants of overall well-being. Other proponents of the

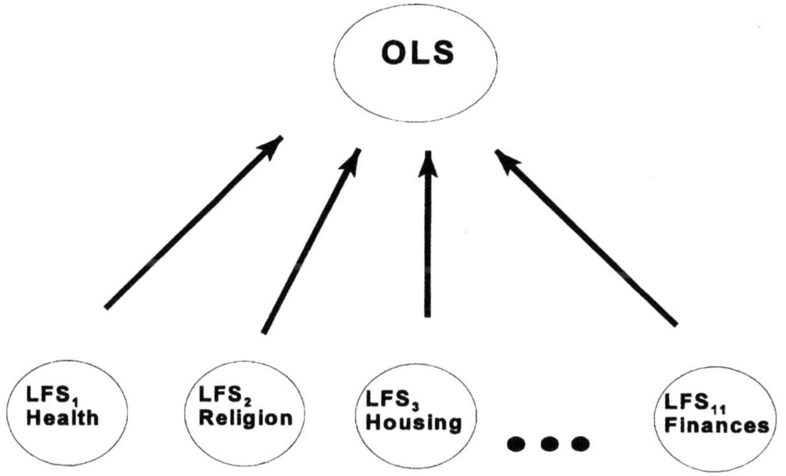

Fig. 3.1 A theoretical representation of a Bottom-Up model. *Note LFS* Life facet satisfaction; *OLS* Overall life satisfaction; *arrows* represent hypothesized causal directions

bottom-up model include Emmons and Diener (1985), Mastekaasa (1984), Near et al. (1980), and Rice et al. (1980). In general, most research conducted on the relationships between overall life satisfaction and life facet satisfaction has taken a BU perspective (Lance et al. 1995).

Top-down model. The *top-down* (TD) model represents an alternative perspective on the LFS-OLS relationship (see Fig. 3.2). Here, OLS is assumed to influence satisfaction in various life facets (Diener 1984; Stones and Kozma 1985). This is a more dispositional theory of satisfaction which suggests that individuals are predisposed towards being satisfied or unsatisfied with their lives in general and, consequently, specific aspects of their lives as well.

For several years, a relatively small group of researchers has argued this perspective by showing that happiness and satisfaction are stable (a) for individuals across situations and across time, and (b) across groups of people that vary dramatically in their financial status. For example, Costa and McCrae (1980) argued that personality differences accounted for subjective well being over a 10 year period. Ten years later, Costa and McCrae (1991) maintained this position and added, "changes in the quality of life lead to increases in happiness only temporarily until the neutral point of comparison has been reset" (p. 143). Also, Watson and Clarke (1984) reported that people with high negative affect ratings tend to be "dissatisfied over time regardless of the situation, even in the absence of any overt or objective source of stress" (pp. 483). Further Diener (1984) argued that the TD approach is supported by the fact that demographic variables account for very little variance in subjective well-being and that personality variables such as self-esteem show consistent relationships with subjective well-being. Additional similar arguments for the TD model have been made by Arvey et al. (1989), Bouchard et al.

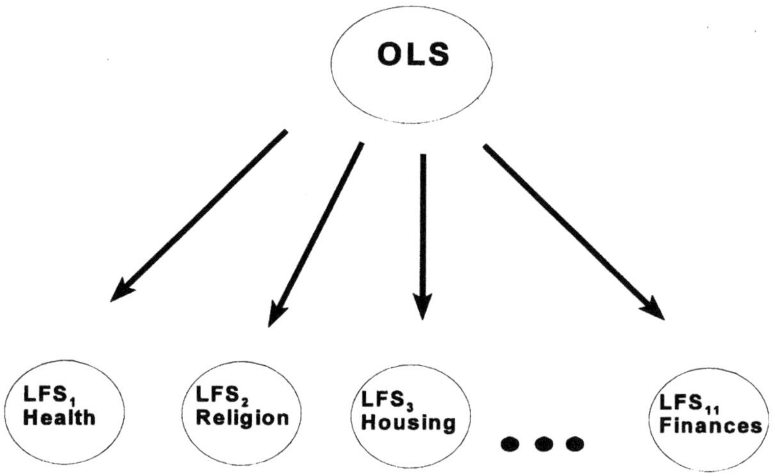

Fig. 3.2 A theoretical representation of a Top-Down model. *Note LFS* Life facet satisfaction; *OLS* Overall life satisfaction; *arrows* represent hypothesized causal directions

(1992), Diener et al. (1993), Levin and Stokes (1989), Staw et al. (1986), Staw and Ross (1985), and Stones and Kozma (1985).

Bidirectional model. Finally, Gerhart (1987, p. 371) argued for an integrated view of the BU and TD models: "It may be more accurate to interpret the predictive power of previous job satisfaction … as indicative of some degree of stability in *both* traits and job attributes…" This perspective is taken with the third model explainin OLS and LFS relationships. Instead of arguing for an exclusively BU or TD relationship between OLS and LFS, a *bidirectional* (BD) view maintains that both influences may be present simultaneously: OLS both results *from* satisfaction in life domains and *influences* satisfaction in those domains contemporaneously (Lance et al. 1989). The BD model is represented in Fig. 3.3.

Diener (1984) argued for such a model in claiming that his results "… point to some portion of happiness being due to personality, but also accentuate the importance of life circumstances" (p. 551). Five years later, the BD model was tested for the first time. Lance et al. (1989) compared the fit of BU, TD, and BD models with three life facets (job satisfaction, marital satisfaction, and satisfaction with social activities) and OLS in a sample of University faculty members in the U.S. They found strongest support for the BD model.

In a second study, Heady et al. (1991) tested the direction of the relationship between subjective well-being and six life facets in an Australian sample. Again, the BD model best accounted for OLS-LFS relationships. In a third study, Sloan (1990) also found that the BD model (vs. the BU and TD models) best accounted for OLS-LFS relationships in a sample of 243 University non-faculty staff members in the U.S. Finally, Lance et al. (1995) examined the relationship of OLS with 11 life facets simultaneously in a sample of 1663 U.S. college students. Again, the BD model provided the best fit to the data.

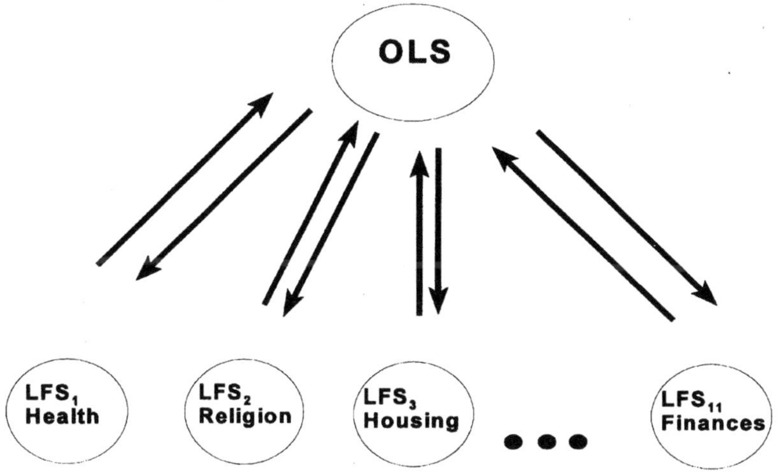

Fig. 3.3 A theoretical representation of a Bidirectional model. *Note LFS* Life facet satisfaction; *OLS* Overall life satisfaction; *arrows* represent hypothesized causal directions

The BD model also has been tested as it relates to OLS—job satisfaction relationships in two additional studies, and reciprocal (i.e., BD) relationships were found (Keon and McDonald 1982; Schmitt and Bedeian 1982; Farkas and Tetrick 1989; James and Jones 1980; James and Tetrick 1986). Other studies have found reciprocal relationships in related domains such as job satisfaction and organizational commitment (Farkas and Tetrick 1989; Lance 1991; Mathieu 1991), and job satisfaction and job perceptions (James and Jones 1980; James and Tetrick 1986). These findings suggest that when reciprocal relationships are tested, they often best explain the relationships under investigation.

Moderating Effects of Culture on OLS-LFS Relationships

While the four studies above comparing the fit of BU, TD, and BD models have, without exception, supported the BD model, they are limited in that their samples were taken from the United States and Australia. As a result, we do not know whether these findings are generalizable to other, non-Western cultures. For example, it is not clear whether the BD model best explains the OLS-LFS relationship for industrialized or English speaking countries only, or if it is a multi-cultural phenomenon. Although ours was largely an exploratory study to determine whether cultural differences in OLS-LFS relationships may exist, there are some reasons to expect that culture may moderate these relationships. For example, in some cultures, success may be defined by the amount of money one has, the type of house and car one can afford, how happy one's family life is, the extent to which one travels the world, and the extent to which one is educated. Thus, a person might strive for a high income, a large house, a spouse and children, etc. towards success and personal satisfaction. This scenario reflects BU rationale for OLS-LFS relationships—the more one is satisfied with one's possessions (housing, transportation), personal situation (health, family, friendships, paid employment, finances), and experiences (recreation, religion, education), the more one is satisfied with life overall.

On the other hand, there are considerable cross-cultural differences in the ways in which individuals classify reality according to differences in the functional relevance of those segments of reality being classified (e.g., Anglin 1995; Bloom 1981; Lakoff 1987), and all cultures may not categorize life satisfaction according to distinct life facets as research indicates that Western English speaking samples have. If individuals do not differentiate between OLS and LFS, or between satisfaction with different aspects of their lives, this could engender the operation of a TD model in which judgments of OLS overshadow more specific judgments of LFSs. Thus, OLS-LFS relationships may vary cross-culturally to the extent that members of different cultures differentiate among and attach varying degrees of significance to individual life facets.

Regardless, investigating OLS-LFS relationships cross-culturally is important not only to further understand the relationship between OLS and LFS, but to assess whether culture moderates this relationship. Exploring cultural differences has practical implications as well. As we become globally linked by increasingly inexpensive and convenient travel, improved communication systems, and advancing technology, we must learn more about each other in order to communicate effectively and work well together.

In summary, the purpose of this study was twofold: (a) to provide additional tests of the structural relationship between OLS and LFS (i.e., BU vs. TD vs. BD models) in eleven life facets, and (b) to explore whether these relationships vary across cultures.

Method

Research Participants and Data Collection

Data reported in this study were collected as part of Michalos' (1991) global study of student well-being. University and college students from 42 countries were asked to complete a 10-page Satisfaction and Happiness Survey (SHS) which contained scales measuring (a) satisfaction and perceived discrepancies with respect to OLS and several distinct life facets, (b) self-esteem, and (c) social support. As described by Michalos (1991), all surveys were translated into the primary language of the host country. Most respondents were students in introductory classes, while others represented a random sample of the complete student population. See Michalos (1991) for a complete description of the scale development and samples' characteristics.

Research participants in this study represented the following countries: Austria, Bahrain, Bangladesh, Belgium, Brazil, Cameroon, Canada, Chile, Egypt, Finland,

Federal Republic of Germany, Greece, India, Israel, Japan, Jordan, Kenya, Korea, Mexico, Netherlands, New Zealand, Norway, Philippines, Portugal, Puerto Rico (a U.S. Territory), Singapore, Republic of South Africa, Spain, Sweden, Tanzania, Thailand, Turkey, United Kingdom, USA, and Yugoslavia.[1] Only those students who were citizens of the country in which they were attending college were included in the study.

Measures

Portions of the SHS reported in this study include measures of (a) satisfaction with life facets and life overall, and (b) Have-Want discrepancy with life facets and with life overall. The eleven life facets we studied were Friendship, Health, Education, Transportation, Religion, Living Partner, Paid Employment, Housing, Finances, Family Relations, and Recreation.

Satisfaction. Research participants were asked to "… consider your life right now …" and rate their satisfaction with each of the 11 facets (LFS) and with their "life as a whole right now" (OLS) using Michalos' (1991) "Delighted-Terrible" scale (1 = "Terrible" to 4 = "Mixed" to 7 = "Delightful;" a "no opinion" option was also provided).

Have-Want discrepancies. As is explained later, these measures were included partly for statistical identification purposes in the BD model. Research participants were asked to "… consider your present life in comparison to your wants or aspirations …" and rate their perceived discrepancy between what they have and what they want (i.e., "… how closely your life now seems to approach your own wants") for each of the 11 life facets and life as a whole. Responses were on a seven point scale: 1 = "Not at all," to 4 = "Half as well as what you want," to 7 = "Matches or is better than what you want." Again, the "no opinion" option was provided. The Have-Want discrepancy scores were direct ratings by the students, and thus were not calculated from separate "Have" and "Want" ratings. Direct perceived discrepancy measures are preferred because difference scores often have inferior psychometric properties (Edwards 1994; Lance et al. 1995).

Tests of BU, TD, and BD Models

We used the LISREL-VII computer program (Joreskog and Sorbom 1989) to conduct structural equation modeling tests of the BU, TD, and BD models and to effect comparative (nested) tests among them.

---

[1]Data were collected before the Bosnian war. The country known as Yugoslavia before 1994 is referred to as Yugoslavia in this study.

Model development. The BU, TD, and BD models of OLS-LFS relationships were compared for each sample (country) to determine which model best fit the data. In order to test reciprocal relationships in the BD model, it was necessary to include the Have-Want discrepancy measures as instrumental variables (James and Singh 1978) for statistical identification purposes. A variable (X) may be considered an instrument if it (a) has a direct, nonminor effect on only *one* of two reciprocally related variables (e.g., Y_1), (b) is not reciprocally related to the variable for which it is acting as an instrument (Y_1), (c) is not causally related to the reciprocally related variable for which it is not serving as an instrument (i.e., Y_2), and (d) is unrelated to both Y_1's and Y_2's disturbance terms (James and Singh 1978). Use of Have-Want discrepancies is justified theoretically because MDT views them as (a) being the immediate direct cause of respective satisfaction judgments, (b) the cause of, rather than being caused by, satisfaction judgments, and (c) leading to satisfaction judgments *within* life domains rather than *across* different domains (e.g., the perceived Have-Want discrepancy regarding Housing would be relevant for a judgment of satisfaction with Housing but not satisfaction with Education).

Models tested. For each sample, three models were tested (see Fig. 3.4 for an example of the BD model). Common elements in these models included (a) treating the Have-Want and Satisfaction variables as manifest variables, (b) designating the Have-Want discrepancy measures as the exogenous variables leading to the endogenous Satisfaction variables, (c) allowing the exogenous variables to correlate

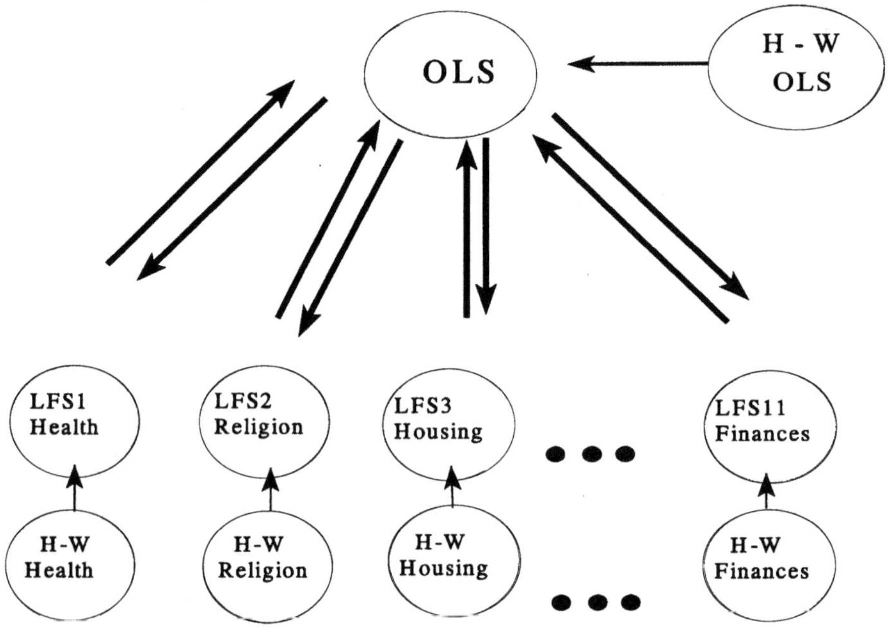

Fig. 3.4 General form of models tested. *Note LFS* Life facet satisfaction; *H-W* Have-Want discrepancy; *OLS* Overall life satisfaction; *arrows* represent hypothesized causal directions

freely, and (d) specifying the residuals (error terms) as mutually uncorrelated. The models differed only in the direction of causation between OLS and LFS. Model I (BU or aggregate model) specified that the life facets were the causal antecedents to OLS. Model II (TD or dispositional model) specified top down influences from OLS to each of 11 life facets. Model III (BD) specified reciprocal relationships between OLS and LFS. Finally, a structural null model (Williams and Holahan 1993) was estimated for comparative purposes in which no causal relationships were estimated between OLS and the LFS measures.

Estimation and fit assessment. Correlation matrices were input for maximum likelihood estimation for each sample by the LISREL—VII program (Joreskog and Sorbom 1989). The model with the best fit for each sample (i.e., BU vs. TD vs. BD) was identified by conducting chi-square difference tests between the BD and BU model, and then again between the BD and TD model. If the BD model did not provide a significantly better fit than did the BU or TD model, then each of these two unidirectional models was compared to the structural null model to determine which of the two provided the greatest increment in fit. This was necessary because the BU and TD models had equal model degrees of freedom; neither model was nested within (a special case of) the other. However, by comparing the BU and TD models to the structural null model, it was possible to determine which of the two provided the best relative fit to the data.

Cluster Analyses

Although as will be discussed later the BD model was found to best represent OLS-LFS relationships for most samples (countries), not all individual OLS-LFS relationships were significantly BD. For example, the Cameroonian sample had a significant BU relationship from satisfaction with Living Partner to OLS; significant TD relationships from OLS to satisfaction with Health, Paid Employment, Housing, Recreation, Religion, and Transportation; and significant BD relationships between OLS and satisfaction with Finances, Family, and Friendships. On the other hand, the Austrian sample had significant BU relationships from satisfaction with Health, Friendships, Living Partner, and Education to OLS; significant TD relationships from OLS to satisfaction with Family, Paid Employment, and Recreation; and significant a BD relationship between OLS and satisfaction with Religion. In fact, each country's pattern of OLS-LFS relationships was unique. To help identify similarities in these patterns, we used Ward's (1963) hierarchical agglomerative clustering method (using binary codes for each OLS-LFS relationship to indicate whether the relationship was null "00," BU "10, TD "01," or BD "11") to define subgroups of samples which shared similar OLS-LFS relationship patterns across life facets. The goal here was to infer what cultural similarities among the countries which had been clustered together empirically might be responsible for similarities in patterns of OLS-LFS relationships.

Results

Tests of BU, TD, and BD Models

We first examined the correlations between the Have-Want discrepancy rating and corresponding Satisfaction rating for each facet (i.e., r_{ij}, where *i* refers to a specific facet) versus the Have-Want rating and *noncorresponding* satisfaction rating for all facets in turn (e.g., r_{ij}, whereas *i* refers to a specific facet and *j* refers to a facet other than *i*) for each of the 11 life facets and OLS. This was necessary to confirm that the discrepancy measures functioned satisfactorily as instrumental variables, that is, that all r_{ii}s were larger than r_{ij}s. This assumption held for all samples but one: the Portuguese sample. Here the correlation between Have-Want Overall and OLS was 0.435 whereas the correlation between Have-Want Religion and Have-Want Transportation and OLS were 0.468 and 0.483, respectively. This rendered OLS with no instrument and as a result, nonrecursive relationships (in the BD model) could not be estimated due to statistical underidentification. Thus, the Portuguese sample was eliminated from further analyses.

The remaining 34 samples were included in the BU, TD, and BD model comparisons. All solutions converged for all samples but the Indian and Singaporean samples. Several model modifications were attempted (e.g., specifying alternative starting values, increasing the problem run time), but convergent solutions could not be obtained. Thus, the Indian and Singaporean samples also were eliminated from analyses. Convergent solutions were obtained for the remaining 32 countries. However it was necessary to remove one or two statistically redundant life facets to achieve a convergent solution in four of the remaining samples. For the Mexican and South African samples, the Finance facet was deleted from analyses. For the Chilean and Kenyan samples, it was necessary to delete both the Finances and Paid Employment facets. The remaining 28 countries contained all 11 life facets and OLS in the analyses.

Table 3.1 shows country (first column), sample sizes (second column), and model degrees of freedom (df) and chi-squared statistics (χ^2) for tests of the BU, TD, and BD models (next three columns). As is often the case with large samples, each of the models could be rejected statistically on the basis of the χ^2 values. Thus realizing that all of the models' fit to the data were imperfect, our intent was to determine which of the theoretically motivated models (i.e., BU vs. TD vs. BD) provided the best *relative* fit to the data (Williams and Holahan 1994). We accomplished this by conducting difference χ^2 tests between nested models.

Difference chi-square tests (rightmost two columns of Table 3.1) showed that (a) the BD model provided a significantly better fit than did the BU model in all 32 samples, and (b) the BD model provided a significantly better fit than did the TD model for all but three samples: the Belgian, Jordanian, and Swedish samples. For these samples, a comparison between the TD model and the structural null model indicated that the TD model significantly improved fit to the data. Thus the TD model was accepted as the best-fitting and most parsimonious model for Belgian,

Table 3.1 Chi-square and chi-square difference tests for 32 samples

Sample	N	BU		TD		BD		BU versus BD		TD versus BD	
		df	x^2	df	x^2	df	x^2	df	x^2	df	x^2
Austria	332	199	621.01	199	600.84	188	556.72	11	64.29	11	44.12
Bahrain	247	199	1160.25	199	1080.29	188	1047.14	11	113.11	11	33.15
Bangladesh	262	199	1359.95	199	1372.32	188	322.56	11	37.39	11	49.76
Belgium	129	199	317.55	199	313.33	188	294.42	11	23.13	11	18.91*
Brazil	274	199	777.53	199	684.94	188	643.81	11	133.72	11	41.13
Cameroon	182	199	898.91	199	862.85	188	802.94	11	95.97	11	59.91
Canada	1516	199	2159.00	199	1932.98	188	1772.78	11	386.22	11	160.20
Chile	260	136	674.82	136	593.05	127	527.27	9	147.55	9	65.78
Egypt	248	199	652.11	199	614.29	188	587.51	11	64.60	11	26.78
Finland	271	199	655.13	199	615.25	188	568.99	11	86.14	11	46.26
Germany	1264	199	640.15	199	663.08	188	573.73	11	66.42	11	89.35
Greece	248	199	729.29	199	676.38	188	624.13	11	105.16	11	52.25
Israel	286	199	588.92	199	537.21	188	491.29	11	97.63	11	45.92
Japan	1209	199	2432.10	199	2289.23	188	2189.58	11	242.52	11	99.65
Jordan	270	199	834.02	199	675.82	188	661.79	11	172.23	11	14.03*
Kenya	272	136	743.86	136	552.73	127	529.66	9	214.20	9	23.07
Korea	392	199	2898.98	199	2757.12	188	2689.06	11	209.92	11	68.06
Mexico	243	166	640.92	166	567.67	156	536.21	10	73.25	10	31.46
Netherlands	346	199	708.72	199	716.05	188	638.44	11	70.28	11	77.61
New Zealand	293	199	823.59	199	843.96	188	770.10	11	53.49	11	73.86
Norway	444	199	1258.91	199	1219.69	188	1157.49	11	101.42	11	62.20
Phillippines	992	199	2597.77	199	2158.11	188	2085.79	11	511.98	11	72.32
Puerto Rico	301	199	724.70	199	654.57	188	626.65	11	98.05	11	27.92

(continued)

Table 3.1 (continued)

Sample	N	BU		TD		BD		BU versus BD		TD versus BD	
		df	x^2	df	x^2	df	x^2	df	x^2	df	x^2
S. Africa	233	166	872.81	166	784.08	156	753.88	10	118.93	10	30.20
Spain	275	199	803.61	199	763.52	188	731.75	11	71.86	11	31.77
Sweden	253	199	416.10	199	372.09	188	364.56	11	51.54	11	7.53*
Tanzania	214	199	894.74	199	715.50	188	686.93	11	207.84	11	28.57
Thailand	582	199	1087.80	199	946.75	188	894.02	11	193.78	11	52.73
Turkey	287	199	586.30	199	596.00	188	539.95	11	46.35	11	56.05
United Kingdom	216	199	682.34	199	691.54	188	606.87	11	75.47	11	84.67
United States	1154	199	2043.19	199	1674.63	188	1530.31	11	512.88	11	144.32
Yugoslavia	330	199	1191.22	199	1060.73	188	983.39	11	207.83	11	77.34

*$p > 0.01$; all other chi-square values are statistically significant at $p < 0.01$

Table 3.2 Statistically significant TD relationships for Belgian, Jordanian, and Swedish samples

Sample	Health	Fin	Fam	PdEmp	Frn	Hous	Liv P	Rec	Rel	Trans	Ed
Belgium				↓		↓			↓		
Jordan	↓	↓	↓		↓	↓	↓	↓	↓	↓	↓
Sweden	↓							↓			↓

Note ↓ statistically significant ($p < 0.05$) TD relationship; *Health* Health, *Fin* Finances, *Fam* Family Relations, *PdEmp* Paid Employment, *Frn* Friendships, *Hous* Housing, *Liv P* Living Partner, *Rec* Recreation Activity, *Rel* Religion, *Trans* Transportation, *Ed* Education

Jordanian, and Swedish samples, whereas the BD model was accepted as the most appropriate model in the remaining samples.

Table 3.2 summarizes the pattern of statistically significant TD relationships found for the Belgian, Jordanian, and Swedish samples. Other than having exclusively TD OLS→LFS relationships, results across these three samples had little in common. Effects of OLS on LFS are sparse in the Belgian and Swedish samples, suggesting that LFS is determined largely by perceived Have-Want discrepancies in the respective domains, and not OLS. For the Jordanian sample on the other hand, OLS had a pervasive effect on LFS in nearly every life domain.

Cluster Analysis

Cluster analysis suggested a seven cluster solution for the 25 samples in which (a) OLS-LFS relationships were estimated for all 11 life facets, and (b) the BD model received the strongest support. These clusters are summarized in Table 3.3, which includes a summary of the direction of the relationship that was supported between each life facet and OLS for each sample. Cluster 1 consisted of Austria, Germany, Netherlands, and New Zealand. A TD relationship from OLS to satisfaction with Family was supported in each of these samples, which also had BU relationships from satisfaction with Education and Living Partner to OLS. Very few (7%) significant BD relationships were found in this cluster. Thirty-four percent of the OLS-LFS relationships in this cluster were significantly BU and 34% were significantly TD. No BD OLS-LFS relationships were found in the German sample and only one each was supported in the remaining three samples. Of all of the clusters, this one was the least "active" in the sense that 22% of the OLS-LFS paths were nonsignificant.

Cluster 2 consisted of Bahrain, Bangladesh, Puerto Rico, and Spain. No facet in this group had a consistently significant BU, TD, or BD relationship with OLS across four samples. Thirty-nine percent of the OLS-LFS relationships were BU, 20% TD, 18% BD, and 23% had no significant relationship between OLS and LFS. The only significant (BU) relationship from satisfaction with Religion to OLS in this cluster was in the Bangladeshi sample. This is noteworthy in that only two of

Table 3.3 Statistically significant OLS-LFS relationships for seven clusters

	Health	Fin	Fam	PdEmp	Frn	Hous	Liv P	Rec	Rel	Trans	Ed
Cluster 1											
Austria	↑		↓	↓	↑		↑	↓	↑↓		↑
Germany	↓		↓	↑	↓		↑	↓	↓		↑
Netherlands	↓		↓		↓	↓	↑	↑	↓	↑↓	↑
New Zealand	↑	↑	↓		↑		↑		↓	↑↓	↑
Cluster 2											
Bahrain	↓	↑	↓	↑↓	↑	↑↓	↑↓	↑		↑	↑↓
Bangladesh	↑			↑		↑↓	↑↓	↑	↑	↓	↑
Puerto Rico	↑		↓		↑	↑↓	↓	↓		↑	↓
Spain	↑	↑↓		↑	↑		↓	↑		↑	↓
Cluster 3											
Brazil	↑	↑↓	↓	↑	↓	↓	↑↓	↓	↑↓	↑	↑↓
Norway	↑	↓			↓	↓	↑↓	↓	↑↓	↑	↓
Tanzania	↓	↑↓	↓		↓	↑	↑↓		↑↓		↓
Cluster 4											
Cameroon	↓	↑↓	↑↓	↓	↑↓	↓	↑	↓	↓	↓	
Canada	↑↓	↑↓	↑↓	↑	↑↓	↓	↑↓	↑↓	↓	↓	↑↓
United States	↑	↑↓	↑↓	↓	↑↓	↑↓	↑↓	↑↓	↓	↑↓	↓
Cluster 5											
Egypt	↑↓	↓	↑	↑↓	↑	↓	↓	↓		↓	↑
Japan	↑↓	↓	↑	↓	↓	↑↓	↓	↑↓	↑↓	↓	↑↓
Korea	↑↓	↓	↑	↑↓	↓	↓	↑↓	↑↓	↑	↓	↓
Cluster 6											
Finland	↑	↓	↑	↓		↓	↓	↓	↓		

(continued)

Table 3.3 (continued)

	Health	Fin	Fam	PdEmp	Frn	Hous	Liv P	Rec	Rel	Trans	Ed
Israel		↑	↑	↓	↓	↓	↑	↑	↓		
Thailand	↓	↑↓	↑	↓	↓	↑↓	↑	↓	↓	↑	↓
Turkey	↑	↑↓	↑		↓		↑	↑↓	↓		↓
Cluster 7											
Greece		↑	↑↓	↑↓	↓	↓	↑	↑↓		↓	↓
Philippines	↑↓	↑↓	↓	↑↓	↓	↓	↑	↑↓	↓	↑↓	
United Kingdom	↓		↑↓	↑↓	↓	↓	↑	↑	↑↓		↑
Yugoslavia	↑↓	↓	↓	↑↓	↑↓	↓	↑↓	↑↓	↓	↑	↓

Note ↑ BU relationship, ↓ TD relationship, and ↑↓ BD relationship; *Health* Health, *Fin* Finances, *Fam* Family Relations, *PdEmp* Paid Employment, *Fri* Friendship, *Hous* Housing, *Liv P* Living Partner, *Rec* Recreation, *Trans* Transportation, *Ed* Education the remaining 24 samples (Egypt and United Kingdom) had nonsignificant OLS—satisfaction with Religion relationships.

Cluster 3 was composed of Brazil, Norway, and Tanzania. Eighteen percent of the OLS-LFS relationships in these countries were BU, 39% TD, and 27% BD. No significant relationships were found for 15% of the OLS-LFS paths. A significant TD relationship from OLS to satisfaction with Friendship, and significant BD relationships between OLS and satisfaction with Living Partner and satisfaction with Religion were found for each of these three samples.

Cluster 4 consisted of Cameroon, Canada, and United States. Only one OLS-LFS relationship in this cluster was not statistically significant. This cluster had a large proportion (52%) of BD relationships between OLS and LFS. Thirty-six percent of the OLS-LFS paths were TD, and 9% were BU. These samples had significant TD relationships from OLS to satisfaction with Religion, and significant BD relationships between OLS and satisfaction with Finance, Family, and Friendships.

Cluster 5 included Egypt, Japan, and Korea. As with the fourth cluster, only one of the possible 33 OLS-LFS relationships was nonsignificant. The remaining significant paths were 18% BU, 45% TD, and 33% BD. A significant BU relationship was found from satisfaction with Family to OLS, and significant TD relationships were found from OLS to satisfaction with Finance and Transportation in all three of these samples. Also, significant BD relationships were found between OLS and satisfaction with Health. This cluster was the only one which shared significant BU, TD, *and* BD relationships between LFS and OLS across samples.

Cluster 6 consisted of Finland, Israel, Thailand, and Turkey. This cluster had relatively few BD relationships (9%). A large proportion of the relationships (43%) were TD whereas 27% of the relationships were BU and 21% of the relationships were nonsignificant. No BD relationships were supported in the Finnish and Israeli samples. All samples in this cluster had a significant BU relationship from satisfaction with Family to OLS, and a significant TD relationship from OLS to satisfaction with Religion.

Finally, Cluster 7 contained Greece, Philippines, United Kingdom, and Yugoslavia. The proportion of TD and BD relationships were evenly divided at 36%. Sixteen percent of the OLS-LFS relationships were BU and the remaining 11% were nonsignificant. All samples shared a significant TD relationship from OLS to satisfaction with Housing and a significant BD relationship between Paid Employment and OLS.

Discussion

For the past several decades, research on OLS-LFS relationships has been conducted primarily from *either* a bottom-up *or* top-down perspective. Recently, a handful of studies have tested possible bidirectional OLS-LFS relationships (e.g., Heady et al. 1991; Lance et al. 1989, 1995; Sloan 1990). Although limited in number, the results of these few studies have indicated that the OLS-LFS relationship is BD.

The first purpose of this paper was to provide additional competitive tests between the BU, TD, and BD models. Overwhelmingly, results supported the BD model, as this model provided the best fit to the data for all but three of the 32 samples examined. In the remaining three samples the TD model received the strongest support. Importantly, the BU model received the *least* support in all 32 samples. This finding runs counter to a majority of satisfaction research whose theoretical assumptions have been rooted in the BU perspective (Diener 1984; Lance et al. 1995; Sloan 1990). Thus findings reported here now provide global support *counter* to the idea that some subjectively weighted composite of LFSs determines OLS, and in support of the idea that OLS-LFS relationships are multidirectional.

The second purpose of this paper was to determine whether culture moderates the OLS-LFS relationship. The fact that the BD model was supported in the overwhelming majority of samples suggests that culture does *not* moderate the OLS-LFS relationship. This is consistent with research reported by Keller (1987), Tanka-Matsumi and Marsella (1976), and Sidanius et al. (1994) who have found that despite diverse cultural backgrounds, findings concerning attitudes, beliefs, and emotions tend to remain invariant. This conclusion is also consistent with previous studies comparing the BU, TD, and BD models.

On the other hand, and at a more micro level, the BD model allows *either* a BU, TD, *or* BD relationship between each life facet and OLS, and some combination of these three OLS-LFS linkages was supported in each sample. Furthermore, no two samples had identical patterns of OLS-LFS relationships across the 11 life facets studied. Thus from this more micro viewpoint, culture acted as a *strong* moderator of the specific pattern of OLS-LFS relationships across the various life facets.

Cluster analyses of these various patterns of OLS-LFS relationships identified seven reasonably homogeneous clusters of samples. What was *not* clear was *why* these clusters of samples exhibited similar patterns of OLS-LFS relationships. Why did the Austrian, German, Dutch, and New Zealander samples have a BU relationship between Living Partner and Education and OLS, when few other countries did? Why did the Cameroonian, Canadian, and American samples have a TD relationship between Friendship and OLS while most other countries did not?

Some clusters consisted of countries which had reasonably transparent cultural commonalities. For example, Cluster 1 included Austria, Germany, and the Netherlands—three geographically proximal countries with common linguistic and historical roots. Cluster 4 included two ethnically diverse, industrialized Western countries—the United States and Canada, and Cluster 5 included two industrialized Far-East nations—Japan and Korea. However, each cluster also contained samples that shared no obvious cultural similarities (e.g., language, geographical location, GNP) with the others. For example, Cluster 4 not only included Canada and the United States, but also Cameroon, and Cluster 5 included Egypt along with Japan and Korea.

Thus the answer to the question "Does culture moderate the OLSLFS relationship?" is not clear. The fact that the BD model received overwhelming support in 29 of the 32 samples studied points to the answer "no." On the other hand, the fact that different patterns of OLS-LFS relationships were found in each sample points to the answer "yes." However, since none of the clusters of samples could be clearly defined by some (set of) cultural factor(s) makes the answer even more difficult. Clearly, additional research is needed on this question. Nevertheless, this study has made an important first step in that it is the first to address this issue.

Limitations and Directions for Future Research

As with most multi-national survey data, one limitation to this study was the extent to which respondents in different countries interpreted the survey items consistently. For example, is it possible that *satisfaction* does not mean the same thing in one culture as it does in another? The question of whether the *meaning* of satisfaction is moderated by culture is an intriguing question. Thus studies are needed of cross-cultural measurement equivalency of satisfaction—related constructs. Vandenberg and Self (1993) present one example of an approach to testing for qualitative differences, response threshold differences, and differences in (latent) mean levels in satisfaction-related constructs across diverse cultures that we suggest for future research.

Second, although there may be no one person better to ask about life satisfaction than the person in question, self report data have often been criticized. However, recent evidence suggests that selfreport method bias is not as serious a threat to measurement as was once believed. For example, Crampton and Wagner's (1994) meta-analysis found that self-report methods contributed little contaminating variance, and concluded "… our results suggest that percept-percept inflation may be more the exception than the rule …" (p. 72). But even if severe method bias was present, there is no reason to suspect that it would bias results in favor of one model of OLS-LFS relations over others.

Third, this study included 11 life facets. No other study has included more life facets in exploring OLS-LFS relationships. However, these 11 facets may not necessarily represent all possible facets that have significant relationships with OLS. In fact, it is possible that for some cultures, important life facets were omitted. For example, safety may be a very salient life domain in less well developed countries, or countries which have experienced long term political/military strife. Thus we suggest that future research include additional life facets that may be peculiarly salient in other cultures.

Finally, the conclusions of this research are restricted to college students and not the entire populations of the nations represented here. Although the BD model has received the strongest support in other Western, non-student samples, these findings may not generalize globally. Nevertheless, results of this study support the ideas that (a) BD OLS-LFS relationships exist globally, (b) and although culture appears as a significant moderator of specific patterns of OLS-LFS relationships across specific life facets, (c) additional research is needed to explain *why*.

Acknowledgements This article is based on a doctoral dissertation completed by the first author under the direction of the second author. We thank Bob Gatewood, Karl Kuhnert, Garnett Stokes, and Kecia Thomas for their helpful comments on an earlier version of this paper.

References

Andrews, F. M. (1991). Stability and change in levels and structure of subjective well-being: USA 1972 and 1988. *Social Indicators Research, 25,* 1–30.

Anglin, J. M. (1995). Classifying the world through language: Functional relevance, cultural significance, and category name learning. *International Journal of Intercultural Relations, 19,* 161–181.

Arvey, R. D., Bouchard, T. J., Jr., Segal, N. L., & Abraham, L. M. (1989). Job satisfaction: Environmental and genetic components. *Journal of Applied Psychology, 74,* 187–192.

Bharaewaj, L., & Wilkening, E. A. (1977). The prediction of perceived well being. *Social Indicators Research, 4,* 421–439.

Bloom, A. (1981). *The linguistic shaping of thought*. Hillsdale, NJ: Erlbaum.

Bouchard, T. J., Arvey, R. D., Keller, L. M., & Segal, N. L. (1992). Genetic influences on job satisfaction: A reply to Crwpanzanw and James. *Journal of Applied Psychology, 77,* 89–93.

Campbell, A., Converse, P. E., & Rodgers, W. L. (1976). *The quality of American life*. New York: Russell Sage Foundation.

Costa, P. T., & McCrae, R. R. (1980). Influence of extroversion and neuroticism on subjective well-being: Happy and unhappy people. *Journal of Personality and Social Psychology, 38,* 668–678.

Costa, P. T., & McCrae, R. R. (1991). Personality as a lifelong determinant of well-being. In C. Malatesta & C. Izard (Eds.), *Affective processes in adult development and aging*. Beverly Hills: Sage Publications.

Crampton, S. M., & Wagner, K. A. (1994). Percept-percept inflation in microorganizational research: An investigation of prevalence and effect. *Journal of Applied Psychology, 79,* 67–76.

Diener, E. (1984). Subjective well-being. *Psychological Bulletin, 95*, pp. 542–575.

Diener, E., E. Sandvik, L. Seidlitz., & Diener, M. (1993). The relationship between income and subjective well-being: Relative or subjective? *Social Indicators Research, 28*, 195–223.

Edwards, J. R. (1994). The study of congruence in organizational behavior research: Critique and a proposed alternative. *Organizational Behavior and Human Decision Processes, 58,* 51–100.

Emmons, R. A. and Diener, E. (1985) Factors predicting satisfaction judgments: A comparative examination. *Social Indicators Research, 16*, pp. 157–167.

Farkas, A. J., & Tetrick, L. E. (1989). A three-wave longitudinal analysis of the causal ordering of satisfaction and commitment on turnover decisions. *Journal of Applied Psychology, 74,* 855–868.

Gauthier, B. (1987). Client satisfaction in program evaluation. *Social Indicators Research, 19,* 229–254.

Gerhart, B. (1987). How important are dispositional factors as determinants of job satisfaction? Implications for job design and other personnel programs. *Journal of Applied Psychology, 72,* 366–373.

Harwood, M. K., & Rice, R. W. (1992). An examination of referent selection processes underlying job satisfaction. *Social Indicators Research, 27,* 1–39.

Headey, B., Holstrom, E., & Wearing, A. (1985). Models of well-being and ill-being. *Social Indicators Research, 17,* 211–234.

Headey, B., VvvoOovvo, R., & Wearing, A. (1991). Top-down versus bottom-up theories of subjective well-being. *Social Indicators Research, 24,* 81–100.
James, L. R., & Jones, A. P. (1980). Perceived job characteristics and job satisfaction: An examination of reciprocal causation. *Personnel Psychology, 33,* 97–135.
James, L. R., & Singh, B. K. (1978). An introduction to the logic, assumptions, and basic analytical procedure of two-stage least squares. *Psychological Bulletin, 85,* 1104–1122.
James, L. R., & Tetrick, L. E. (1986). Confirmatory analytic tests of three causal models relating job perceptions to job satisfaction. *Journal of Applied Psychology, 71,* 77–82.
Joreskog, K., & Sorbom, D. (1989). *LISREL 7: A guide to the program and applications.* Chicago: SPSS Inc.
Keller, R. T. (1987). Cross-cultural influences on work and nonwork contributors to life quality. *Group and Organizational Studies, 12,* 304–318.
Keon, T. L. & McDonald, D. (1982) Job satisfaction and life satisfaction: An empirical evaluation of their interrelationship. *Human Relations 35,* 167–180.
Lakoff, G. (1987). *Women, fire, and dangerous things: What categories reveal about the mind.* Chicago, IL: University of Chicago Press.
Lance, C. E. (1991). Evaluation of a structural model relating job satisfaction, organizational commitment and precursors to voluntary turnover. *Multivariate Behavioral Research, 26,* 137–162.
Lance, C. E., LautenscOlager, G. J., Sloan, C. E., & Varca P. E. (1989). A comparison between bottom-up, top-down, and bidirectional models of relationships between global and life facet satisfaction. *Journal of Personality 57,* 601–624.
Lance, C. E., Mallard, A. G. C., & Michalos, A. C. (1995). Tests of the causal directions of global-life facet satisfaction relationships. *Social Indicators of Research, 34,* 69–92.
Levin, R. J., & Stokes, J. P. (1989). Dispositional approach to job satisfaction: Role of negative affectivity. *Journal of Applied Psychology, 74,* 752–758.
Mastekaasa, A. (1984). Multiplicative and additive models of job and life satisfaction. *Social Indicators Research, 14,* 141–163.
Mathieu, J. E. (1991). A cross-level nonrecursive model of the antecedents of organizational commitment and satisfaction. *Journal of Applied Psychology, 76,* 607–618.
Michalos, A. C. (1985). Multiple discrepancies theory (MDT). *Social Indicators Research, 8,* 385–442.
Michalos, A. C. (1986). An application of multiple discrepancies theory (MDT) to seniors. *Social Indicators Research, 18,* 349–373.
Michalos, A. C. (1991) *Global report on student well-being, Vol. I: Life satisfaction and happiness.* New York: Springer.
Neapolitan, J. (1988). General symbolic definitions and subjective well-being. *Sociological Spectrum, 8,* 153–168.
Near, J. P., Rice, R. W., & Hunt, R. G. (1980). Work and extra-work correlates of life and job satisfaction. *Academy of Management Review, 5,* 415–429.
Rice, R. W., McFarlin, D. B., & Bennett, D. E. (1989). Standards of comparison and job satisfaction. *Journal of Applied Psychology, 74,* 591–598.
Rice, R. W., McFarlin, D. B., Hunt, R. G., & Near, J. P. (1980). Organizational work and the perceived quality of life: Toward a conceptual model. *Academy of Management Review, 10,* 296–310.
Schmitt, N., & Bedeian, A. G. (1982). A comparison of LISREL and two-stage least squares analysis of a hypothesized life-job reciprocal relationship. *Journal of Applied Psychology, 67,* 806–817.
Sidanius, J., Pratto, R., & Rabinowitz, J. L. (1994) Gender, ethnic status, and ideological asymmetry. *Journal of Cross-Cultural Psychology 25,* 194–216.
Sloan, C. E. (1990). *Relations between global life and domain satisfaction: The role of domain scope and criticality* (Unpublished doctoral dissertation, University of Georgia, Athens).
Strnssen, M. A., & Stoats, S. R. (1988). Hope and happiness: A comparison of some discrepancies. *Social Indicators Research, 20,* 45–58.

Staw, B. M., Bell, N. E., & Claussen, J. A. (1986). The dispositional approach to job attitudes: A lifetime longitudinal investigation. *Administrative Science Quarterly, 31,* 56–77.

Staw, B. M., & Ross, J. (1985). Stability in the midst of change: A dispositional approach to job attitudes. *Journal of Applied Psychology, 70,* 469–480.

Stones, M. J., & Kozma, A. (1985) Structural relationships among happiness scales: A second order factorial study. *Social Indicators Research 17*, 19–28.

Tanka-Matsumi, J., & Marsella, A. J. (1976). Cross-cultural variation in the phenomenological experience of depression. *Journal of Cross-Cultural Psychology, 7,* 379–399.

Vandenberg, R. J., & Self, R. M. (1993). Assessing newcomers' changing commitments to the organization during the first 6 months of work. *Journal of Applied Psychology, 78,* 557–568.

Ward, J. H. (1963). Hierarchical grouping to optimize an objective function. *Journal of the American Statistical Association, 58,* 236–244.

Watson, D., & Clarke, L. A. (1984) Negative affectivity: The disposition to experience aversive emotional states. *Psychological Bulletin 96*, 465–490.

Williams, L. J., & Holahan, P. J. (1994) Parsimony-based fit indices for multiple- indicator models: Do they work? *Structural Equations Modeling 1*, 161–189.

Wright, S. J. (1985). Health satisfaction: A detailed test of the multiple discrepancies theory. *Social Indicators Research, 17,* 299–313.

Chapter 4
Determinants of Health and the Quality of Life in the Bella Coola Valley

Alex C. Michalos, Harvey V. Thommasen, Rua Read, Nancy Anderson and Bruno D. Zumbo

Introduction

The aim of this investigation is to obtain some baseline self reported data on the health status and overall quality of life of a sample of residents of the Bella Coola Valley of British Columbia aged 17 years or older, and to measure the impact of a set of designated health determinants on their health and quality of life. The structure of the essay is as follows. The next section contains a description of the sampling technique and questionnaire. Following that, there is a section describing

Michalos, A.C., Thommasen, H.V., Read, R., Anderson, N., & Zumbo, B.D.: 2005. Determinants of health and the quality of life in the Bella Coola Valley. Social Indicators Research, 72, pp. 1–50. © Springer 2005.

A.C. Michalos (✉)
University of Northern British Columbia, Prince George, BC, Canada
e-mail: michalos@brandonu.ca

H.V. Thommasen
University of Northern British Columbia, Prince George, BC V2N 4Z9, Canada
e-mail: thommash@unbc.ca

R. Read
Faculty of Medicine, University of British Columbia, Vancouver, BC V6T 1Z4, Canada

N. Anderson
Faculty of Medicine, University of British Columbia, Bella Coola Medical Clinic, Box 220, Bella Coola, BC V0T 1C0, Canada

B.D. Zumbo
Measurement, Evaluation and Research Methodology Program, University of British Columbia, 2125 Main Mall, Vancouver, BC V6T 1Z4, Canada
e-mail: bruno.zumbo@ubc.ca

A.C. Michalos, *Connecting the Quality of Life Theory to Health, Well-Being and Education*, DOI 10.1007/978-3-319-51161-0_4

the demographic composition of the sample. Descriptive statistics for the measures of health status, health-related behaviour, health care and (domain specific and global) quality of life are given in the next four sections. Bivariate relationships among the dependent variables alone and then among the independent and dependent variables are reviewed in the next two sections, respectively. Multivariate relationships among all our measures are examined in the next section, followed by a short overview section and conclusion.

Sample Area, Sampling Technique and Questionnaire

The Bella Coola Valley is in northwestern British Columbia. There are four rural and remote communities in the Valley, namely, Bella Coola, Hagensborg, Firvale and Stuie, containing an estimated 2332 people. Approximately 40% of the residents are of aboriginal descent, most of which belong to the Nuxalk nation. The Nuxalk people are Salish-speaking and have lived in the British Columbia Central Coast area for many years. The hospital in Bella Coola is one of the 10 most isolated physician-staffed health facilities in British Columbia. The closest referral hospital is over 450 km by road (Williams Lake) or a 2 h flight to Vancouver. Bella Coola is serviced by three physicians at any given time. In any given year, these physicians can expect 8000 clinic visits, 2500 emergency room visits, 400 admissions to hospital and 20–30 obstetrical deliveries (Thommasen et al. 1999).

In the period from August to November 2001, a number of procedures were used to try to get every resident aged 17 years or older of the Bella Coola Valley of British Columbia to fill out an 11-page questionnaire. A questionnaire was mailed out to everyone who had attended the Bella Coola Medical Clinic who were known to live in the Bella Coola Valley. Questionnaires were also distributed at the Clinic, the emergency department of the Bella Coola Hospital, and in two local grocery stores. Booths were set up at the grocery stores and at the Clinic where research assistants administered the questionnaire to people who might not normally respond to a mail-out survey, including elderly people and those with literacy problems. Questionnaires were also hand-delivered on the local reserve and picked up later. Finally, an attempt was made to pick up a few more stragglers by mailing out a one-page questionnaire mainly with some quality of life items.

The first three and a half pages contained the 36-item Medical Outcomes Study Short Form (SF-36) profile (Ware et al. 1993). These were followed by 13 items from the United States Centers for Disease Control and Prevention, Behavioural Risk Factor Surveillance System (BRFSS) (CDC 2000). There are 14 items in the BRFSS, the first of which is a general health question that is also the first question in SF-36. Seven items measuring socializing activities and social support came next, followed by 12 items forming an Index of Life Stress and 10 items forming an Index of Good Family Life (selected from Hudson 1982). There were six questions about community health issues, e.g., Alcohol abuse is a problem here. Then there were 12 questions about health-related behaviours, i.e., on tobacco smoking, drinking alcoholic beverages, eating and sleeping routines, use of over-the-counter and prescription drugs, free time physical activities and physical activities at work. Eleven items were devoted to health care issues, e.g., rating personal and most people's health care, frequency of seeking medical and dental care in the past year, and distances travelled to receive care. Following these, there was a page containing our standard set of 19 quality of life items, e.g., happiness and satisfaction with life as a whole, and satisfaction with specific domains of life like one's housing, friendships and financial security. The last two pages had basic demographic questions, supplemented by five items about respondents' experiences in residential schools and an item about household pets.

Sample Characteristics

By the end of June we had received 687 useable full-length questionnaires and 281 one-pagers. The 687 full-length questionnaires form the working dataset for this analysis, which represents about 40% of the estimated 1736 residents 17 years or older in the Valley. Of the 686 respondents who identified their gender, 57% (394) were females. Fifty-five percent (370) of those who answered the marital status question were married. The average age was 48, and the range ran from 17 to

Table 4.1 Sample composition compared to 1996 census

	N	%	1996%
Gender			
Male	292	42.6	52.0
Female	394	57.4	48.0
Total	686	100.0	100.0
Age			
17–34	152	22.9	42.0[a]
35–49	219	33.0	39.0
50–64	180	27.1	19.0
65–90	113	16.4	10.0
Total	664	100.0	100.0
Ethnic background			
Nuxalk	107	16.1	na
Other Aboriginal	130	19.6	38.0[b]
All others[c]	426	64.3	62.0
Total	663	100.0	100.0
Marital status			
Now married	370	54.7	49.0[d]
Live-in/common law partner	110	16.2	na

(continued)

Table 4.1 (continued)

	N	%	1996%
Single	91	13.4	35.0
Divorced	22	3.2	9.0
Separated	35	5.2	4.0
Widowed	49	7.2	3.0
Total	677	100.0	100.0
Highest level of education			
Elementary school incomplete	27	4.0	na
Elementary school complete	28	4.1	9.0[e]
Secondary school incomplete	134	19.5	24.0
Secondary school complete	132	19.2	15.0
Some trade/tech/business/ community college	83	12.1	na
Diploma/cert. from trade/etc.	112	16.3	30.0[f]
Some university	59	8.6	12.0
University degree, any level	95	13.8	10.0
Total	670	100.0	100.0
Primary employment status			
Unemployed	87	13.0	9.0
Employed full-time	204	30.4	64.0[g]
Employed part-time	131	19.5	na
Retired	111	16.5	na
Homemaker	65	9.7	na
Student	13	1.9	na
Other	60	8.9	27.0[h]
Total	671	100.0	100.0

[a]15–34 years old
[b]All Aboriginal
[c]Mostly Canadian, British and European
[d]Includes common law partners
[e]Less than grade 9
[f]Some trade + trade certificates and diplomas
[g]Includes full- and part-time employed
[h]Includes everyone not in labour force, i.e., retired homemakers and students

90. Fifty-nine (9%) had some university education, with 95 (14%) holding a university degree. Two hundred and four (30%) were employed full-time and 131 (20%) part-time. A household income question turned out to be useless because only 122 people responded to it. Regarding cultural or ethnic background, 107 (16%) were Nuxalk, 130 (20%) came from other aboriginal or metis backgrounds and the remaining 426 (64%) were from non-aboriginal backgrounds (mostly Canadian, British and European). In another study, we will examine aboriginal and non-aboriginal similarities and differences more extensively. Table 4.1 gives a more detailed summary of the total sample.

Health Status Measures

The SF-36 profile is sometimes referred to as the 'gold standard' for health status measurement and its norms for several populations provide useful benchmarks for other developed countries (Ware and Sherbourne 1992; McHorney et al. 1993, 1994; Ware et al. 1993, 1994). Table 4.2 summarizes its basic elements.

The SF-36 scale works best as a health profile measure with eight dimensions, rather than as a single summative measure. SF-36 profile scores are designed such that 0 represents the worst and 100 represents the best state of health. Using a panel study of 3445 patients, McHorney et al. (1994) found that the internal-consistency reliability (Cronbach's $\propto$) for each of the eight concepts measured in the SF-36 with this panel ranged from 0.78 to 0.93, with a mean of 0.85.

In the next three tables we summarize the eight SF-36 profile scores for the respondents in the Bella Coola Valley taken all together and for males and females, and compare their scores with scores from Prince George, Aberdeen, the United States, Sweden and a sample of people 55 years old or older from the Northern Interior Health Region (NIHR) of British Columbia.

Table 4.2 Content of the SF-36 questionnaire

Concepts	Number of items	Meaning of low scores	Meaning of high scores
Physical functioning	10	Limited a lot in performing all physical activities including bathing or dressing due to health	Performs all types of physical activities including the most vigorous without limitations due to health
Role physical	4	Problems with work or other daily activities as a result of physical health	No problems with work or other daily activities as a result of physical health
Bodily pain	2	Very severe and extremely limiting pain	No pain or limitations due to pain
General health	5	Evaluates personal health as poor and believes it is likely to get worse	Evaluates personal health as excellent
Vitality	4	Feels tired and worn out all of the time	Feels full of pep and energy all of the time
Social functioning	2	Extreme and frequent interference with normal social activities due to physical or emotional problems	Performs normal social activities without interference due to physical or emotional problems
Role emotional	3	Problems with work or other daily activities as a result of emotional problems	No problems with work or other daily activities as a result of emotional problems
Mental health	5	Feelings of nervousness and depression all of the time	Feels peaceful, happy, and calm all of the time
Reported health transition	1	Believes general health is much worse now than one year ago	Believes general health is much better now than one year ago

Source Ware et al. (1993, p. 3:5)

Table 4.3 SF-36 comparisons of country and city scores[a]

	BC valley	PG 1998	PG 1999	Aberdeen	USA	Sweden	NIHR seniors
PF	82.3	87.2	87.7	79.2	84.2	87.9	69.1
RP	67.5	81.8	76.6	76.5	81	83.2	61.1
BP	54.6	60.9	72.2	76.9	75.2	74.8	61.4
GH	55.5	73.7	71.7	68.7	72	75.8	64.8
VT	54.0	58.4	58.4	61.2	60.9	68.8	57.5
SF	50.0	83.5	81.8	78.6	83.3	88.6	80
RE	75.1	80.7	78.1	75	81.3	85.7	80.4
MH	62.4	74.5	75.2	73.7	74.7	80.9	77.3

Sources Garratt et al. (1993), Ware et al. (1993), Sullivan et al. (1995), Han et al. (1998), Michalos et al. (2000, 2001), Michalos and Zumbo (2003). [a]Bella Coola Valley, March 2002, $N = 687$, ages 17–90; Prince George, November 1998, $N = 719$, ages 17–92; Prince George, November 1999, $N = 438$, ages 17–86; Aberdeen, $N = 542$, ages 18 and older; USA, $N = 2474$, ages 18 and older; Sweden, $N = 8930$, ages 15 and older; Northern Interior Health Region, October 1999, $N = 875$, ages 55–95

Table 4.3 lists the scores for our respondent group as a whole. The scores range from 82.3 for Physical Functioning to 50.0 for Social Functioning, with a mean of 62.7. This mean score is lower than those of all the other six group samples. If we take these means of the eight scores as broadly indicating the health of the seven samples listed in Table 4.3, then it is fair to say that the respondents in our Bella Coola Valley sample are relatively less healthy than those in the other five samples. In fact, ignoring the seniors sample, there is only one comparison in which the Valley sample score is higher than another. The Valley score of 82.3 for physical functioning is higher than the 79.2 score for Aberdeen. Otherwise, ignoring the seniors sample, the Valley sample scores for every dimension are lower than all others in the same row.

After making the comparisons with the other population groups and finding the Valley scores so much lower, we thought the latter might be biased downward because of its relatively higher percentage of older people. Generally, as age increases, mean SF-36 health dimension scores decrease (Ware et al. 1993, pp. 10:14–17). So, we included the NIHR seniors' figures as another comparison group. As Table 4.3 shows, there are only two scores in the Valley figures (Physical Functioning and Role Physical) that are higher than their counterparts in the NIHR seniors' figures, and the mean score for the eight dimensions of the latter is higher (69.0) than that of the former (62.7).

In their factor analyses of the eight dimension scores, Ware et al. (1993, p. 9:22) found two fairly distinct factors with three dimensions in each. The physical health factor included physical functioning, role physical and bodily pain, while the mental health factor included mental health, role emotional and social functioning. The other two dimensions of SF-36 were moderately related to both factors. Inspection of the Valley scores in Table 4.3 reveals that for the group as a whole,

Table 4.4 SF-36 Comparisons of city and country male scores[a]

	BC valley	PG 1998	PG 1999	USA	NIHR seniors
PF	82.4	87.1	88.3	87.2	72
RP	66.7	83.6	80	86.6	62
BP	53.4	61.9	74.5	76.9	65.2
GH	54.7	74	72.4	73.5	63.4
VT	54.1	60.2	59.6	63.6	59.7
SF	50.8	85.3	82.5	85.2	80.5
RE	76.2	81.5	78.4	83.3	81.1
MH	63	75.5	76	76.4	78.6

Sources Ware et al. (1993), Michalos et al. (2000, 2001), Michalos and Zumbo (2003)
[a]Bella Coola Valley, N = 292, ages 17–90; Prince George, November 1998, N = 365, ages 17–82; Prince George, November 1999, N = 202, ages 17–86; USA, N = 1055, ages 18 and older; Northern Interior Health Region, October 1999, N = 283, ages 55–97

the average physical health score (68.1) was superior to the average mental health score (62.5).

Table 4.4 lists the scores for males in the five groups for which we had data. The scores for Bella Coola Valley male respondents range from 82.4 for physical functioning to 50.8 for social functioning, with a mean of 62.7. Again, this mean is lower than that of the other four sample means for males. This time, ignoring the seniors' sample, across every dimension, there is no case in which Valley scores are higher than any others. Still, there are only two dimensions (physical functioning and role physical) in which the Valley scores are higher than the seniors' scores. The mean score for male physical health (67.5) is higher than that for mental health (63.3).

Table 4.5 lists the scores for females in the five groups. The scores for Bella Coola Valley female respondents range from 82.1 for physical functioning to 49.4 for social functioning, with a mean of 62.7. So, on average our female respondents

Table 4.5 SF-36 comparisons of city and country female scores[a]

	BC valley	PG 1998	PG 1999	USA	NIHR seniors
PF	82.1	87.3	87.1	81.5	67.6
RP	68.1	79.8	73.8	77.8	60.7
BP	55.5	59.7	70.2	73.6	59.5
GHc	56.1	73.4	71.2	70.6	65.5
VT	54	56.5	57.3	58.4	56.4
SF	49.4	81.7	81.1	81.5	79.8
RE	74.3	79.8	77.8	79.5	80.1
MH	61.9	73.5	74.5	73.3	76.7

Sources Ware et al. (1993), Michalos et al. (2000, 2001), Michalos and Zumbo (2003)
[a]Bella Coola Valley, N = 394, ages 17–88; Prince George, November 1998, N = 352, ages 17–92; Prince George, November 1999, N = 236, ages 20–86; USA, N = 1412, ages 18 and older; Northern Interior Health Region, October 1999, N = 592, ages 55–95

are just as healthy as our males. Again, ignoring the seniors' scores, across every dimension, the Valley scores are lower than all others. As in the male case, the Valley female scores were higher than the seniors' scores for physical functioning and role physical. The mean score for female physical health (68.6) is also higher than that for mental health (61.9). Curiously then, while the overall average scores for the eight dimensions are the same for men and women, on average the women have higher physical health scores and lower mental health scores than the men.

Since 1993 the United States Centres for Disease Control and Prevention (CDC) have been developing a set of indicators to be used in tracking the population health status of residents of all 50 States (CDC 2000). The whole system is known as the Behavioural Risk Factor Surveillance System (BRFSS). There were four items in the original core of the system and 10 were added to it in January 1995. Table 4.6 lists results from seven surveys for the original four items from the BRFSS that provide good summaries of people's health from different perspectives. Specifically, the items measure self-reported general health on a 5-point scale from excellent to poor, the number of days in the past 30 that the respondent experienced "not good health" physically, the number of days that were mentally "not good" and the number on which "not good" physical or mental health prevented the respondent from engaging in his or her usual activities.

Except for the American survey, all of the other surveys were based on mailout questionnaires to adults 18 years of age or older in British Columbia. Four of the surveys came from random samples of from 2000 to 2500 households, with three in the city of Prince George and one in the city of Quesnel. The province-wide British Columbia sample was based on two independent surveys taken in November 1999

Table 4.6 Mean scores for physical and mental not good health days, limited activity days, general health; 7 surveys

Indicator	BC valley	Quesnel May 2000	PG April 2000	PG November 2000	PG May 2001	BC November 1999	13 USA states 1995–1997
Sample size	687	642	607	437	695	1468	42632
Phys. H. not good days	6.5	3.7	3.4	4.1	3.2	3.9	3.1
Ment. H. not good days	5.5	4.2	3.5	3.2	3.1	4.2	2.8
Limit, act. days	4.1	2.8	2.1	1.5	2.2	2.3	1.7
General health	2.8	2.5	2.4	2.2	2.2	2.4	na

Sources CDC (2000), Michalos et al. (2000, 2003), Institute for Social Research and Evaluation surveys (2000–2001)

Table 4.7 Mean scores for additional five CDC items

Indicator: days in the past 30 in which you felt,	Bella Coola valley	13 USA States 1995–1997
Sad, blue or depressed	5	3
Worried, tense or anxious	6.7	5.2
You did not get enough sleep	9.5	7.6
Pain limited your usual activities	5	2.6
Very healthy and full of energy	16.4	19

Source CDC (2000)

with the intention of comparing views of relatively arbitrarily selected "northerners" (people living north of the town of Hundred Mile House) and "southerners" in the province. For this article the two samples were combined into one. This combined sample is not representative of the whole province because it has about twice as many "northerners" as "southerners".

Table 4.6 lists the sample sizes for each of the seven surveys and the mean scores for each of the four items for each survey. The first column of the exhibit reveals that on average the Bella Coola Valley sample had more "not good" physical and mental health days, and more limited activity days than the other samples. Respondents in the Valley averaged 6.5 days in the past 30 in which their health was physically not good, 5.5 days when it was mentally not good and 4.1 days when their health limited their usual daily activities. Because the raw scores for the general health item ran from 1 indicating 'excellent' to 5 indicating 'poor', the Valley mean sample score of 2.8 was the worst of the six, and the Prince George scores of November 2000 and May 2001 (2.2) were the best. Eleven percent of the Valley respondents described their general health as "excellent" and another 27% said it was "very good".

Table 4.7 lists five other items from the CDC collection that were included in our questionnaire. The formats are the same as above, with respondents asked to indicate the number of days in the past 30 in which they felt one way or another. The first four are negative. On average, respondents felt sad on 5.0 of the past 30 days, worried on 6.7 days, did not get enough sleep on 9.5 days and had their usual activities limited by pain on 5.0 days. In general, they felt "very happy and full of energy" on 16.4 of the past 30 days. Compared to the American sample for 13 States, on average, respondents in the Bella Coola Valley sample reported more unhealthy days.

Health-Related Behaviour and Exposure

Tables 4.8, 4.9, 4.10 and 4.11 review health-related behaviour and exposure issues, including some comparisons with the 1998 Prince George survey. Table 4.8 lists the percentages of respondents who were tobacco smokers and/or were exposed to secondhand smoke. There were 66.5% reporting that they never smoked, compared

Table 4.8 Smoking behaviour and exposure

	BCV (%)	PG 1998 (%)
Frequency of smoking tobacco		
Never	66.5	77.1
Occasionally	10.2	6
Daily	13.1	8
Hourly	10.2	8.9
Frequency of exposure to second-hand smoke at home		
Never	68.7	68.5
Occasionally	13.7	15.8
Daily	11.6	10.1
Hourly	6.0	5.6
Frequency of exposure to second-hand smoke outside home		
Never	20.4	8.6
Occasionally	64.4	74.4
Daily	12.1	15.2
Hourly	3.1	1.8

Source Michalos et al. (2000)

Table 4.9 Drinking[a] alcoholic beverages behaviour

	BCV (%)	PG1998 (%)
Frequency of drinking		
Never	33.8	12.3
Less than once a month	17.1	22.5
Once a month	5	7.7
2–3 times a month	13	16.6
Once a week	6.4	9.4
2–3 times a week	12.4	16.1
4–6 times a week	6.9	10.5
Every day	5.4	5
Average # drinks per sitting		
1 or 2 drinks	63.6	71.3
3 or 4 drinks	21	21.7
5 or more drinks	15.4	7

Source Michalos et al. (2000)

[a]'Drink' means one bottle or can of beer or a glass of draft, one glass of wine or a wine cooler, or one straight or mixed drink with one and a half ounces of hard liquor

Table 4.10 Mean number of times per week in the past month that respondents engaged in various kinds of physical activities in their leisure time for 15 min or more

Free time activities	Mean # of times
Strenuous exercise (e.g., running, jogging, long distance cycling, singles tennis)	1
Moderate exercise (e.g., easy cycling, volleyball, easy swimming, folk dancing)	2.3
Mild exercise (e.g., yoga, golf, gardening, easy walking)	5.5

Table 4.11 Percent describing the physical activity required for their paid or unpaid work

Work activities	%
Work requires heavy physical labour (e.g., digging, lifting heavy things)	13.2
Work requires moderately physical labour (e.g., climbing stairs, carrying things)	17
Work requires moving about but no lifting or carrying heavy things	36.5
Work is mainly sitting	15

to 77.1% in the Prince George survey. In the Valley, 68.7% said they were never exposed to second-hand smoke at home, compared to 68.5% in Prince George. Twenty percent (20.4%) of the Valley respondents and only 8.6% of the Prince George respondents said they were never exposed to second-hand smoke outside their homes.

Table 4.9 lists the percentages of respondents who drank alcoholic beverages. In the Valley, 33.8% of respondents said that they never drank alcoholic beverages, compared to only 12.3% in the Prince George survey and 8.8% in the 1996–1997 Canadian National health Survey (FPTC 1999, p. 174). Of those who drank, 63.6% of Valley respondents reported that on average they had one or two drinks per sitting, compared to 71.3% in Prince George. At the other end of the scale, 15.4% of Valley respondents said that they drank five or more drinks per sitting on average, while only 7.0% of Prince George respondents drank that much. So, the Bella Coola Valley sample had fewer drinkers, a smaller percent of moderate drinkers and a bigger percent of heavy drinkers than the Prince George sample.

Table 4.10 shows that on average, in their leisure time, Valley respondents engaged in strenuous physical exercise over 15 min in duration about once a week in the past month, moderate exercise about twice a week and mild exercise about five and a half times a week. In their work time, about 13.2% were engaged in heavy physical labour, 17.0% in moderately physical labour, 36.5% in light physical labour and 15.0% mainly in sitting (Table 4.11).

Health Care

Table 4.12 lists results of several questions related to respondents' views about health care and aspects of their own care, including a column of scores from the 1998 Prince George survey for comparison. On a 5-point scale from 1 = poor to 5 = excellent, the mean respondent rating for their own health care services was 3.4, practically the same as their mean rating (3.3) for the health care services of most people. These were surprising scores because usually for such pairs of questions, respondents reveal an ego-centric bias by rating their own care higher than most peoples' (Michalos 1991). The 1998 Prince George scores for the same questions were more typical, i.e., 3.1 for own versus 2.6 for others.

In the Valley, 59.9% of respondents said they had a family physician, compared to 95.7% in Prince George. Still, on average Valley respondents had seen a physician in the past year more often than respondents in Prince George. The former had seen a physician 5.6 times per year, compared to 3.8 times for the latter. The Valley respondents had also been in hospital more often than the Prince George respondents, 1.4 times compared to 0.4 times per year. We did not have a distance travelled question in our earlier survey, but on average Valley respondents travelled 67.9 km the last time they needed routine medical care and 579.0 km the last time they needed specialist care.

Although 61.4% of Valley respondents and 88.3% of Prince George respondents had a dentist, members of the two groups saw a dentist equally often, 1.6 compared to 1.7 times per year.

Generally speaking, then, although most of our measures indicate that the health status of the Bella Coola Valley respondents was lower than that of the Prince

Table 4.12 Views about and aspects of health care

Health care issue	BCV	PG 1998
Mean rating of respondents' own health care services[a]	3.4	3.1
Mean rating of health care services for most people[a]	3.3	2.6
Percent having a family physician	59.9	95.7
Number of times seen a physician in the past year	5.6	3.8
Number of times been in hospital in the past year	1.4	0.4
Distance traveled for routine medical care last time it was needed (km)	67.9	na
Distance traveled for specialist care last time it was needed (km)	579	na
Percent having a dentist	61.4	88.3
Number of times seen a dentist in the past year	1.6	1.7

Source Michalos et al. (2000)

[a]Ratings on 5-point scale with 1 = poor, 2 = fair, 3 = average, 4 = good and 5 = excellent

George respondents, the former evaluate their health care and that of most others to be at least as good as the latter evaluate their own and most others' care. Although Valley respondents do not have family physicians and dentists at the same rate as Prince George respondents, the former contact a physician more often than the latter and contact a dentist equally often.

Quality of Life Measures

Table 4.13 lists results for 19 measures of the quality of people's lives, including 15 measures of specific domains (e.g., housing, job, family relations) and four global measures (e.g., overall happiness, satisfaction with life as a whole). All of the items were formatted in 7-point scales running from 1 = very dissatisfied (or very unhappy), through 4 = evenly balanced, to 7 = very satisfied (or very happy). Besides the Bella Coola Valley sample, the exhibit also includes comparison figures from a survey in Prince George in May 2001, in Quesnel in May 2000 and in

Table 4.13 Mean satisfaction and happiness levels

How satisfied are you with:	BCV	PG May 2001	Quesnel May 2000	Jasper July 1997
Your house, apartment	5.4	5.6	5.6	5.7
Your neighborhood	5.7	5.5	5.4	5.7
Your family relations	5.7	5.9	5.9	5.8
Your living partner	5.8	6.2	6.3	5.4
Your job	5.1	5.2	5.4	4.6
Your life as a whole	5.5	5.7	na	5.9
Your friendships	5.7	5.8	5.8	6.0
Your health	4.9	5.4	5.5	5.8
Your religion/spiritual fulfilment	5.2	5.2	5.4	4.5
Your overall standard of living	5.4	5.4	5.3	5.7
Your financial security	4.4	4.6	4.7	4.9
Your recreation activities	4.6	5.1	4.8	na
Your self-esteem	5.2	5.5	5.7	5.8
Your personal safety around home	5.8	5.6	na	na
Federal government officials	3.3	2.9	3.6	3.0
Provincial government officials	3.3	2.6	3.7	3.0
Local government officials	3.6	3.4	4.1	na
Your overall quality of life	5.5	5.7	5.5	5.9
Your overall happiness	5.5	5.8	5.6	5.8
N	687	695	642	447

Sources Zumbo and Michalos (2000), Michalos and Zumbo (2000), Michalos (2002)

Jasper, Alberta in July 1997. The average score for the Valley respondents was 5.0, ranging from 3.3 for satisfaction with both federal and provincial government officials to 5.8 for satisfaction with living partners and with personal safety around home. The average scores for the samples from Prince George, Quesnel and Jasper were 5.1, 5.2 and 5.2, respectively.

Summing the scores for the global items (i.e., happiness, life satisfaction, overall quality of life and standard of living), we may construct a general measure of Subjective Well-Being Index (SWB) that has a good Cronbach internal reliability score of $\alpha = 0.86$. The Valley resident SWB mean score is 21.4, compared to 22.4 for the Prince George sample and 22.5 for the Jasper sample (Because the Quesnel survey lacked a life satisfaction item, a SWB score could not be calculated for that sample).

Considering only the rank ordering of only the domain satisfaction scores for the four samples, one finds some interesting similarities and differences at both ends of the satisfaction scales. For the samples from the Valley, Prince George and Quesnel, living partner satisfaction scores were ranked highest, while for the Jasper sample, it was friendship satisfaction. Curiously, the Valley personal safety satisfaction score was the same as the living partner satisfaction score. Family relations satisfaction scores ranked second for all four samples, although these scores were tied with neighborhood and friendship satisfaction scores in the Valley, and with health and personal selfesteem in Jasper. At the other end of the scale, in every sample government officials at all levels had the lowest satisfaction ratings. Local officials always faired a bit better than federal and provincial officials. Apart from government officials, which routinely serve as a sort of public punching bag in most surveys, lowest levels of satisfaction scores are reported for financial security in the Valley, Prince George and Quesnel. In Jasper, apart from government officials, the lowest scores are reported for religion or spiritual fulfilment.

Bivariate Relationships: Dependent Variables

There is some flexibility about the interpretation of several of the variables included in our data set. In different analyses they might be regarded as independent (predictors) or dependent variables. Broadly speaking, we classified variables as independent if they belonged to the British Columbia Provincial Health Officer's (1994) list of determinants of health and dependent if they had been validated as relatively general measures of health status or overall (global) quality of life. In some analyses we use health status indicators as predictors of overall quality of life, because the concept of the 'quality of life' is more comprehensive than the concept of 'health' (Michalos and Zumbo 2003). Table 4.14 provides an overview of how we view the most important ones. As the exhibit shows, we have some independent variables for four of the five broad categories of determinants identified by the Provincial Health Officer. In particular, we have no measures of the physical environment in the Valley. It should also be noted that four of the items listed among the predictor

Table 4.14 Independent and dependent variables

Independent (predictors, determinants)
Biological influences
Age, gender, body mass index, ethnic background
Social/economic environment
Education level, Social Support Index, Good Family Index, Stress Index No. of Pets in house, Community Problems Index, No. of people in household, Marital Status, No. of Volunteer meetings, No. religious services
Health behaviours
Smoking frequency, second-hand smoke exposure, drinking frequency drinking amount, eating breakfast, skipping meals, No. of drugs taken sleep lost, vigorous free time activities, physical activities at work
Health services
Personal health care, most people's health care, No. of times seeing doctor, No. of times in hospital, No. of times seeing dentist, distance to doctor, distance to specialist
Dependent
Health variables
8 dimensions of SF-36
Physical Health Index
Mental Health Index
General Health Single Item
No. of Good Health Days in the past 30
No. of Good Health Days Physically in the past 30
No. of Good Health Days Mentally in the past 30
Overall quality of life variables
Happiness
Satisfaction with life as a whole
Satisfaction with quality of life
Satisfaction with standard of living
Subjective Well-Being Index

variables in Table 4.14 are most likely consequences rather than antecedents of ill health, namely, number of over-the-counter or prescription drugs taken, number of visits to doctors and dentists, and number of times in hospital.

Before we undertook any regression analyses to examine the relative impact of our potential predictors on our dependent variables, we looked at several correlations with an aim to eliminating variables that had little or no significant relation to our primary dependent variables. Because measured bivariate relationships are often influenced by other variables that are not explicitly included in the correlation, a correlation coefficient often provides a maximum measure of the shared variance between two variables. Table 4.15 lists the Pearson Product Moment Correlations that are statistically significant at the 0.05 level or better for 19 variables, including all of the primary dependent variables. Reading from left to right across the top row and from top to bottom down the first column, we have correlation coefficients for the 8 dimensions of SF-36. Ignoring self-correlations, there were 28 unique others to examine, 9 of which were not significant. We were surprised to find five negative correlations and looked very hard to find some anomaly in our coding or in the raw data, without success. The vitality dimension was negatively correlated with

Table 4.15 Correlations among dependent variables, significant $p \leq 0.05$[a]

	PF	RP	BP	GH	Vt	SF	RE	MH	He	GHD	HDP	HDM	Hap	LS	SQL	SSL	SWB	PHI	MHI
PF	1.00																		
RP	0.57	1.00																	
BP	0.31	0.40	1.00																
GH	0.13	0.10	ns	1.00															
Vt	−0.13	−0.13	−0.08	ns	1.00														
SF	ns	−0.12	ns	ns	0.08	1.00													
RE	0.33	0.47	0.19	0.13	ns	−0.13	1.00												
MH	ns	0.12	ns	0.09	0.31	ns	0.22	1.00											
He	0.48	0.53	0.28	0.33	−0.11	−0.10	0.38	0.12	1.00										
GHD	0.37	0.59	0.35	ns	ns	ns	0.54	0.17	0.53	1.00									
HDP	0.48	0.63	0.39	ns	−0.08	−0.09	0.36	0.09	0.53	0.85	1.00								
HDM	0.20	0.36	0.23	0.09	ns	ns	0.58	0.25	0.39	0.75	0.44	1.00							
Hap	0.24	0.26	0.19	0.11	ns	ns	0.39	0.11	0.30	0.39	0.24	0.46	1.00						
LS	0.11	0.23	0.13	ns	ns	ns	0.36	0.10	0.29	0.39	0.18	0.49	0.60	1.00					
SQL	0.17	0.27	0.20	0.11	ns	ns	0.33	0.09	0.34	0.40	0.28	0.48	0.61	0.65	1.00				
SSL	0.11	0.24	0.14	0.10	ns	ns	0.30	0.12	0.28	0.31	0.19	0.35	0.48	0.59	0.64	1.00			
SWB	0.21	0.29	0.19	0.14	ns	ns	0.39	0.13	0.36	0.41	0.25	0.50	0.77	0.83	0.85	0.80	1.00		
PHI	0.78	0.91	0.65	0.10	−0.13	−0.10	0.45	0.11	0.55	0.59	0.64	0.36	0.29	0.22	0.28	0.23	0.31	1.00	
MHI	0.31	0.42	0.18	0.15	0.08	0.14	0.94	0.45	0.35	0.51	0.33	0.59	0.38	0.35	0.31	0.28	0.39	0.42	1.00

[a]*PF* Physical Functioning, *RP* Role Physical, *BP* Bodily Pain, *GH* General Health (Index), *V* Vitality, *SF* Social Functioning, *RE* Role Emotional, *MH* Mental Health, *He* Single Item General Health, *GHD* #Good Health Days in past 30, *HDP* Good Health Days Physically, *HDM* Good Health Days Mentally, *Hap* Happiness, *LS* Life Satisfaction, *SQL* Satisfaction with quality of life, *SSL* Satisfaction with standard of living, *SWB* Subjective Well-Being Index, *PHI* SF-36 Physical Health Index, *MHI* SF-36 Mental Health Index

physical functioning and role physical ($r = -0.13$ each) and Bodily Pain ($r = -0.08$), Social functioning was negatively correlated with role physical ($r = -0.12$) and with role emotional ($r = -0.13$). The three dimensions most closely associated were physical functioning and role physical ($r = 0.57$), and role physical with role emotional ($r = 0.47$) and bodily pain ($r = 0.40$).

Each of the eight dimensions of SF-36 was significantly correlated with our single item measure of general health (He in the exhibit), and two of the correlations were negative, namely, vitality ($r = -0.11$) and social functioning ($r = -0.10$). Role physical had the strongest positive correlation with general health ($r = 0.53$). Five of the eight dimensions were correlated with the number of good health days, with role physical ($r = 0.59$) and role emotional ($r = 0.54$) having the strongest relationships. Seven of the eight dimensions were correlated with Good physical health days, with role physical having the strongest association ($r = 0.63$). Vitality and social functioning were negatively related to good physical health days at $r = -0.08$ and -0.09, respectively. Six of the eight dimensions were positively correlated with good mental health days, with role emotional having the strongest association ($r = 0.58$).

Happiness was positively but moderately associated with six of the eight dimensions, with role emotional leading the pack at $r = 0.39$. Life satisfaction had 5 significant positive relations out of the 8 possible, and for each dimension, the relation was weaker than it was for happiness, e.g., physical functioning was correlated with happiness and life satisfaction at $r = 0.24$ and 0.11, respectively. Satisfaction with the overall quality of life was positively correlated with the same 6 SF-36 dimensions that were positively correlated with happiness, with some stronger and some weaker correlations. Role emotional had the strongest correlation with satisfaction with the overall quality of life at a modest $r = 0.33$. Satisfaction with one's standard of living also had six positive correlations, all very similar to those of life satisfaction, although the strongest relationship was only $r = 0.30$, for role emotional. Rolling our four global quality of life variables together into our index of subjective well-being, we found six SF-36 dimensions positively correlated with it, all fairly modest. The strongest association was with role emotional at $r = 0.39$.

Following up the suggestion of Ware et al. (1993) to use the mean of the scores for physical functioning, role physical and bodily pain as a Physical Health Index, we correlated these index scores with the eight dimensions of SF-36. The second last row of Table 4.15 shows that six of the eight dimensions were positively associated with this index, and its component role physical had a very robust relationship of $r = 0.91$ with it. Vitality and social functioning were negatively correlated with the index at $r = -0.13$ and -0.10, respectively. A Mental Health Index was formed by calculating the mean of social functioning, role emotional and mental health scores, and it was found to be positively associated with all 8 dimensions, especially strongly with its component role emotional at $r = 0.94$. The two general indexes for physical and mental health were correlated at $r = 0.42$.

Examining the column under the single item general health measure (He), one finds the Physical Health Index of SF-36 had the strongest relationship with it at

$r = 0.55$. Under good health days, apart from its two components (good physical and good mental health days), the physical health Index of SF-36 had the strongest relationship at $r = 0.59$. The correlation between the Physical Health Index and Good physical health days is even stronger, at $r = 0.64$. Good mental health days is most closely associated with the Mental Health Index from SF-36, at $r = 0.59$. Happiness is most closely associated with life satisfaction and satisfaction with the overall quality of life, at $r = 0.60$ and $r = 0.61$, respectively, apart from the Index of subjective Well-Being, of which it is a component. Satisfaction with the overall quality of life is correlated with life satisfaction at $r = 0.65$ and with satisfaction with one's standard of living at $r = 0.64$. The latter has a very strong relation to the Index of Subjective Well-Being at $r = 0.80$, of which it is a component. Finally, Subjective Well-Being is moderately associated with the Physical Health and Mental Health Indexes at $r = 0.31$ and $r = 0.39$, respectively.

Bivariate Relationships: Determinants and Dependent Variables

Table 4.16 gives the results of correlating 31 potential health determinants from Table 4.14 with the single item measure of general health (He), the SF-36 indexes of physical health (PHI) and mental health (MHI), good health days (GHD), happiness (Hap), life satisfaction (LS) and the Subjective Well-Being Index (SWB). Six potential determinants had no statistically significant association ($p \leq 0.05$) with any of the seven dependent variables, namely, the Index of Community Problems, number of people (adults, children and total) in a household, gender, distance to a specialist and number of visits to a dentist. So, these are omitted from the table. As indicated earlier, the causal arrows most likely run from numbers of over-the-counter or prescription drugs and visits to doctors and hospitals in reverse order from the other items listed as predictors in Table 4.16, although for some of the latter items (e.g., number of hours of sleep per night) the causal arrows probably run in both directions.

The diverse relationships between the determinants and health versus broader quality of life measures are thought-provoking. Some determinants are significantly related to respondents' health and overall quality of life in the same directions and in similar amounts, while others vary in directions and amounts. For example, age is negatively related to general health and Physical Health, but positively related to life satisfaction. Since the squared correlation coefficient is a measure of the amount of variation explained by either variable in the pair (i.e., the coefficient of determination), and since it is relatively easy to get statistical significance in a sample of nearly 700 people, one cannot be very impressed to find that 1% of the variation in life satisfaction is determined by respondents' age. After all, that leaves 99% determined by something else. As a matter of fact,

Table 4.16 Correlations among selected health determinants and dependent variables, significant $p \leq 0.05$

	He	PHI	MHI	GHD	Hap	LS	SWB
Age	−0.20	−0.34	ns	ns	ns	0.12	ns
Aboriginal descent/not	0.26	0.12	0.15	0.13	ns	ns	0.11
Body mass index	−0.26	−0.14	−0.10	−0.10	ns	ns	ns
Education level	0.30	0.22	0.10	0.10	ns	ns	ns
Social Support Index	0.17	0.18	0.21	0.22	0.33	0.30	0.33
Good Family Index	0.19	0.19	0.21	0.21	0.34	0.39	0.40
Stress Index	ns	0.08	−0.14	−0.14	−0.10	−0.19	−0.13
No. of pets at home	ns	ns	−0.09	−0.09	−0.11	−0.11	−0.14
No. of voluntary meetings	0.22	0.17	0.20	0.25	0.17	ns	0.20
No. of religious services	−0.09	−0.11	ns	ns	0.09	0.08	ns
Smoking frequency	−0.13	ns	−0.09	−0.18	−0.13	−0.11	−0.14
Drinking frequency	0.15	0.17	ns	ns	ns	ns	ns
Drinking amount	ns	0.12	ns	ns	−0.13	−0.16	−0.12
Skipping meals	−0.17	−0.09	−0.14	−0.19	−0.16	−0.17	− 0.13
Eating breakfast	ns	ns	0.09	0.12	0.10	0.16	0.16
No. of drugs taken per week	−0.30	−0.35	−0.27	−0.32	−0.22	−0.19	−0.21
Hours of sleep per night	0.25	0.20	0.15	0.25	0.14	0.18	0.20
Vigorous leisure activities	0.21	0.20	ns	0.13	ns	ns	ns
Rating your health care	0.19	ns	0.15	0.18	0.19	0.27	0.28
Rating most people's H.C.	0.18	0.09	0.19	0.22	0.20	0.26	0.26
No. of times seeing doctor	−0.31	−0.29	−0.31	−0.32	−0.16	−0.13	−0.16
No. of times in hospital this year	−0.12	−0.12	−0.11	−0.10	ns	ns	ns
Distance to GP	ns	−0.10	−0.14	−0.10	−0.13	−0.09	−0.12

> Stock et al. (1983) undertook the most extensive review of research on the relation between age and subjective well-being, and concluded on the basis of 221 estimates from 119 different American sources published before 1980 that 'the amount of variance in SWB explained by age…never rises above 1%' (p. 297) (Michalos 1991, p. 60).

On the other hand, it is not unimportant to find that 12% of the variation in Physical Health Index scores is determined by age.

The entry listed as 'aboriginal descent/not' in Table 4.16 refers to a dichotomous variable constructed by putting Nuxalk and other people of aboriginal descent into one class and everyone else into another. Positive correlations, then, indicate that not being of aboriginal descent contributes to better health and quality of life. As the row scores show, five of the seven dependent variables are positively associated with ethnic background thus defined. We found no statistically significant relationship between the latter variable and happiness or life satisfaction, contrary to what we found and reported for a Prince George sample in Michalos and Zumbo (2001).

Education is positively related to the four health measures but not to the quality of life measures. The Social Support Index and the Good Family Index are positively related to all seven dependent variables, with the latter reaching $r = 0.39$ for life satisfaction and $r = 0.40$ for subjective well-being. The Stress Index was not significantly related to general health, but it was positively related to the Physical Health Index and negatively related to the other five dependent variables. We found no significant relationships between any of the seven dependent variables and respondents' numbers of pet dogs, cats, fish or birds, but respondents' total number of pets was negatively related to five of the seven dependent variables. Only general health and the Physical Health Index were not significantly associated with respondents' total number of pets.

There was a positive correlation between six of the seven dependent variables and the frequency with which respondents participated in activities sponsored by voluntary associations; life satisfaction was the only unaffected dependent variable. Frequency of attending religious services was modestly negatively associated with general health and the Physical Health Index, but positively associated with happiness and life satisfaction. Frequency of smoking was negatively associated with every dependent variable except the Physical Health Index. Frequency of drinking was positively associated with general health and the Physical Health Index, but nothing else. However, the amount of drinking at each sitting was negatively associated with the three quality of life measures, and positively associated with the Physical Health Index.

Frequency of skipping meals was negatively associated with all seven dependent variables, and frequency of eating breakfast was positively associated with five of the seven. Frequency of eating breakfast was unrelated to general health and the Physical Health Index. There was a negative association between the total number of drugs respondents took per week and each of the seven dependent variables. In fact, although the exact numbers were omitted from Table 4.16, there was a negative association between each of the seven dependent variables and the number of sleeping pills taken per week, and also the number of pain killers taken per week. The number of tranquilizers taken per week was negatively associated with the four health measures and happiness, while the number of stimulants taken per week was negatively associated with the three quality of life measures and good health days.

Respondents' hours of sleep per night were positively associated with all seven dependent variables. Frequency of vigorous leisure activities was positively correlated with general health, good health days and the Physical Health Index, but to nothing else. Respondents' ratings of their own health care were positively associated with six of the seven dependent variables, everything but the Physical Health Index. Surprisingly, respondents' ratings of most people's health care, apart from their own, were positively associated with all seven dependent variables. As one might have expected, number of times respondents saw a doctor in the past year were negatively related to all seven dependent variables, with the health-related associations all stronger than the quality of life associations. Number of times respondents were in hospitals in the past year were negatively associated with the health-related variables but had no significant relationships to the quality of life variables. Respondents' distance to their family doctors was negatively associated with every dependent variable except general health.

Explaining Health and the Quality of Life: Multivariate Relationships

Tables 4.17, 4.18, 4.19, 4.20, 4.21, 4.22 and 4.23 summarize results of systematically regressing each of our seven dependent variables (i.e., the single item general health, SF-36 Physical Health Index, SF-36 Mental Health Index, good health days, happiness, life satisfaction and Subjective Well-Being Index) on the set of 31 health determinants listed in Table 4.14 as well as measures of satisfaction in 13 domains of life (i.e., satisfaction with one's house, neighbourhood, family relations, living partner, job, friendships, religion, financial security, recreation activities, self-esteem, personal safety and three levels of government (using the mean of the 3)). Of all the potential predictors, the only ones that appear in any particular exhibit are those that had at least one significant relationship to the dependent variable considered in that exhibit. The strategy of the analysis for each dependent variable was the same and the structure of each exhibit is the same. Each of the seven numerical columns gives results of applying stepwise regression with mean substitution for missing values using the following sets of potential determinants: biological, social/economic, health behaviour, health services, all health variables, domain satisfaction (without health satisfaction), and all significant variables from the previous six regressions. We are interested in measuring:

1. the total explanatory power (R^2) of each set of determinants for each dependent variable;
2. the relative explanatory power (β value) of each determinant in the context of each set of predictors for each dependent variable;
3. the similarities and differences obtained in all the explanations of the four global measures of health status and the three global measures of overall quality of life.

We will comment on the results of each exhibit in turn and then provide some overview remarks in the next section.

Table 4.17 (column 2) shows that three biological determinants explain 14% of the variation in the scores of the single item measure of general health. In the context of the set of biological determinants employed, respondents' ethnic background (being non-aboriginal) was most influential ($\beta = 0.25$). Five social/economic determinants could also account for 14% of the variance in general health scores (column 3), with respondents' highest levels of education most influential ($\beta = 0.27$). Five health behaviours accounted for 13% of the variance in general health scores (column 4), with respondents' number of hours of sleep per

Table 4.17 Explaining general health by health determinants and domain satisfaction, $N = 686$

	Biological determinants	Social/economic determinants	Health behaviour determinants	Health services determinants	All health determinants	Domain sat. determinants	All significant determinants
% Variance expl.	14	14	13	3	24	12	29
Predictors	β	β	β	β	β	β	β
BMI	−0.17	a	a	a	−0.13	a	−0.13
Age	−0.20	a	a	a	−0.14	a	−0.20
Aboriginal/not	0.25	a	a	a	0.15	a	0.14
Education	a	0.27	a	a	0.13	a	0.16
No. of vol. Meetings	a	0.11	a	a	b	a	b
Good Family Index	a	0.14	a	a	0.12	a	0.07
No. of relig. meetings	a	−0.09	a	a	b	a	b
Social Support Ind.	a	0.11	a	a	0.07	a	b
Vigor. Leisure	a	a	0.15	a	0.08	a	b
Hours sleep/night	a	a	0.19	a	0.14	a	0.11
2nd home smoke exp.	a	a	−0.14	a	−0.12	a	−0.11
Drink frequency	a	a	0.14	a	b	a	b
Skipping meals	a	a	−0.12	a	−0.08	a	b

(continued)

Table 4.17 (continued)

	Biological determinants	Social/economic determinants	Health behaviour determinants	Health services determinants	All health determinants	Domain sat. determinants	All significant determinants
Own health care	a	a	a	0.19	b	a	b
Financial sec. sat.	a	a	a	a	a	0.10	b
Government sat.	a	a	a	a	a	−0.08	b
Recreation sat.	a	a	a	a	a	0.20	0.15
Self-esteem sat.	a	a	a	a	a	0.15	0.18

[a]Not in equation, [b]significance level too low to enter equation

Table 4.18 Explaining SF-36 Physical Health Index by health determinants and domain satisfaction, $N = 686$

	Biological determinants	Social/economic determinants	Health behaviour determinants	Health services determinants	All health determinants	Domain sat. determinants	All significant determinants
% Variance expl.	14	11	8	1	20	7	23
Predictors	β	β	β	β	β	β	β
Age	−0.36	a	a	a	−0.28	a	−0.34
Aboriginal/not	0.17	a	a	a	0.08	a	b
Education	a	0.18	a	a	0.09	a	0.13
Good Family Index	a	0.14	a	a	0.13	a	b
Stress Index	a	0.09	a	a	b	a	b
Social Support Ind.	a	0.13	a	a	0.08	a	b
No. of vol. meetings	a	0.07	a	a	b	a	b
No. of relig. meetings	a	−0.10	a	a	b	a	b
Vigor. Leisure	a	a	0.15	a	0.07	a	b
Hours sleep/night	a	a	0.17	a	0.12	a	0.08
Drink frequency	a	a	0.15	a	0.07	a	0.09
Distance to GP	a	a	a	−0.09	b	a	b
Recreation sat.	a	a	a	a	a	0.18	0.12

(continued)

Table 4.18 (continued)

	Biological determinants	Social/economic determinants	Health behaviour determinants	Health services determinants	All health determinants	Domain sat. determinants	All significant determinants
Government sat.	a	a	a	a	a	−0.09	b
Religion sat.	a	a	a	a	a	−0.12	b
Family sat.	a	a	a	a	a	0.08	0.10
Self-esteem sat.	a	a	a	a	a	0.13	0.13

[a]Not in equation, [b]significance level too low to enter equation

Table 4.19 Explaining SF-36 Mental Health Index by health determinants and domain satisfaction, $N = 686$

	Biological determinants	Social/economic determinants	Health behaviour determinants	Health services determinants	All health determinants	Domain sat. determinants	All significant determinants
% Variance expl.	2	9	4	4	12	15	20
Predictors	β	β	β	β	β	β	β
Aboriginal/not	0.15	a	a	a	0.10	a	b
No. of vol. meetings	a	0.13	a	a	0.09	a	0.12
No. of relig. meetings	a	−0.08	a	a	b	a	−0.10
Good Family Index	a	0.15	a	a	0.14	a	b
Stress Index	a	−0.13	a	a	−0.10	a	b
Social Support Ind.	a	0.15	a	a	0.15	a	0.09
Hours sleep/night	a	a	0.12	a	0.10	a	b
2nd home smoke exp.	a	a	−0.10	a	−0.11	a	−0.14
2nd outside smoke exp.	a	a	0.08	a	0.08	a	0.10
Skipping meals	a	a	−0.11	a	b	a	b
Most people's health C	a	a	a	0.17	b	a	0.08
Distance to GP	a	a	a	−0.10	−0.12	a	b

(continued)

Table 4.19 (continued)

	Biological determinants	Social/economic determinants	Health behaviour determinants	Health services determinants	All health determinants	Domain sat. determinants	All significant determinants
Recreation sat.	a	a	a	a	a	0.08	b
Living partner sat	a	a	a	a	a	0.10	0.08
Self-esteem sat.	a	a	a	a	a	0.30	0.32

[a]Not in equation, [b]significance level too low to enter equation

Table 4.20 Explaining good health days by health determinants and domain satisfaction, $N = 686$

	Biological determinants	Social/economic determinants	Health behaviour determinants	Health services determinants	All health determinants	Domain sat. determinants	All significant determinants
% Variance expl.	1	9	10	4	16	15	21
Predictors	β	β	β	β	β	β	β
Aboriginal/not	0.13	a	a	a	b	a	b
No. of vol. meetings	a	0.16	a	a	0.13	a	0.13
Good Family Index	a	0.13	a	a	0.12	a	b
Stress Index	a	−0.12	a	a	−0.07	a	b
Social Support Ind.	a	0.16	a	a	0.13	a	0.10
Vigor. Leisure	a	a	0.09	a	0.08	a	b
Hours sleep/night	a	a	0.20	a	0.18	a	0.16
Skipping meals	a	a	−0.12	a	−0.08	a	b
Smoking freq.	a	a	−0.14	a	−0.12	a	−0.11
Most people's H.C.	a	a	a	0.21	b	a	b
Recreation sat.	a	a	a	a	a	0.20	0.14
Self-esteem sat.	a	a	a	a	a	0.25	0.22

[a]Not in equation, [b]significance level too low to enter equation

Table 4.21 Explaining happiness by health determinants and domain satisfaction, $N = 686$

	Biological determinants	Social/economic determinants	Health behaviour determinants	Health services determinants	All health determinants	Domain sat. determinants	All significant determinants
% Variance expl.	0	18	5	5	20	36	39
Predictors	β	β	β	β	β	β	β
No. of relig. meetings	a	0.09	a	a	b	a	b
Good Family Index	a	0.26	a	a	0.24	a	0.11
Social Support Ind.	a	0.26	a	a	0.26	a	0.12
Hours sleep/night	a	a	0.12	a	0.10	a	b
Smoking freq.	a	a	−0.08	a	−0.09	a	−0.06
Skipping meals	a	a	−0.11	a	b	a	b
Amount drinking	a	a	−0.10	a	−0.11	a	b
Most people's H.C.	a	a	a	0.19	b	a	b
Distance to GP	a	a	a	−0.09	b	a	b
Living Partner sat.	a	a	a	a	a	0.16	0.12
Friendships sat.	a	a	a	a	a	0.20	0.16

(continued)

Table 4.21 (continued)

	Biological determinants	Social/economic determinants	Health behaviour determinants	Health services determinants	All health determinants	Domain sat. determinants	All significant determinants
Recreation sat.	a	a	a	a	a	0.09	0.08
Self-esteem sat.	a	a	a	a	a	0.34	0.32

[a]Not in equation, [b]significance level too low to enter equation

Table 4.22 Explaining life satisfaction by health determinants and domain satisfaction, $N = 686$

	Biological determinants	Social/economic determinants	Health behaviour determinants	Health services determinants	All health determinants	Domain sat. determinants	All significant determinants
% Variance expl.	2	20	7	7	24	61	62
Predictors	β	β	β	β	β	β	β
Age	0.13	a	a	a	b	a	b
BMI	−0.09	a	a	a	b	a	b
Good Family Index	a	0.30	a	a	0.30	a	0.08
Social Support Ind.	a	0.21	a	a	0.20	a	b
Stress Index	a	−0.15	a	a	−0.10	a	b
Education	a	−0.09	a	a	−0.10	a	b
Hours sleep/night	a	a	0.15	a	0.13	a	0.05
Skipping meals	a	a	−0.12	a	b	a	b
Eating breakfast	a	a	0.09	a	0.09	a	b
Amount drinking	a	a	−0.13	a	−0.13	a	b
2nd outside smoke exp.	a	a	−0.09	a	b	a	b
Own health care	a	a	a	0.26	b	a	b
Living partner sat.	a	a	a	a	a	0.16	0.17

(continued)

Table 4.22 (continued)

	Biological determinants	Social/economic determinants	Health behaviour determinants	Health services determinants	All health determinants	Domain sat. determinants	All significant determinants
Friendships sat.	a	a	a	a	a	0.29	0.29
Job sat.	a	a	a	a	a	0.09	0.09
Financial sec. sat.	a	a	a	a	a	0.09	0.08
Religion sat.	a	a	a	a	a	0.06	0.06
Family sat.	a	a	a	a	a	0.09	b
Self-esteem sat.	a	a	a	a	a	0.34	0.34

[a]Not in equation, [b]significance level too low to enter equation

Table 4.23 Explaining Subjective Well-Being Index by health determinants and domain satisfaction, $N = 686$

	Biological determinants	Social/economic determinants	Health behaviour determinants	Health services determinants	All health determinants	Domain sat. determinants	All significant determinants
% Variance expl.	1	22	7	7	26	59	61
Predictors	β	β	β	β	β	β	β
Aboriginal/not	0.11	a	a	a	b	a	b
Good Family Index	a	0.31	a	a	0.31	a	0.10
Social Support Ind.	a	0.22	a	a	0.22	a	0.06
Stress Index	a	−0.08	a	a	b	a	0.07
No. of vol. meetings	a	0.10	a	a	0.08	a	0.06
No. of pets in the house	a	−0.08	a	a	−0.08	a	b
Hours sleep/night	a	a	0.19	a	0.15	a	0.08
Eating breakfast	a	a	0.10	a	0.10	a	b
2nd home smoke exp.	a	a	−0.09	a	b	a	b
Amount drinking	a	a	−0.08	a	−0.09	a	b
Own health care	a	a	a	0.28	b	a	b
Living Partner sat.	a	a	a	a	a	0.11	0.12

(continued)

Table 4.23 (continued)

	Biological determinants	Social/economic determinants	Health behaviour determinants	Health services determinants	All health determinants	Domain sat. determinants	All significant determinants
Friendships sat.	a	a	a	a	a	0.23	0.22
Job sat.	a	a	a	a	a	0.07	0.08
Recreation sat.	a	a	a	a	a	0.06	b
Safety near home sat.	a	a	a	a	a	0.07	0.07
Financial security sat.	a	a	a	a	a	0.18	0.18
Family sat.	a	a	a	a	a	0.08	b
Self-esteem sat.	a	a	a	a	a	0.32	0.34

[a]Not in equation, [b]significance level too low to enter equation

night most influential ($\beta = 0.19$). One health services determinant explained 3% of the variance in general health scores (column 5), namely, respondents' ratings of their own health care ($\beta = 0.19$). Using the 14 statistically significant health determinants together, we found a narrower set of 10 significant predictors could account for 24% of the variance in general health scores. Explanatory power is so evenly spread among the 10 predictors in this narrower set that it is difficult to identify a dominant one. However, the most influential three are ethnic (non-aboriginal) background ($\beta = 0.15$), age ($\beta = -0.14$) and hours of sleep per night ($\beta = 0.14$). Levels of satisfaction in four of the 13 distinct domains of life explained 12% of the variance in general health scores (column 6), with respondents' satisfaction with their recreation activities most influential ($\beta = 0.20$). Finally, using all the significant health and domain satisfaction determinants together, we were able to explain 29% of the variation in general health scores (column 7). In that regression, nine predictors remained statistically significant, with age ($\beta = -0.20$) and satisfaction with one's own self-esteem ($\beta = 0.18$) most influential.

Table 4.18 (column 2) shows that two biological determinants explain 14% of the variation in the scores of the SF-36 Physical Health Index. In the context of the set of biological determinants employed, respondents' age was most influential ($\beta = -0.36$). Six social/economic determinants could account for 11% of the variance in SF-36 Physical Health Index scores (column 3), with respondents' highest levels of education most influential ($\beta = 0.18$). Three health behaviours accounted for 8% of the variance in SF-36 Physical Health Index scores (column 4), with respondents' number of hours of sleep per night most influential ($\beta = 0.17$). One health services determinant explained 1% of the variance in SF-36 Physical Health Index scores (column 5), i.e., the distance respondents had to travel to get routine health care ($\beta = -0.09$). Using the 12 statistically significant health determinants together, we found a narrower set of eight significant predictors accounted for 20% of the variance in SF-36 Physical Health Index scores, with respondents' age dominating the set ($\beta = -0.28$). Levels of satisfaction in five of the 13 distinct domains of life explained 7% of the variance in SF-36 Physical Health Index scores (column 6), with respondents' satisfaction with their recreation activities most influential ($\beta = 0.18$). Finally, using all the significant health and domain satisfaction determinants together, we were able to explain 23% of the variation in SF-36 Physical Health Index scores (column 7). In that regression, seven predictors remained statistically significant, with age ($\beta = -0.34$) most influential, followed by respondents' highest levels of education and satisfaction with their own self-esteem ($\beta = 0.13$ for each variable).

Table 4.19 (column 2) shows that one biological determinant explained 2% of the variation in the scores of the SF-36 Mental Health Index, i.e., respondents' (non-aboriginal) ethnic background ($\beta = 0.15$). Five social/economic determinants could account for 9% of the variance in SF-36 Mental Health Index scores (column 3), with respondents' Good Family and Social Support Indexes most influential ($\beta = 0.15$ for each index). Four health behaviours accounted for 4% of the variance in SF-36 Mental Health Index scores (column 4), with respondents' number of hours of sleep per night most influential (β = 0.12), followed closely by the frequency with which they skip meals (β = −0.11). Two health services determinants also explained 4% of the variance in SF-36 Mental Health Index scores (column 5), with respondents' ratings of the health care most people in the community get being most influential (β = 0.17). Using the 12 statistically significant health determinants together, we found a narrower set of nine significant predictors accounted for 12% of the variance in SF-36 Mental Health Index scores, with respondents' Social Support Index (β = 0.15) and Good Family Index (β = 0.14) most influential. Levels of satisfaction in three of the 13 distinct domains of life explained 15% of the variance in SF-36 Mental Health Index scores (column 6), with respondents' satisfaction with their own self-esteem most influential (β = 0.30). Finally, using all the significant health and domain satisfaction determinants together, we were able to explain 20% of the variation in SF-36 Mental Health Index scores (column 7). In that regression, eight predictors remained statistically significant, with respondents' satisfaction with their own self-esteem dominating the lot (β = 0.32).

Table 4.20 (column 2) shows that one biological determinant explained 1% of the variation in good health days scores, i.e., respondents' (non-aboriginal) ethnic background (β = 0.13). Four social/economic determinants could account for 9% of the variance in good health days scores (column 3), with respondents' Social Support Index and frequency of participating in activities sponsored by voluntary associations most influential (β = 0.16 for each predictor). Four health behaviours accounted for 10% of the variance in good health days scores (column 4), with respondents' numbers of hours of sleep per night most influential (β = 0.20). One health services determinant explained 4% of the variance in good health days scores (column 5), i.e., respondents' ratings of the health care most people in the community get (β = 0.21). Using the 10 statistically significant health determinants together, we found a narrower set of eight significant predictors accounted for 16% of the variance in good health days scores, with respondents' number of hours of sleep per night most influential (β = 0.18). Levels of satisfaction in two of the 13 distinct domains of life explained 15% of the variance in good health days scores (column 6), with respondents' satisfaction with their own selfesteem most influential (β = 0.25). Finally, using all the significant health and domain satisfaction determinants together, we were able to explain 21% of the variation in good health days scores (column 7), with respondents' satisfaction with their own self-esteem leading the lot (β = 0.22).

Table 4.21 (column 2) shows that the biological determinants did not explain any of the variation in happiness scores. Three social/economic determinants could account for 18% of the variance in happiness scores (column 3), with respondents' Social Support and Good Family Indexes most influential (β = 0.26 for each predictor). Four health behaviours accounted for 5% of the variance in happiness scores (column 4), with respondents' number of hours of sleep per night most influential (β = 0.12). Two health services determinants also explained 5% of the variance in happiness scores (column 5), with respondents' ratings of the health care most people in the community get being most influential (β = 0.19). Using the nine statistically significant health determinants together, we found a narrower set of five significant predictors accounted for 20% of the variance in happiness scores, with respondents' Social Support Index most influential ($\beta = 0.26$). Levels of satisfaction in four of the 13 distinct domains of life explained 36% of the variance in happiness scores (column 6), with respondents' satisfaction with their own self-esteem most influential ($\beta = 0.34$). Finally, using all the significant health and domain satisfaction determinants together, we were able to explain 39% of the variation in happiness scores (column 7), with respondents' satisfaction with their own self-esteem dominating the lot ($\beta = 0.32$).

Table 4.22 (column 2) shows that two biological determinants explain 2% of the variation in life satisfaction scores, with respondents' age most influential ($\beta = 0.13$). Four social/economic determinants could account for 20% of the variance in life satisfaction scores (column 3), with respondents' Good Family Index most influential ($\beta = 0.30$). Five health behaviours accounted for 7% of the variance in life satisfaction scores (column 4), with respondents' number of hours of sleep per night most influential ($\beta = 0.15$). One health services determinant explained 7% of the variance in life satisfaction scores (column 5), namely, respondents' ratings of their own health care ($\beta = 0.26$). Using the 12 statistically significant health determinants together, we found a narrower set of seven significant predictors accounted for 24% of the variance in life satisfaction scores, with respondents' Good Family Index dominating the set ($\beta = 0.30$). Levels of satisfaction in seven of the 13 distinct domains of life explained 61% of the variance in life satisfaction scores (column 6), with respondents' satisfaction with their own self-esteem most influential ($\beta = 0.34$), followed by satisfaction with their friendships ($\beta = 0.29$). Finally, using all the significant health and domain satisfaction determinants together, we were able to explain 62% of the variation in life satisfaction scores (column 7). In that regression, eight predictors remained statistically significant, again with respondents' satisfaction with their own self-esteem most influential ($\beta = 0.34$), followed by satisfaction with their friendships ($\beta = 0.29$).

Table 4.23 (column 2) shows that one biological determinant explained 1% of the variation in Subjective Well-Being Index scores, with respondents' ethnic (non-aboriginal) background most influential ($\beta = 0.11$). Five social/economic determinants accounted for 22% of the variance in Subjective Well-Being Index scores (column 3), with respondents' Good Family Index most influential ($\beta = 0.31$). Four health behaviours accounted for 7% of the variance in Subjective Well-Being Index scores (column 4), with respondents' number of hours of sleep per night most influential ($\beta = 0.19$). One health services determinant explained 7% of the variance in Subjective WellBeing Index scores (column 5), namely, respondents' ratings of their own health care ($\beta = 0.28$). Using the 11 statistically significant health determinants together, we found a narrower set of seven significant predictors accounted for 26% of the variance in Subjective Well-Being Index scores, with respondents' Good Family Index dominating the set ($\beta = 0.31$). Levels of satisfaction in eight of the 13 distinct domains of life explained 59% of the variance in Subjective Well-Being Index scores (column 6), with respondents' satisfaction with their own selfesteem most influential ($\beta = 0.32$), followed by satisfaction with their friendships ($\beta = 0.23$). Finally, using all the significant health and domain satisfaction determinants together, we were able to explain 61% of the variation in Subjective Well-Being Index scores (column 7). In that regression, 11 predictors remained statistically significant, again with respondents' satisfaction with their own self-esteem most influential ($\beta = 0.34$), followed by satisfaction with their friendships ($\beta = 0.22$).

Overview of Variance Explained and Most Influential Determinants

Table 4.24 lists the percent of variance explained in each of the seven dependent variables by each cluster of health determinants and the cluster of domain satisfaction scores. The four clusters of health determinants explained from 12% (SF-36 Mental Health Index) to 24% (general health) of the variance in the dependent global health variables, and from 20% (happiness) to 26% (Subjective Well-Being Index) of the variance in the dependent global quality of life variables. Adding domain satisfaction scores to the total set of predictors allowed us to explain from 20% (SF-36 Mental Health Index) to 29% (general health) of the variance in the dependent global health variables, and from 39% (happiness) to 62% (life satisfaction) in the dependent global quality of life variables. Thus, the four clusters of health determinants explained from 60 to 87% of the explained variance in the dependent global health variables, but only from 39% (life satisfaction) to 51% (happiness) of the explained variance in the dependent global quality of life variables. Although the health-related determinants may seem to be relatively weak predictors of the dependent global quality of life variables, they are relatively stronger than might have been expected from previous research (e.g., Michalos 2003). One should not forget, of course, that the importance of social support and good family relationships to a good quality of life as well as to good health has been documented in dozens of studies over the past 30 years (Michalos 1986, 1991). Thus, by including measures of social support and good family relationships in our

Table 4.24 Percent of variance explained by health determinants and domain satisfaction

	Gen. health	SF-36 PHI	SF-36 MHI	GHD	Happiness	Life satisf.	SWB
Bio. det.	14	14	2	1	0	2	1
Soc/econ. D	14	11	9	9	18	20	22
Health beh.	13	8	4	10	5	7	7
Health serv. D	3	1	4	4	5	7	7
All health D	24	20	12	16	20	24	26
Domain sat. D	12	7	15	15	36	61	59
All sig. det	29	23	20	21	39	62	61
Health/all	0.83	0.87	0.60	0.76	0.51	0.39	0.43

Table 4.25 Most influential predictors

	Gen.H.	PHI	MHI	GHD	Hap	Life Sat	SWB
Biol. D	Eth[a]	Age	Eth	Eth	0	Age	Eth
Soc/E D	Ed	Ed	GF/SS	SS/V	GF/SS	GF	GF
Health B	Sleep	Sleep	Sleep	Sleep	Sleep	Sleep	Sleep
Health S	Own HC	Dist GP	Most HC	Most HC	Most HC	Own HC	Own HC
All H	Eth	Age	SS	Sleep	SS	GF	GF
Dom Sat	Rec. Sat	Rec. Sat	SE	SE	SE	SE	SE
All Det	SE	Age	SE	SE	SE	SE	SE

[a]*Eth* ethnic background, *0* no significant impact, *Ed* highest level of education, *GF* Good Family Index, *SS* Social Support Index, *V* number of volunteer activities, Own *HC* rating of respondents' own health care, Most *HC* rating of most people's health care, Dist *GP* distance traveled to get routine health care, *Rec. Sat* satisfaction with one's recreation activities, *SE* satisfaction with one's own self-esteem

set of health determinants, we practically guaranteed that the latter would be relatively strongly predictive of dependent global quality of life.

Table 4.25 lists the most influential predictors of each of the seven dependent variables from each cluster of health determinants and the cluster of domain satisfaction scores. Inspection of the b values in Tables 4.17, 4.18, 4.19, 4.20, 4.21, 4.22 and 4.23 reveals several cases in which there are tied scores in some clusters and often a single percentage point difference among several other scores. So, one should read the entries in Table 4.25 with caution and not make too much out of them, although they are thought-provoking. Given four dependent global health variables and exactly the same initial array of potential health determinants, one might have expected greater similarity in the entries in Table 4.25, not to mention Tables 4.17, 4.18, 4.19 and 4.20. Even granting that the two SF-36 Indexes are not quite global health indicators, one might have expected greater similarity of results. Given three dependent global quality of life variables and exactly the same initial array of potential predictors, one might also have expected greater similarity of results, although there is more similarity in the entries for those dependent variables than for the dependent health variables in Table 4.25 as well as in Tables 4.21, 4.22 and 4.23.

Conclusion

The aim of this investigation was to obtain some baseline selfreported data on the health status and overall quality of life of a sample of residents of the Bella Coola Valley of British Columbia aged 17 years or older, and to measure the impact of a set of designated health determinants on their health and quality of life. In the period from August to November 2001, a variety of procedures were used to ensure that all eligible residents of the Valley received a copy of our questionnaire.

Questionnaires were mailed out to each household, and distributed from the local medical clinic and central shopping areas. By June, 687 useable questionnaires were obtained for our working dataset. The average age of respondents was 48 (range 17–90), 57% were female and 36% had an aboriginal or metis ethnic background.

Health status was measured by SF-36 and the U.S. Centres for Disease Control healthy days items. Thirty-one items were used to measure the Provincial Health Officer's designated determinants of health in four clusters, namely, biological, social and economic, health behaviours and health services determinants. Quality of life was measured by satisfaction levels in 13 specific domains of life (e.g., family, financial security), four global items (e.g., happiness, life satisfaction) and one global Subjective Well-Being Index. Besides obtaining baseline figures on all our measures for the Valley, we made some comparisons among our figures and those from other areas, e.g., Prince George, BC. Most of the measures indicated that the health status and quality of life of Bella Coola Valley residents were lower than those of Prince George residents.

For the sample as a whole, SF-36 scores on the eight dimensions ran from 82.3 (physical functioning) to 50.0 (social functioning), with a mean of 62.7. The average physical health score was higher than the average mental health score for the whole group, and for males and females separately, although women generally had higher physical health scores and lower mental health scores than men. Residents in the Valley averaged 6.5 days in the past 30 in which their health was physically not good, 5.5 days when it was mentally not good and 4.1 days when their health limited their usual daily activities. Eleven percent of respondents described their general health as "excellent" and another 27% said it was "very good". Sixty-seven percent reported that they never smoked and 33.8% said they never drank alcoholic beverages. On a 5-point scale from 1 = poor to 5 = excellent, the mean respondent rating for their own and most people's health care services was 3.4 and 3.3, respectively. Sixty percent said they had a family physician and on average respondents had seen a physician 5.6 times in the past year.

On a 7-point scale from 1 = very dissatisfied to 7 = very satisfied, respondents had average life satisfaction and satisfaction with the overall quality of life scores of 5.5. For specific domains of life, the lowest mean level of satisfaction was reported for federal and provincial government officials (3.3) and the highest was reported for living partners and personal safety around home (5.8).

Regarding bivariate relations, each of the eight dimensions of SF-36 was significantly correlated with a single item measure of general health, and 5 of the 8 were significantly correlated with the number of good health days. Happiness and the Subjective Well-Being Index were positively but moderately correlated with 6 of the 8 dimensions, and life satisfaction was positively correlated with 5. Age was negatively related to general health, but positively related to life satisfaction. Not being of aboriginal descent was positively related to all of the four global health indicators and to the Subjective Well-Being Index. Education was positively related to the four global health measures but not to the three global quality of life measures. The Social Support and Good Family Indexes were positively related to all seven global measures. There was a positive correlation between six of the seven global measures and the frequency with which respondents participated in activities sponsored by voluntary organizations. Frequency of smoking was negatively associated with every global dependent variable except the Physical Health Index. Frequency of skipping meals was negatively associated and average hours of sleep per night was positively associated with all seven global measures.

Turning to multivariate relationships, the four clusters of health determinants explained from 12% (SF-36 Mental Health Index) to 24% (general health) of the variance in the dependent global health variables, and from 20% (happiness) to 26% (Subjective Well-Being Index) of the variance in the dependent global quality of life variables. Adding domain satisfaction scores to the total set of predictors allowed us to explain from 20% (SF-36 Mental Health Index) to 29% (general health) of the variance in the dependent global health variables, and from 39% (happiness) to 62% (life satisfaction) in the dependent global quality of life variables. By including measures of social support and good family relationships in our set of health determinants, we practically guaranteed that the latter would be relatively strongly predictive of dependent global quality of life.

Acknowledgements We would like to thank Julie Orlando, Dieter Ayers, Carol Thommasen, Andy Bottomley, Bill Tallio, Steve Murray and Rhonda Elliott for their help with various parts of this research.

References

CDC. (2000, November). *Centers for disease control and prevention, measuring healthy days.* Atlanta, Georgia.

FPTC. (1999). *Federal, provincial and territorial advisory committee on population health.* Statistical Report on the health of Canadians, statistics Canada, Ottawa, Cat. #82–570-X1E. Retrieved March, 2000, http://www.statcan.ca.

Garratt, A. M., Ruta, D. A., Abdullha, M. I., Buckingham, J. K., & Russell, I. T. (1993). The SF-36 health survey questionnaire: An outcome measure suitable for routine use within the NHS? *British Medical Journal, 306,* 1440–1444.

Han, T. S., Tijhuis, M. A. R., Lean, M. E. J., & Seidell, J. C. (1998). Quality of life in relation to over-weight and body fat distribution. *American Journal of Public Health, 88*(12), 1814–1821.

Hudson, W. W. (1982). *The clinical measurement package: A field manual.* Homewood, IL: Dorsey Press.

McHorney, C. A., Ware, J. E., & Raczek, A. E. (1993). The MOS 36-item short-form health survey (SF-36): II. Psychometric and clinical tests of validity in measuring physical and mental health constructs. *Medical Care, 31*(3), 247–263.

McHorney, C. A., Ware, J. E., Lu, J. F. R., & Donald Sherbourne, C. (1994). The MOS 36-item short-form health survey (SF-36): III. Tests of data quality, scaling assumptions, and reliability across diverse patient groups. *Medical Care, 32*(1), 40–66.

Michalos, A. C. (1986). Job satisfaction, marital satisfaction and the quality of life: A review and a preview. In F. M. Andrews (Ed.), *Research on the quality of life* (pp. 57–83). Ann Arbour: Institute for Social Research, University of Michigan.

Michalos, A. C. (1991) Global report on student well-being: Volume 1, Life satisfaction and happiness. New York: Springer.

Michalos, A. C. (2002). Policing services and the quality of life. *Social Indicators Research, 61,* 1–18.
Michalos, A. C., & Zumbo, B. D. (2000). *Quality of life in Quesnel, British Columbia*. UNBC: Institute for Social Research and Evaluation.
Michalos, A. C., & Zumbo, B. D. (2001). Ethnicity, modern prejudice and the quality of life. *Social Indicators Research, 53,* 189–222.
Michalos, A. C., & Zumbo, B. D. (2003). Leisure activities, health and the quality of life. In A. C. Michalos (Ed.), *Essays on the quality of life* (pp. 217–238). Kluwer Academic Publishing.
Michalos, A. C., Zumbo, B. D., & Hubley, A. (2000). Health and the quality of life. *Social Indicators Research, 51,* 245–286.
Provincial health Officer. (1994). *A Report of the health of British Columbians: Provincial health officer's annual report 1994*. Victoria, BC: Ministry of health and Ministry Responsible for Seniors.
Stock, W. A., Okun, M. A., Haring, M. J., & Witter, R. A. (1983). Age differences in subjective well-being: A meta-analysis. *Evaluation Studies Review Annual, 8,* 279–302.
Sullivan, M., Karlsson, J., & Ware, J. E. (1995). The Swedish SF-36 health survey—1. Evaluation of data quality, scaling assumptions, reliability and construct validity across general populations in Sweden. *Social Science and Medicine, 41*(10), 1349–1358.
Thommasen, H. V., Newbery, P., & Watt, W. D. (1999). Medical history of central coast of British Columbia. *B.C. Medical Journal 41*(9), 464–470.
Ware, J. E., & Donald Sherbourne, C. (1992). The MOS 36-item short-form health survey (SF-36): I. Conceptual framework and item selection. *Medical Care, 30*(6), 473–483.
Ware, J. E., Kosinsky, M., & Keller, S. D. (1994). *SF-36 Physical and mental health summary scales: A user's manual*. Boston, MA: The Health Institute, New England Medical Center.
Ware, J. E., Snow, K. K., Kosinski, M., & Gandek, B. (1993). *SF-36 health survey: Manual and interpretation guide*. Boston, MA: The health Institute, New England Medical Center.
Zumbo, B. D., & Michalos, A. C. (2000). Quality of life in Jasper Alberta. *Social Indicators Research, 49,* 121–145.

Chapter 5
Health and Quality of Life of Aboriginal Residential School Survivors, Bella Coola Valley, 2001

Sylvia S. Barton, Harvey V. Thommasen, Bill Tallio, William Zhang and Alex C. Michalos

Introduction

The Indian residential school system no longer exists in Canada, but the legacy lives on in the form of significant pain and suffering among residential school survivors and their families. As late as the mid- 1960s, an estimated 10,000 Aboriginal students were attending 60 Indian residential schools across Canada. In British Columbia there were 19 Indian residential schools in operation, at various

---

Barton, S.S., Thommasen, H.V., Tallio, B., Zhang, W., & Michalos, A.C.: 2005. Health and quality of life of aboriginal residential school survivors, Bella Coola Valley. Social Indicators Research, 73, pp. 295–312. © Springer 2005.

S.S. Barton · W. Zhang
University of Northern British Columbia, 3333 University Way, Prince George, British Columbia V2N 4Z9, Canada
e-mail: bartons@unbc.ca

W. Zhang
e-mail: wzhang@unbc.ca

H.V. Thommasen
UBC Faculty of Medicine, 4202 Davie Avenue, Prince George, British Columbia V2M 4G7, Canada
e-mail: thommas@pgonline.com; thommash@unbc.ca

B. Tallio
Nuxalk Nation, Health and Wellness, Bella Coola, British Columbia, Canada
e-mail: billtallio@belco.bc.ca

A.C. Michalos (✉)
University of Northern British Columbia, Prince George, BC, Canada
e-mail: michalos@brandonu.ca

A.C. Michalos, *Connecting the Quality of Life Theory to Health, Well-Being and Education*, DOI 10.1007/978-3-319-51161-0_5

times and locations, with as many as 1500 children in these schools. From almost every Aboriginal community in British Columbia, children as young as three to age eighteen were removed from their homes, mostly forcibly, and placed in boarding schools, where they stayed isolated from their family, community, culture, and the rest of Canadian society (Miller 1996; Brasfield 2001; Ward 2001). It was not until 1984 that the last residential school in British Columbia, St. Mary's, closed (Miller 1996).

The residential school experience has affected Aboriginal peoples in destructive ways and continues to have a drastic impact on families. The practice of separating children from their parents has resulted in suffering related to the loss of family structure, cohesion, and quality of family life. Children who attended these schools, in particular, suffered from the loss of culture, identity, and language as residential school life altered the traditional ways of Aboriginal peoples and broke up traditional ways of Aboriginal family life. In addition to physical, sexual, mental, emotional, and spiritual abuse, many children who attended residential schools were exposed to unhealthy environmental conditions, as well as malnutrition. Low self-esteem and self-concept problems emerged as children were taught that their own culture was inferior and uncivilized, and it is believed that as a result, many residential school survivors suffer from low self-respect, and long-term emotional and psychological effects (Wade 1995; Royal Commission on Aboriginal Peoples 1996; Kelm 1998; Milloy 1999; Brasfield 2001; Ward 2001).

While it is generally assumed that the majority of Aboriginal peoples have had negative residential school experiences, and that there is a relationship between residential school experience and longterm poor health status, data to support these assumptions are lacking. A recent National First Nations and Inuit Health Survey, for example, found no statistically significant difference in the prevalence rates of selected chronic health problems between adults, age 45 or older, who had attended residential schools and adults who had not attended residential schools, after controlling for age (Reading 1999). These investigators hypothesized that confounding health determinants, such as socioeconomic factors and problems inherent with the use of survey methods most likely accounted for a lack of association between residential school attendance and long-term physical, or mental illness and disability.

Aboriginal residential school survivors without alternative sources of self-esteem and happiness, such as family relations, jobs, and recreation may view the effects of residential schooling as a contributor to poor health status. How would Aboriginal residential school survivors rate their health and overall quality of life in comparison to Aboriginal non-residential school attendees? Is self-esteem implicated? Do survivors of residential schooling experience higher rates of chronic illness, such as heart disease and diabetes? The objective of this study was to make comparisons between Aboriginal residential school survivors' perceptions of health status and overall quality of life, and Aboriginal non-residential school attendees, as well as between non-Aboriginals.

Methods

The study was based on a comparative analysis design in order to make comparisons between Aboriginal residential school survivors' perceptions of health status and overall quality of life, and Aboriginal non-residential school attendees, as well as between non-Aboriginals. The data for this study used 33 questions derived from the 2001 Determinants of Health and Quality of Life Survey (Michalos et al. 2004). The Determinants of Health and Quality of Life Survey was a regional survey that collected information on self-reported data on the health status and overall quality of life of all residents of the Bella Coola Valley, aged 17 years or older, from August to November, 2001. The Bella Coola Valley is in southwestern British Columbia, Canada, and includes four rural and remote communities. According to the 2001 census, 43% of the population of the Bella Coola Valley belong to the Nuxalk Nation, who reside predominantly in and around the Bella Coola township.

Specifically, the survey measured the influence of a set of designated health determinants on respondents' health and quality of life, utilizing health status measures from the SF-36 questionnaire (Ware et al. 1993) and the US Centers for Disease Control (CDC 2000; Michalos and Zumbo 2000) healthy days items; measures from the BC Provincial Health Officer's Annual Report (1994), which designated determinants of health; and measures of quality of life by satisfaction levels, global items, and the Subjective Well-Being Index (Zumbo and Michalos 2000). These items created a summated rating index that was estimated to produce good health and quality of life metric qualities among adults. The Likert-type items were easy to read and comprehend, and could be completed quickly. Reliability and validity coefficients have been established and deemed acceptable as a result of repeated use throughout northern British Columbia, as well as globally (Michalos 1986, 1991; Michalos and Zumbo 2000, 2001; Michalos et al. 2000).

First, this data set of 687 residents provided the 33 questions (secondary data set) related to age, gender, Aboriginal status, education, residential school attendance, happiness, self-rating of health, pain, stress, and self-rating of health care services that was used in this study, as outlined in Table 5.1.

Second, a detailed, retrospective review of all 2001 Bella Coola Medical Clinic charts, which included demographic information (age, gender, aboriginal status), number of times a physician was seen in the past year, and the presence of chronic diseases was completed, enabling cohort matching of the survey with the charts. In addition, definitions of chronic health problems were constructed prior to data collection, which culminated in a total of ten descriptions based on the 2003 Inner Central Coast Pilot Project, Summary of Health and Population Indicators for the Bella Coola Valley (Bella Coola Medical Clinic). Forty-seven Aboriginal residential school survivors were identified from the survey and matched, based on age and gender, with Aboriginal non-residential school attendees to form a cohort (n = 60), as well as with non-Aboriginals (n = 94). Approval of a Canadian university institutional ethics review board was obtained. In order to protect

Table 5.1 Thirty-three questions

Four questions related to age, gender, aboriginal status, and highest level of education
Five questions pertained to residential school attendance: Did you attend residential school? —yes or no Where did you attend residential school? —name What years did you attend residential school? —number of years Looking back, how happy were you at residential school? —very unhappy (1) to very happy (7) At the present time, how happy does it make you feel to think about residential school? —very unhappy (1) to very happy (7)
One question pertained to happiness: Considering your life as a whole, how happy would you say you are now? —very unhappy (1) to very happy (7)
One question pertained to self-rating of general health, which was also the first question in the SF-36 instrument: How would you rate your health in general now? —excellent (1) to poor (5)
Two questions pertained to bodily pain: How much bodily pain have you had during the past 4 weeks? —none (1) to very severe (6) How much did pain interfere with your normal week during the past 4 weeks? —not at all (1) to extremely (5)
One question pertained to a self-rating of the respondent's current life stress level (Hudson 1982): How stressful would you rate your life as a whole? —very non-stressful (1) to very stressful (7)
One question pertained to a self-rating of the respondent's personal health care he or she received in the Bella Coola Valley: All things considered, how would you rate the health care services you get here? —poor (1) to excellent (5)
Eighteen questions pertained to overall quality of life: How satisfied are you with your residence, neighbourhood, family relations, living partner, job, life as a whole, friendships, health, spiritual, overall standard of living, financial security, recreation activities, self-esteem, personal safety, federal government, provincial government, local government, and overall quality of life? —very dissatisfied (1) to very satisfied (7)

respondents' privacy, only one investigator anonymously matched the three cohorts' survey responses with patients' medical charts.

In the context of this data set, analysis was conducted using the Statistical Package for the Social Sciences (SPSS) for Windows. Tests and measures consisted of a series of descriptive, univariate, and Pearson Chi-square equations comparing health status and quality of life outcome measures, physician visits, and chronic disease prevalence rates between the cohorts. Descriptive statistics, including means, standard deviations, and skewness were computed for all variables. Univariate analysis of variance was used on the visit data and Pearson Chi-square (Asymp. Sig. [2-sided]) statistics were used on the remaining data (Tabachinick and Fidell 1996). A comparison of different combinations of outcomes between the cohorts allowed for the representation of a more detailed picture of health status and overall quality of life between Aboriginal residential school survivors and Aboriginal non-residential school attendees, as well as between non-Aboriginals. Thus the results were interpreted by comparing the differences made by each variable between the cohort of Aboriginal residential school survivors and the cohort of all others, as well as between the three cohorts (Aboriginal residential school survivors, Aboriginal non-residential school attendees, and non-Aboriginals).

Results

Proportion of Aboriginal Residential School Survivors

According to the survey, of the 176 Aboriginal respondents who completed the survey (43% response rate), 47 respondents stated that they had attended a residential school (27%), 111 respondents had not attended a residential school (63%), and 18 respondents did not answer the question (10%). The youngest respondent who had attended residential school was 35 years old.

Comparisons Between Aboriginal Residential School Survivors and Others

Table 5.2 indicates the mean values for responses to the survey questions and yearly physician visits for Aboriginal residential school survivors and for all those who did not attend residential school. Significant differences were found for self-health, health care, satisfaction with health, years of education, life as a whole, self-esteem, pain interference, happiness, overall quality of life, neighborhood, financial security, and spirituality questions, as well as for yearly number of doctor visits.

Table 5.3 indicates the mean values for responses to the survey questions and yearly physician visits for Aboriginal residential school survivors, Aboriginal non-residential school attendees, and non-Aboriginals. The only variable to yield a statistically significant difference when scores were compared between the cohort of Aboriginal residential school survivors and the cohort of Aboriginal non-residential school attendees, was self-health rating, which was lower for Aboriginal residential school survivors. A comparison of the scores between all three cohorts identified numerous statistically significant differences, which included self-health rating, health care rating, life as a whole, over all quality of life, and satisfaction with health. Thus both the Aboriginal residential school survivors and the Aboriginal

Table 5.2 Comparing residential school survivors to others

	Attended residential school mean ± SD (# answering)	Others Mean ± SD (# answering)	*p*-Value
Age (years)	63.5 ± 12.3 (n = 47)	61.2 ± 11.6 (n = 154)	
Sex (F = 1)	F = 25; M = 22; T = 47	F = 83; M = 71; T = 154	
Aboriginal (Yes = 1)	n = 47	n = 60 Aboriginal; 94 Other	
Attended RS (D8) (Yes = 1)	n = 47	n = None	
Self-health rating (SF1)	3.7 ± 0.9 (n = 47)	2.8 ± 1.0 (n = 154)	<0.001
Health care (HC1)	3.1 ± 1.1 (n = 47)	3.7 ± 1.0 (n = 152)	0.002
Health (QL8)	4 ± 2.0 (n = 45)	5.0 ± 1.6 (n = 151)	0.003
Education (D7)	2.2 ± 1.7 (n = 43)	3.5 ± 2.0 (n = 150)	0.008
Life as whole (QL6)	5 ± 2.0 (n = 45)	5.7 ± 1.4 (n = 151)	0.008
Self-esteem (QL13)	4.9 ± 2.1 (n = 45)	5.5 ± 1.4 (n = 147)	0.01
Pain interferes (SF8)	2.4 ± 1.3 (n = 45)	2.0 ± 1.1 (n = 151)	0.011
Happiness (QL19)	5 ± 1.8 (n = 46)	5.7 ± 1.4 (n = 153)	0.013
Overall QOL (QL18)	4.9 ± 1.6 (n = 45)	5.6 ± 1.4 (n = 149)	0.017
Neighbourhood (QL2)	5.2 ± 1.8 (n = 45)	6.0 ± 1.4 (n = 149)	0.027
Financial security (QL11)	4.0 ± 2.0 (n = 44)	4.9 ± 1.8 (n = 150)	0.03
Spirituality (QL9)	5.1 ± 2.0 (n = 43)	5.6 ± 1.6 (n = 137)	0.036
Number of Physician visits	6.9 ± 6.0 (n = 47)	5.1 ± 5.1 (n = 154)	0.048
Friendships (QL7)	5.4 ± 1.9 (n = 45)	6.0 ± 1.3 (n = 150)	0.055
Recreation (QL12)	4.0 ± 1.9 (n = 41)	4.8 ± 1.7 (n = 147)	0.074
Bodily pain (SF7)	3.4 ± 1.4 (n = 46)	2.8 ± 1.3 (n = 150)	0.076
Overall standard of living (QL10)	5.1 ± 1.9 (n = 45)	5.7 ± 1.4 (n = 150)	0.118
Residence (QL1)	5.1 ± 2.1 (n = 42)	5.6 ± 1.7 (n = 150)	0.146
Job (QL5)	5 ± 1.7 (n = 23)	5.3 ± 1.7 (n = 91)	0.175
Federal government (QL15)	3.6 ± 1.6 (n = 41)	3.1 ± 1.7 (n = 130)	0.294
Personal safely (QL14)	5.8 ± 1.4 (n = 44)	5.9 ± 1.3 (n = 146)	0.41
Family relations (QL3)	5.6 ± 1.6 (n = 44)	6.1 ± 1.3 (n = 147)	0.555
Provincial government (QL16)	3.7 ± 1.7 (n = 39)	3.3 ± 1.7 (n = 135)	0.623

(continued)

Table 5.2 (continued)

	Attended residential school mean ± SD (# answering)	Others Mean ± SD (# answering)	*p*-Value
Stress (ST 12)	4.2 ± 1.7 (n = 45)	4.1 ± 1.7 (n = 147)	0.684
Living partner (QL4)	5.8 ± 1.6 (n = 30)	6.2 ± 1.4 (n = 118)	0.688
Local government (QL17)	3.7 ± 1.7 (n = 38)	3.6 ± 1.6 (n = 128)	0.796

Table 5.3 Comparison of scores between the three cohorts

Mean ± SD	RS-A	Non-RS-A	Non-A
Age (years)	63.5 ± 12.3 (n = 47)	58.1 ± 10.2 (n = 60)	63.2 ± 12 (n = 94)
Total years residential school	4.7 ± 2.9 (n = 34)		
How happy then (D ll)	2.9 ± 2.1 (n = 46)		
How happy now (D12)	2.7 ± 1.9 (n = 45)		
Education (D7)	2.2 ± 1.7 (n = 43)	2.5 ± 1.8 (n = 56)	4.1 ± 1.8[a] (n = 94)
Self health rating (SF1)	3.7 ± 0.9 (n = 47)	3.1 ± 1.2[b] (n = 60)	2.7 ± 0.9[a] (n = 94)
Health care (HC1)	3.1 ± 1.1 (n = 47)	3.4 ± 1.1 (n = 59)	3.9 ± 0.8[a] (n = 93)
Happiness (QL19)	5.0 ± 1.8 (n = 46)	5.8 ± 1.3 (n = 59)	5.5 ± 1.5[b] (n = 94)
Bodily pain (SF7)	3.4 ± 1.4 (n = 46)	3.0 ± 1.4 (n = 58)	2.7 ± 1.3[b] (n = 92)
Pain interferes (SF8)	2.4 ± 1.3 (n = 45)	2.2 ± 1.2 (n = 58)	1.9 ± 1.0[b] (n = 93)
Stress (ST 12)	4.2 ± 1.7 (n = 45)	4.0 ± 1.7 (n = 57)	4.2 ± 1.7 (n = 90)
Satisfaction with			
Neighbourhood (QL2)	5.2 ± 1.8 (n = 45)	5.8 ± 1.5 (n = 58)	6.1 ± 1.4[a] (n = 91)
Life as a whole (QL6)	5.0 ± 2.0 (n = 45)	5.7 ± 1.5 (n = 59)	5.8 ± 1.3[c] (n = 92)
Health (QL8)	4.0 ± 2.0 (n = 45)	4.6 ± 1.6 (n = 58)	5.2 ± 1.6[c] (n = 93)
Financial security (QL11)	4.0 ± 2.0 (n = 44)	4.3 ± 2.1 (n = 58)	5.2 ± 1.6[c] (n = 92)
Overall QOL (QL18)	4.9 ± 1.6 (n = 45)	5.5 ± 1.6 (n = 58)	5.7 ± 1.3[c] (n = 91)
Residence (QL1)	5.0 ± 2.2 (n = 43)	5.1 ± 2.0 (n = 58)	6.0 ± 1.5[b] (n = 92)
Family relations (QL3)	5.6 ± 1.6 (n = 44)	6.1 ± 1.2 (n = 57)	6.0 ± 1.4 (n = 90)
Living partner (QL4)	5.8 ± 1.6 (n = 30)	6.1 ± 1.6 (n = 46)	6.3 ± 1.2 (n = 72)
Job (QL5)	5.0 ± 1.7 (n = 23)	4.8 ± 2.1 (n = 33)	5.7 ± 1.3 (n = 58)
Friendships (QL7)	5.4 ± 1.9 (n = 45)	5.9 ± 1.4 (n = 59)	6.0 ± 1.3[b] (n = 91)
Spirituality (QL9)	5.1 ± 2.0 (n = 43)	5.6 ± 1.8 (n = 55)	5.6 ± 1.4[b] (n = 82)
Overall standard of living (QL10)	5.1 ± 1.9 (n = 45)	5.4 ± 1.6 (n = 59)	5.8 ± 1.3[b] (n = 91)
Recreation (QL12)	4.0 ± 1.9 (n = 41)	4.6 ± 1.9 (n = 57)	4.9 ± 1.5[b] (n = 90)
Self-esteem (QL13)	4.9 ± 2.1 (n = 45)	5.5 ± 1.4 (n = 58)	5.5 ± 1.4[b] (n = 89)
Personal safely (QL14)	5.8 ± 1.4 (n = 44)	5.7 ± 1.5 (n = 58)	6.0 ± 1.2[b] (n = 88)

(continued)

Table 5.3 (continued)

Mean ± SD	RS-A	Non-RS-A	Non-A
Federal government (QL15)	3.6 ± 1.6 (n = 41)	2.9 ± 1.9 (n = 49)	3.3 ± 1.6 (n = 81)
Provincial government (QL16)	3.7 ± 1.7 (n = 39)	3.1 ± 1.9 (n = 50)	3.4 ± 1.5 (n = 85)
Local government (QL17)	3.7 ± 1.7 (n = 38)	3.4 ± 1.9 (n = 46)	3.7 ± 1.5 (n = 82)
Number of physician visits	6.9 ± 6.0 (n = 47)	7.2 ± 6.1 (n = 60)	3.7 ± 3.8 (n = 94)

RS-A Residential School Aboriginal; *Non-RS-A* Non-Residential School Aboriginal; *Non-A* Non-Aboriginal
[a]Comparison with RS-A (Residential School Aboriginal) significant at $p \leq 0.001$
[b]Comparison with RS-A (Residential School Aboriginal) significant at $p \leq 0.05$
[c]Comparison with RS-A (Residential School Aboriginal) significant at $p \leq 0.01$

non-residential school attendees reported poorer health on most of the outcome measures compared with non-Aboriginals. The significant differences reported for Aboriginal versus non-Aboriginal groups on the following items were matched in the Prince George sample described in Michalos and Zumbo (2001): satisfaction with one's own health, self-esteem, neighborhood, financial security, recreation, residence, family relations, living partner, life as a whole, overall quality of life, and overall happiness.

Table 5.4 summarizes chronic disease prevalence rates. The prevalence of chronic disease was similar between both the Aboriginal residential school

Table 5.4 Chronic disease prevalence rates

	RS-A	Non-RS-A	Non-A
Total #	47	60	94
Diabetes	34% (n = 16)	27% (n = 16)	6% (n = 6)[a]
Chronic obstructive			
Pulmonary disease	4% (n = 2)	2% (n = 1)	4% (n = 4)
Hypertension	30% (n = 14)	28% (n = 17)	32% (n = 30)
Coronary artery disease	6% (n = 3)	12% (n = 7)	14% (n = 8)
Depression/anxiety	17% (8)	12% (n = 7)	26% (n = 24)
Cancer	4% (n = 2)	7% (n = 4)	5% (n = 5)
Osteoarthritis	15% (n = 7)	23% (n = 14)	17% (n = 16)
Inflammatory arthritis	6% (n = 3)	12% (n = 7)	2% (n = 2)
Chronic back/neck pain	17% (n = 8)	12% (n = 7)	12% (n = 11)
Musculoskeletal problem	19% (n = 9)	15% (n = 9)	10% (n = 9)

RS-A Residential School Aboriginal; *Non-RS-A* Non-Residential School Aboriginal; *Non-A* Non-Aboriginal
[a]Comparison with RS-A (Residential School Aboriginal) significant at $p \leq 0.001$
[b]Comparison with RS-A (Residential School Aboriginal) significant at $p \leq 0.05$
[c]Comparison with RS-A (Residential School Aboriginal) significant at $p \leq 0.01$

survivors and the Aboriginal non-residential attendees. Noteworthy is the finding that the prevalence rate of diabetes was higher in both Aboriginal cohorts when compared to the non-Aboriginal cohort, all age-matched cohorts ($p < 0.001$).

Discussion

It is a fact that a well-known and longstanding inequality in health and social status affects indigenous peoples in Canada and around the world. This study has identified that Aboriginal peoples residing in the Bella Coola Valley, regardless of whether they attended residential school or not, experience similar inequality in health status and quality of life in comparison to non-Aboriginals residing in the same location. In addition, the prevalence rate of chronic disease was identified to be similar among both Aboriginal groups. Specifically, the prevalence rate of diabetes was identified to be much higher in both Aboriginal groups in comparison to the non-Aboriginal group. Although there has been a huge improvement in the health status of Aboriginal peoples, there is still substantial progress to be made in achieving a level of health and quality of life comparable to other Canadians.

Residential Schooling and Aboriginal Peoples in the Bella Coola Valley

Aboriginal peoples in the Bella Coola Valley, regardless of whether they attended residential school or not, are continuing to experience the negative effects of residential school: the historical policy of separation that resulted in the disintegration of traditional Aboriginal families. Such influences can continue to live on from residential school survivors through to second, third, and fourth generations.

Of the 176 people of Aboriginal ancestry who completed the survey, 47 stated they had attended a residential school (27%). The relatively small number of people attending residential school is somewhat contrary to the popular belief that all Aboriginal peoples in British Columbia attended residential school. The findings are, however, consistent with a recent Indian Affairs Annual Report, that indicated an average of 7100 (38%) Aboriginal students attended residential schools each year between 1890 and 1965, compared to an annual average of 11,400 (62%) who attended day schools over the same period. In 1960, for example, 40,637 Aboriginal students were enrolled in government schools across Canada. Of those students, 9109 (22%) were in residential schools, 22,049 (54%) were attending federal day schools, and another 9479 (23%) were attending regular, provincial public schools (Foot 2001).

It was not possible to tell from the survey data whether or not the Aboriginal respondents, who did not attend residential school, had parents who attended residential school. It became apparent during the study that when residential schools prevailed, they were being used as 'child protection' facilities. Children, who were judged to be living in difficult family situations or extreme poverty, were relocated to residential schools. Thus for some Nuxalk Nation people in the Bella Coola Valley, the residential school experience also included a complex home environment that preceded the act of sending children off to residential school.

Inequality in Health Confounded with Residential School Effects

The study indicated that both Aboriginal residential school survivors and Aboriginal non-residential school attendees have lower health and quality of life survey scores compared to non-Aboriginals. Interestingly, when Aboriginal residential school survivors were compared to Aboriginal non-residential school attendees, the only variable to yield a statistically significant difference was the self-health rating, which indicated that residential school survivors reported lower self-health scores. Perhaps with a larger sample, statistical significant differences could be identified for such measures as self-rated pain, happiness, and self-esteem. This finding, however, appears consistent with the results of the First Nations and Inuit Regional Health Survey. This survey found no statistically significant differences in the prevalence of specific long-term health problems between those who had attended residential schools and those who had not (Reading 1999).

It could be surmised from this Bella Coola Valley study that the 'residential school years' were extremely difficult for both Aboriginal peoples who attended residential school, as well as for those who remained in their own communities. A recent review of mortality for the Nuxalk Nation people revealed that 52% of all deaths in the Bella Coola township, between 1917 and 1983, involved people who were under 25 years of age (Edwards 1992). The majority of deaths were due to infection, such as tuberculosis and pertussis (whooping cough), but there were also a significant number of deaths related to suicides, accidents, and drownings. High alcohol consumption was found to be a factor in a significant proportion of deaths.

Over the past twenty years, there has been a huge improvement in the health status of Aboriginal peoples in British Columbia. Nuxalk Nation people's health, like other Aboriginal nations in the province, has improved significantly, especially related to infant mortality, unintentional injuries, suicide, as well as most other causes of death. It is suggested that although many health indicators currently lag behind the British Columbia population, Aboriginal peoples could achieve a level of health comparable to other British Columbians over the next 10 years. There is still a lot of work to be done before Aboriginal communities, including the Nuxalk Nation of Bella Coola, achieve the same level of health as enjoyed by most other British Columbians, but huge gains are materializing (British Columbia Provincial Health Officer 2002).

Residential School Syndrome

Brasfield (2001) describes a syndrome complex known as "Residential School Syndrome", which affects a significant minority of Aboriginal residential school survivors. The symptomology resembles post-traumatic stress disorder (PTSD). Studies have indicated that people suffering from PTSD are likely to suffer from pain, fatigue, and somatization (American Psychiatric Association 1994). Features of residential school syndrome include: recurrent intrusive memories, nightmares, occasional flashbacks, avoidance of anything that might be reminiscent of the residential school experience, relationship dysfunction, diminished interest and participation in cultural activities, sleep difficulties, anger management difficulties, and a persistent tendency to abuse alcohol or sedative medication drugs (MacMillan et al. 1996; Young 1994).

It was speculated from the study that lower self-reported health scores for Aboriginal residential school survivors may suggest a higher prevalence of post-traumatic stress disorder exists among members of this group. As Ing (1991) states, "... the current generation of elders and others who survived the system suffered traumatic losses in the areas of self-esteem, parenting skills, and language; that those losses are both psychological and cultural; and that, consequently, those traumatic experiences will be transmitted in some form to the next generations" (p. 86). Thus residential school syndrome interrupted normal child development by restricting experience and interrupting expertise of essential life skills. And in adults, it is associated with increased probability of educational failure, marital instability, and unemployment. A study of post- traumatic stress disorder among residential school survivors would be revealing.

Limitations

Inferences drawn from this comparative cohort analysis are limited because of nonrandom, convenience sampling. Issues that should be considered by the reader when interpreting the findings, include the possibility that because residential school experiences are historical, positive life experiences might have influenced respondents' perceptions of health and quality of life over time. In addition, the health and quality of life survey was developed in studies of non-Aboriginals; therefore, the expected relationship between perceptions of self-rated health and quality of life might be different when applied to Aboriginal peoples born and living in Canada.

Conclusions

This study contributes to an understanding of Aboriginal residential school survivors who reported poorer self-rated health compared with Aboriginal people who did not attend residential school. It also provides empirical data about Aboriginal residential school survivors when compared to non-Aboriginal Bella Coola Valley residents, the former reporting poorer health and lower satisfaction scores. These low scoring variables included years of education, life as a whole, selfesteem, pain interference, happiness, overall quality of life, neighborhood, financial security, and spirituality questions, as well as yearly number of doctor visits. The samples were based on 47 Aboriginal residential school survivors who were identified from the survey and matched, based on age and gender, with Aboriginal non-residential school attendees to form a cohort (n = 60), as well as with non-Aboriginal (n = 94).

This study highlights that 25 of the 26 variables compared found no significant differences between Aboriginal residential school survivors and Aboriginal non-residential school attendees. It is possible that our samples were too small or that the tests lacked power. Perhaps there were influences unaccounted for, but we found evidence contrary to the received view of the devastation of the residential school experience. Further research is needed to determine if, and to what extent, residential schooling is influencing Aboriginal health and quality of life through second, third, and fourth generations.

Acknowledgements We would like to express thanks to the staff at the Bella Coola Medical Clinic, Dr. Rua Read, Dr. Nancy Anderson, and Steve Murray for their assistance in distributing and collecting quality of life surveys. We would also like to acknowledge Dr. R. McIlwain, Director of the United Church Health Services, for his support of this project.

References

American Psychiatric Association. (1994). *Diagnostic and statistical manual of mental disorders* (4th ed.). Washington, DC.

Brasfield, C. R. (2001). Residential school syndrome. *British Columbia Medical Journal, 43*(2), 78–81.

British Columbia Provincial Health Officer. (1994). *A report on the health of British Columbian: Provincial health officer's annual report 1993*. Victoria, BC: Ministry of Health and Ministry Responsible for Seniors.

British Columbia Provincial Health Officer (2002). The health and well-being of Aboriginal people in British Columbia. In *A report on the health of British Columbians: Provincial health officer's annual report 2001*. Victoria, BC: Ministry of Health and Ministry Responsible for Seniors.

CDC. (2000). *Centers for disease control and prevention, measuring healthy days*. Atlanta, Georgia: CDC.

Edwards, G. W. (1992). Development of a Native Community Health Information System (NCHIS) for Indian and inuit communities in Canada, a working resource for self-informed and self-determined primary health care and community development by Canadian first nations. In L. Scott (Ed.), *Building Partnerships in Community Health through Applied Technology.*

Proceedings of the 4th National and 2nd International Conference on Information Technology and Community Health (pp. 33–40). British Columbia: University of Victoria.
Foot, R. (2001). Research Defends Residential Schools, National Post Newspaper Article, March 17.
Hudson, W. W. (1982). *The clinical measurement package: A field manual*. Illinois: Dorsey Press.
Ing, N. R. (1991). II. The policy of separation and the disintegration of traditional native families. *Canadian Journal of Native Education, 18*(Supplement), 71–86.
Kelm, M. (1998). *Colonizing bodies: Aboriginal health and healing in British Columbia 1900-1950*. Vancouver: University of British Columbia Press.
MacMillan, H. L., MacMillan, A. B., Offord, D. R., & Dingle, J. L. (1996). Aboriginal health. *Canadian Medical Association Journal, 155*(11), 1569–1578.
Michalos, A. C. (1986). Job satisfaction, marital satisfaction and the quality of life: A review and a preview. In F. M. Andrews (Ed.), *Research on the quality of life* (pp. 57–83). Ann Arbour: Institute for Social Research, University of Michigan.
Michalos, A. C. (1991). *Global report on student well-being: Volume 1, life satisfaction and happiness*. New York: Springer.
Michalos, A. C., Thommasen, H. V., Read, R., Anderson, N., & Zumbo, B. D. (2004). Determinants of health and the quality of life in the Bella Coola Valley. Social Indicators Research, tbp.
Michalos, A. C., & Zumbo, B. D. (2000). *Quality of life in Quesnel, British Columbia*. Prince George: Institute for Social Research and Evaluation, University of Northern British Columbia.
Michalos, A. C., & Zumbo, B. D. (2001). Ethnicity, modern prejudice and the quality of life. *Social Indicators Research, 53,* 189–222.
Michalos, A. C., Zumbo, B. D., & Hubley, A. (2000). Health and the quality of life. *Social Indicators Research, 51,* 245–286.
Miller, J. R. (1996). *Shingwauk's vision: A history of native residential schools*. Toronto: University of Toronto Press.
Milloy, J. S. (1999). *A national crime: The Canadian government and the residential school system, 1879 to 1986*. Winnipeg: University of Manitoba Press.
Reading, J. (1999). An Examination of Residential Schools and Elder Health. First Nations and Inuit Regional Longitudinal Survey. The Assembly of First Nations Resource Centre, 613-241-6789, Ottawa.
Royal Commission on Aboriginal Peoples. (1996). *The report of the royal commission on aboriginal peoples*. Ottawa: Minister of Supply and Services, Canada, Communications Group.
Tabachinick, B., & Fidell, L. (1996). *Using multivariate statistics* (3rd ed.). New York: Harper Collins College Publishers.
Wade, A. (1995). Resistance knowledges: Therapy with aboriginal persons who have experienced violence. In P. H. Stephenson, S. J. Elliott, L. T. Foster, & J. Harris (Eds.), *Persistent spirit: Towards understanding aboriginal health in British Columbia* (pp. 167–206). Victoria: Western Geographical Press.
Ward, K. J. (2001). Provincial Residential School Project. http://www.prsp.bc.ca.
Ware, J. E., Snow, K. K., Kosinski, M., & Gandek, B. (1993). *SF-36 health survey: Manual and interpretation guide*. Boston, Massachusetts: The Health Institute, New England Medical Center.
Young, T. K. (1994). *The health of native Americans: Toward a biocultural epidemiology*. United Kingdom: Oxford University Press.
Zumbo, B. D., & Michalos, A. C. (2000). Quality of life in Jasper, British Columbia. *Social Indicators Research, 49,* 121–145.

Chapter 6
Comparing Self-rated Health, Satisfaction and Quality of Life Scores Between Diabetics and Others Living in the Bella Coola Valley

Angela Grigg, Harvey V. Thommasen, Hugh Tildesley and Alex C. Michalos

Introduction

Diabetes has been described as a "burgeoning worldwide epidemic." The most recent available Canadian data indicate that in 1998/1999, the physician-diagnosed prevalence of diabetes in people who were 20 years of age and older was approximately 1.05 million (Canadian Diabetes Association 2003). This number translates to 4.8% of the total Canadian population. Yet, previous estimates suggest that the true proportion may actually be greater than 7%. In any case, these statistics are alarming: Not only are they associated with huge financial costs to the Canadian healthcare system, but they are also an indication of the tremendous potential that exists for deterioration in Canadians' quality of life. Having diabetes substantially increases one's risk of developing blindness, end stage renal disease, lower limb

Grigg, A., Thommasen, H.V., Tildesley, H., & Michalos, A.C.: 2006. Comparing self-rated health, satisfaction and quality of life scores between diabetics and others living in the Bella Coola Valley. Social Indicators Research, 76, pp. 263–281. © Springer 2006.

A. Grigg
Community Medicine Program, University of Northern British Columbia,
Prince George, BC V2N 4Z9, Canada

H.V. Thommasen
UBC Faculty of Medicine, 4202 Davie Avenue, Prince George, BC V2M 4G7, Canada
e-mail: thommas@pgonline.com

H. Tildesley
Department of Medicine, Diabetes Teaching and Training Centre,
UBC, St. Paul's Hospital, Vancouver, BC, Canada

A.C. Michalos (✉)
University of Northern British Columbia, Prince George, BC, Canada
e-mail: michalos@brandonu.ca

A.C. Michalos, *Connecting the Quality of Life Theory to Health, Well-Being and Education*, DOI 10.1007/978-3-319-51161-0_6

amputations, and dying from coronary artery disease, stroke, or peripheral vascular disease (Murphy 2000; Wilson et al. 1991).

Quality of life studies among people with type 2 diabetes highlight several common findings. First, increasing age among people with type 2 diabetes appears to be associated with worse self-reported physical and social functioning, as measured by the SF-36 (Camacho et al. 2002; Jacobson et al. 1994; Johnson et al. 1996). However, other studies of people in the general population (Fugl-Meyer et al. 2002) and people with mental illnesses (Mercier et al. 1998) have found that increasing age is significantly associated with greater satisfaction with several aspects of life. Insulin use among people with type 2 diabetes is associated with worse self-reported physical and social functioning, and with more limitations in role functioning due to physical health problems (Camacho et al. 2002; Johnson et al. 1996).

People with type 2 diabetes who use insulin appear to have worse self-perceived health (Johnson et al. 1996) and they report being less satisfied with and more negatively impacted by their current diabetes treatment regimens (Jacobson et al. 1994) compared to those not using insulin.

Number of diabetes-related complications has also been associated with reports of less satisfaction with current diabetes treatment regimen, worse role functioning due to physical health problems (Jacobson et al. 1994), and worse emotional well-being, as well as with greater role limitations due to emotional health problems (Johnson et al. 1996) among people with type 2 diabetes.

Our review of the literature on the broad topic of quality of life among people with type 2 diabetes did not reveal any study that operationalized quality of life as happiness, or even as satisfaction with life as a whole or with overall quality of life. As well, no studies appear to have investigated the relative impact that diabetes has on either self-rated health or quality of life, *separate* from other potential influences. For instance, if a woman is aging, Aboriginal, and overweight or obese—all risk factors for developing diabetes—what additional impact might developing diabetes have on her self-rated health and quality of life that wasn't perhaps already being felt?

The present study investigates the individual impacts that diabetes, gender, race—broadly categorized as *Aboriginal* or *all others*—age, and Body mass index (BMI), have on the self-rated health, healthcare services, stress, satisfaction with various domains of life, and quality of life of residents of a rural British Columbia community. Each of these analyses is intended to contribute to the overall goal of determining the relative impact that diabetes has. Among the subpopulation of people with type 2 diabetes, the influences of insulin use, extent of compliance with diabetes treatment regimen, and extent of diabetes-associated morbidity on the above items will also be investigated. Following the example of Michalos et al. (2000), quality of life will be operationalized as happiness, satisfaction with life as a whole, and satisfaction with overall quality of life (Michalos et al. 2000).

Methods

A Health and Quality of Life Questionnaire was offered to all adults (age 17 and up) living in the Bella Coola Valley of British Columbia between August 2001 and May 2002. Details of this survey are reported elsewhere (Michalos et al. In press). Twenty-one questions of this questionnaire form the basis of this research paper. The first question is a self-rating general health question which is also the first question in SF-36 (Ware et al. 1993). The next is a self-rating question on the respondent's current life stress level (Hudson 1982). Next, the respondent is asked to rate the personal health care he or she receives in the Bella Coola Valley. Then the respondent is asked to rate 16 quality of life items, including happiness, satisfaction with life as a whole, health, spiritual fulfilment, overall quality of life, overall standard of living, as well as residence, neighbourhood, family relations, living partner, job, friendships, financial security, recreational activities, self-esteem, and personal safety around home. Lastly, there were two demographic questions on gender (male or female) and age (years). These quality of life questions have been part of numerous surveys distributed throughout the north and world; so comparisons can be readily made (Michalos 1986, 1991, 2002, 2003; Michalos and Zumbo 2000, 2001; Michalos et al. 2000).

Table 6.1 summarizes the survey items, their abbreviations, Likert score ranges, and the specification of Likert score ranges. An identification number was given to

Table 6.1 Overview of survey questions and number of pair respondents

	Abbrev	Likert #	Specification of likert #
Survey item			
Self-rated health	SF1	1–5	Excellent to poor
Self-rated stress	ST12	1–7	Unstressful to stressful
Self-rated health care services	HC1	1–5	Poor to good
Satisfaction with			
House, apartment, home	QL1	1–7	Dissatisfied to satisfied
Neighborhood	QL2	1–7	Dissatisfied to satisfied
Family relations	QL3	1–7	Dissatisfied to satisfied
Living partner	QL4	1–7	Dissatisfied to satisfied
Job	QL5	1–7	Dissatisfied to satisfied
Life as whole	QL6	1–7	Dissatisfied to satisfied
Friendships	QL7	1–7	Dissatisfied to satisfied
Health	QL8	1–7	Dissatisfied to satisfied
Religion, spiritual fulfillment	QL9	1–7	Dissatisfied to satisfied
Overall standard living	QL10	1–7	Dissatisfied to satisfied
Financial security	QL11	1–7	Dissatisfied to satisfied
Recreational activities	QL12	1–7	Dissatisfied to satisfied
Self-esteem	QL13	1–7	Dissatisfied to satisfied
Personal safety around home	QL14	1–7	Dissatisfied to satisfied
Overall quality of life	QL15	1–7	Dissatisfied to satisfied
Happiness	QL16	1–7	Unhappy to happy

each questionnaire sent out. Dr. Thommasen was the only one able to link this number to the 2001 clinic patient list. This information was used for the purposes of re-mailing, and for linking survey responses to clinic charts. All recipients were asked to read an informed consent form or were read an informed consent form prior to completion of a questionnaire. Questionnaire answers were entered into an electronic EXCEL spreadsheet from which results were summarized and graphs of the data were later made (Harvey 1994).

At the same time the Health and Quality of Life questionnaire was being offered to residents of the Bella Coola Valley, Dr. H. Thommasen did three retrospective reviews of clinic charts. The first chart review was done in July–August 2001 to determine who was still living in the Bella Coola Valley. After excluding clinic charts of people not living within the Bella Coola Valley and not currently living in the Bella Coola Valley, 2329 patients made up the September 2001 Clinic population list—approximately 104% of the May 2001 census estimate (British Columbia Vital Statistics Agency 2003a, b). After defining the Bella Coola Medical Clinic population, clinic charts were once again reviewed in the spring of 2004 for the following information: age, sex, aboriginal status, number of clinic visits, height, weight, presence or absence of diabetes and other chronic diseases. From the chart review 127 diabetics were identified. Diabetic charts were then reviewed for the following information—date of diagnosis and duration of diabetes (years); blood glucose and glycoslyated hemoglobin (HgA1c) levels over time; presence or absence of diabetes related morbidities (coronary artery disease, peripheral vascular disease, nephropathy, retinopathy, or neuropathy); diabetic management recommendations with respect to medications (oral hypoglycaemic agents and insulin); whether or not that patient received diabetic education teaching, saw an internist, saw a dietician. A morbidity scoring system was developed (see Appendix A). Finally, a compliance scoring system was also developed. Bella Coola's Nurse Practitioner, who works closely with residents who have diabetes, was asked to provide a crude rating of each person's compliance with his or her current diabetes treatment regimen. Compliance was ranked on a scale ranging from 1 (*low*) to 3 *(high)*.

Chart derived information was entered into an electronic EXCEL spreadsheet from which results were summarized and graphs of the data were later made (Harvey 1994). Lastly, identification numbers on each returned Health and Quality of Life questionnaire were linked to the 2001 Bella Coola Clinic population list so that survey responses could be linked to chart review information. Names and addresses were removed from this linked data set, and passed on to statisticians and other researchers for further analyses.

Differences in the outcomes between diabetics and non-diabetics, as well as the differences between ethnic groups (aboriginal vs. others), between age groups, between sexes (male vs. female), and between weight groups were evaluated using Pearson's chi-square or One Way ANOVA tests with a significance p-value ≤ 0.05 for each outcome measure (Snedecor and Cochran 1980).

Results

Survey Response Rates

A total of 971 questionnaires were returned, of which 968 were useable for the purposes of this project. An estimated 1734 Bella Coola adult residents were eligible to complete our questionnaire. So the estimated response to this survey was 56% (968/1734). Of the 968 questionnaires, 964 were linked to names on the Bella Coola Clinic patient list.

Comparison of responder to non-responder populations reveals that a proportionately greater number of women, older people, people who were not aboriginal, and diabetics answered the survey questions as compared to younger people, men, aboriginal people, and people who are not diabetic, respectively.

Comparison of diabetic responders to non-responders reveals no differences between the two groups with respect to age, weight, BMI, HbA_{1c} values, years with diagnosed diabetes, morbidity scores, compliance scores, gender distribution, race distribution, proportion taking either oral hypoglycemic agents or insulin, or number of physician visits in 2001. Only one parameter differed between the two diabetic groups, namely, the mean total number of health facility visits among those who participated in the survey was greater than that of those who did not participate ($M = 21.99$, $SD = 17.53$ and $M = 14.61$, $SD = 13.24$, respectively), $t\,(125) = 2.15$, $p < 0.05$.

Table 6.2 presents mean self-rated health, health care services, stress, and quality of life scores for people without diabetes and those with diabetes. We were interested in comparing the scores of participants who didn't have diabetes with those who had diabetes that was associated with either low, medium, or high levels of morbidity. However, the latter two categories were combined due to small numbers. Participants without diabetes tended to rate their health significantly better than participants with diabetes that was associated with either level of morbidity, $F\,(2924) = 29.74$, $p < 0.001$. Participants with diabetes that was associated with medium-to-high morbidity appear to have thought, on average, that the stress in their lives was fairy evenly balanced ($M = 4.54$, $SD = 1.93$), participants without diabetes and with diabetes that was associated with low morbidity appear to have thought that their lives were at least a little stressful ($M = 3.50$, $SD = 1.55$ and $M = 3.42$, $SD = 1.30$, respectively). These differences were significant, $F\,(2940) = 6.24$, $p < 0.001$. Meanwhile, participants both without diabetes and with diabetes that was associated with either low or medium-to-high morbidity appear to have thought, on average, that the health care services they received were better than average ($M = 3.44$, $SD = 1.11$; $M = 3.53$, $SD = 1.22$; and $M = 3.72$, $SD = 1.25$, respectively), and there was no evidence that any of their mean scores for this item were significantly different, $F\,(2951) = 1.10$, $p > 0.05$. No mean quality of life score for participants in any category fell below 4.0 (*evenly balanced*). However, compared to participants without diabetes, those who had diabetes that was associated with low morbidity were, on average, significantly less

Table 6.2 Self-rated health, health care services, stress, and quality of life

Survey item	Without diabetes			With diabetes					
				Morbidity category					
				Low (1.0–2.0)			Medium to high (2.5–4.0)		
	M	*SD*	*n*	*M*	*SD*	*n*	*M*	*SD*	*n*
Current health***	3.29	1.02	833	2.58	0.82	67	2.19	0.88	27
Health care services	3.44	1.11	859	3.53	1.22	66	3.72	1.25	29
Life stress*	3.50	1.55	851	3.42	1.30	64	4.54	1.93	28
Domain-specific quality of life indicators *Satisfaction with*									
House, apartment***	5.37	1.68	854	5.09	1.98	66	6.56	0.93	27
Neighborhood	5.70	1.52	852	5.53	1.50	66	6.32	1.16	28
Family relations	5.72	1.47	848	5.54	1.55	65	6.32	1.12	28
Living partner	5.87	1.60	719	5.96	1.76	45	6.11	1.23	18
Job	4.98	1.69	684	5.30	1.82	40	5.58	1.73	12
Friendships	5.61	1.43	847	5.89	1.40	65	5.73	1.66	26
Health**	4.93	1.60	843	4.32	1.57	63	4.36	1.78	28
Religion, spirituality	5.14	1.62	782	5.41	1.70	61	5.83	1.23	23
Financial security	4.36	1.84	839	4.06	2.02	65	5.00	1.98	25
Recreation activities	4.51	1.71	831	4.14	1.86	63	4.96	1.98	23
Self-esteem	5.15	1.54	836	5.02	1.64	66	5.62	1.58	26
Personal safety	5.74	1.40	842	5.67	1.26	64	6.17	1.27	24
Global quality of life indicators *Satisfaction with*									
Life as a whole	5.41	1.47	846	5.53	1.57	66	5.69	1.49	26
Overall standard of living	5.36	1.47	846	5.24	1.58	66	5.54	1.63	26
Overall quality of life	5.48	1.39	851	5.32	1.55	66	5.41	1.58	27
Overall happiness	5.49	1.58	863	5.43	1.46	67	5.54	1.42	28

Notes Current health and health care services were rated on 5-point scales (1 = *poor,* 3 = *good,* 5 = *excellent,* and 1 = *poor,* 3 = *average,* 5 = *excellent,* respectively). All other indicators were rated on 7-point scales (1 = *very stressful/dissatisfied/unhappy,* 4 = *evenly balanced,* 7 = *very unstressful/satisfied/happy)*
$^{*}p < 0.05$. $^{**}p \leq 0.008$. $^{***}p \leq 0.001$

satisfied with their health ($M = 4.93$, $SD = 1.60$ and $M = 4.32$, $SD = 1.57$, respectively), $F\ (2931) = 5.86$, $p < 0.008$.

Insulin use. Regardless of whether they used insulin, participants with diabetes appeared to think, on average, that their current health was less than good ($M = 2.00$, $SD = 0.82$ and $M = 2.54$, $SD = 0.84$ for participants who did and did not use insulin, respectively). Despite this similarity, participants who used insulin rated their current health significantly lower than those who did not use insulin, $t\ (92) = 2.18$, $p < 0.05$. Meanwhile, both groups appeared to think, on average, that the health care services they received were somewhere between average and good

(M = 3.77, SD = 1.17 and M = 3.56, SD = 1.24 for participants who did and did not use insulin, respectively), and that their lives were at least a little stressful (M = 3.33, SD = 1.44 and M = 3.83, SD = 1.61 for participants who did and did not use insulin, respectively). Of all the mean quality of life scores, the only one that fell below 4.0 (*evenly balanced*) was satisfaction with health for participants who took insulin.

Compliance with diabetes treatment regimen. Regardless of the extent to which they complied with their recommended diabetes treatment regimens, participants with diabetes appear to have thought, on average, that their current health was somewhat less than good (M = 2.29, SD = 0.86; M = 2.41, SD = 0.78; M = 2.87, SD = 0.82 for participants in the low, medium, and high compliance categories, respectively); that the healthcare services they received were somewhere between average and good (M = 3.52, SD = 1.13; M = 3.59, SD = 1.32; M = 3.71, SD = 1.30 for participants in the low, medium, and high compliance categories, respectively), and that their lives were at least a little stressful (M = 3.67, SD = 1.44; M = 3.90, SD = 1.80; M = 3.75, SD = 1.62 for participants in the low, medium, and high compliance categories, respectively). Nevertheless, of all the survey items, the only one for which there was evidence of an effect by extent of compliance as categorized for the present study was current health, F (291) = 3.80, $p < 0.05$. Differences between means tests (Bonferroni) revealed that the worst mean rating of current health for participants in the lowest compliance category compared to that for participants in the highest compliance category was the only significant contributor to this finding. Satisfaction with health had the lowest mean score for participants in the low compliance category (M = 4.07, SD = 1.54), while satisfaction with financial security had the lowest mean score for participants in both the medium (M = 4.11, SD = 1.70) and the high (M = 4.48, SD = 2.33) compliance categories. As these data indicate, there was no instance for which satisfaction with any quality of life item fell below 4.0 (evenly balanced).

Self-rated health. The way participants rated their current health was significantly influenced in univariate analyses by whether they had diabetes, as well as what their races, ages, and BMIs were. Stepwise regression analysis revealed that, when these variables were considered concurrently, each one was retained as a significant predictor of how participants rated their current health, F (4884) = 34.42, $p < 0.001$. Together, they accounted for approximately 14% of the variation in current health ratings. Presence of diabetes was most influential, accounting for 6% of this variation, followed by race, age, and BMI (βs = −0.14, −0.22, −0.19, and −0.098, respectively). In a practical sense, this means that having diabetes, being Aboriginal, being over 45 years old, and having a BMI equal to or greater than 25.0 each predicted lower self-rated health, but even when these characteristics were considered concurrently, approximately 86% of the influence came from other things.

Satisfaction with health. It has also been noted that participant satisfaction with their health was significantly influenced in univariate analyses by whether they had diabetes and what their ages were. However, stepwise regression analysis revealed that only the presence of diabetes (β = −0.073) was retained as a significant predictor when these two factors were considered concurrently, $F(1916) = 4.96$, $p < 0.05$. That is, participants who had diabetes associated with low morbidity tended to be less satisfied with their health than others. However, this accounted for only a mere 0.5% of the variation in how satisfied participants were with their health: 99.5% was left up to other things.

Satisfaction with overall quality of life. Since satisfaction with overall quality of life among the total sample of survey participants was significantly influenced in univariate analyses by both their ages and their races—that is, whether they were Aboriginal or part of the group of all others—stepwise regression analysis was used to determine the relative importance of the latter in predicting the former. Interestingly, only race ($\beta = -0.10$) was retained as a significant predictor, $F(1937) = 8.69$, $p < 0.008$. That is, being Aboriginal was associated with significantly less self-reported satisfaction with overall quality of life. However, this explained only 0.9% of the variation in participants' satisfaction, which means that approximately 99.1% was explained by factors other than their races, ages, genders, BMIs, or even whether they had diabetes.

Discussion

Recent studies have shown that keeping blood sugar levels within normal range reduces chances of developing at least some of the complications associated with having diabetes (American Diabetes Association 2001; Diabetes Control and Complications Trial Research Group 1993; Thompson 1997; Tildesley 1997; UKPDS 1998, 2000). Consequently, an important aspect of Type 2 diabetes treatment is lowering blood sugar levels through diet, exercise, and medications (Brown 1996; Hu and Stampfer 2001; Pan and Li 1997; Schneider 1992; Vaaler 2000). Comprehensive management of diabetic patients also includes monitoring glycosylated hemoglobin, blood pressure, and lipids, encouraging smoking cessation, and the prophylactic use of acetylsalicylic acid (ASA) (American Diabetes Association 2001; Expert Committee of the Canadian Advisory Board 1998). Whenever possible, diabetic patients should receive dietary advice from a registered dietician. If adequate blood sugar levels have not been reached on a regimen that includes appropriate use of diet, exercise and oral agents, then insulin therapy should be initiated to improve diabetic control. The rationale is that if insulin is started early enough, endogenous insulin secretion might transiently or partly recover, reducing overall insulin requirements (Berger 1999; Ilkova 1997; Lindstorm 1999).

Unfortunately, in the real world it is extremely difficult to get diabetic patients to adhere to diet plans, to lose weight, to engage in exercise programs, to take hypoglycaemic, antihypertensive, cholesterol lowering agents, or to accept insulin. Perhaps by understanding how diabetic patients view their health and quality of life, one can get insights into why it is so difficult to engage diabetics in long-term treatment plans. For example, if a diabetic patient is very satisfied with his or her overall quality of life, or is very happy in life, he or she may not feel motivated to change things, adopt behaviours, or take medications which may impact happiness or overall quality of life. Denial may be an issue. If a diabetic feels that he or she is not really unhealthy, that may be a reason for why he or she does not wish to change behaviour. If our aim is to encourage people with diabetes to adopt and maintain recommended diabetes self-care behaviours, there is a need to further understand how they view their disease and its impact on their lives.

As Gafvels et al. (1993) noted, "self-perceived health has been suggested to play an important role in the adherence to diabetic management and metabolic control (Gafvels et al. 1993)." We have shown in the present study that regardless of the extent of their associated morbidity, people with diabetes recognize, on average, that their current health is less than good. In fact, as has been found in other studies, people with diabetes rated their health significantly less favorably, on average, than people without diabetes (Stewart et al. 1989). However, Aboriginals, people over 65 years old, and obese people—that is, people who had BMIs that were 30.0 or greater—also appeared to think, on average, that their current health was less than good. These results are consistent with those of other studies that have found a deterioration in self-reported physical functioning associated with being Aboriginal (British Columbia Provincial Health Officer 2002), as well as with increasing age (Jacobson et al. 1994; Johnson et al. 1996) and BMI (Lean et al. 1999).

When presence of diabetes, race, age, and BMI were considered concurrently, each one remained a significant predictor of how participants rated their current health. Together, these factors accounted for approximately 14% of the variation in participants' current health ratings. Nevertheless, presence of diabetes was most influential, accounting for 6% of this variation, followed by race, age, and BMI.

Considering this, it seemed worthwhile to focus on the impact that having diabetes had on participants' *satisfaction* with their health. Certainly, it seems plausible that, even though a person may recognize that his or her current health is not good, he or she may not feel motivated to maintain or improve it if they are already satisfied with it. In the present study, participants' satisfaction with their health was significantly influenced by whether they had diabetes and by what their ages were. However, when these two factors were considered concurrently, having diabetes was retained as a significant predictor of their satisfaction with their health. Specifically, participants who had diabetes that was associated with a low level of morbidity tended to be less satisfied with their health than others, both without diabetes or with diabetes that was associated with a medium to high level of morbidity. Jacobson et al. report "worries about the future of diabetes are possibly stimulated by the start of a pharmacological treatment but recede once the anticipated injections begin (Jacobson et al. 1994)." Perhaps a similar phenomenon accounts for the lower scores among those with lower morbidity as these would typically be recently diagnosed diabetics.

One might expect that poor self-rated health and diminished satisfaction with health might lead to improved self-care. However, in the present study, participants with diabetes who were the least compliant with their treatment regimens actually rated their current health significantly lower than those who were the most compliant.

Interestingly, people with diabetes, regardless of the extent of their associated morbidities, were no more likely to be unhappy or dissatisfied with their lives as a whole or with the overall quality of their lives compared to people without diabetes. In fact, only race and age had any influence. Compared to all others, Aboriginal people rated their satisfaction with the overall quality of their lives significantly lower and, compared to 46- to 64-year-olds, 65- to 94-year-olds were significantly more satisfied with the overall quality of their lives and their lives as a whole. As well, compared to 17- to 45-year-olds, 65- to 94-year-olds were significantly more satisfied with their lives as a whole. These findings are consistent with those of other studies of people in the general population (Fugl-Meyer et al. 2002) and people with mental illnesses (Mercier et al. 1998) that have found that increasing age is significantly associated with greater satisfaction with several aspects of life.

Among people with diabetes, however, those who used insulin do report significantly less satisfaction with the overall quality of their lives than those who don't use insulin. Certainly, this finding is not surprising, and is consistent with those of other studies. For instance, Jacobson et al. (1994) reported that, among their sample of 240 people who had either type 1 or type 2 diabetes, those who used insulin were significantly less satisfied with, and reported a significantly greater negative impact from, their diabetes treatment regimens. As well, they found that people who were being treated with diet alone had better general health perceptions (Jacobson et al. 1994).

So, if our aim is to encourage people with diabetes to adopt and maintain recommended diabetes self-care behaviours, doing so will likely not result in improvements in current health or quality of life self-ratings—especially if insulin is being used to control blood sugar. Based on the findings in our study, quality of life self-ratings may actually decrease once insulin is initiated. This may explain why diabetic patients are very reluctant to begin insulin despite current recommendations that they be started on it. As Watkins et al. (2000) found, it may actually be individuals' levels of understanding of the common aspects of a diabetes treatment regimen and their perceptions of how much control they have over diabetes—for instance, feeling that they are able to keep their blood sugar in good control, keep their weight under control, do the things they need to do for diabetes, and handle their feelings about their diabetes—that are the most significant predictors of their acceptance of recommended treatment regimens (Watkins et al. 2000).

Conclusion(s)

After accounting for age, race, and weight, we found that diabetics report significantly poorer self-rated health, and lower satisfaction with health scores compared to people without diabetes. Participants with diabetes who were the least compliant with their treatment regimens actually rated their current health significantly lower than those who were the most compliant. People with diabetes were, however, no more likely to be unhappy or dissatisfied with their lives as a whole or with the overall quality of their lives compared to people without diabetes. Among people with diabetes, those who used insulin reported significantly less satisfaction with the overall quality of their lives than those who didn't use insulin.

Acknowledgements We want to thank William Zhang and Jonathan Berkowitz for always being available to answer questions about statistics. We also wish to acknowledge the staff at the Bella Coola Medical Clinic for survey assistance, Steve Murray for his assistance in distributing and collecting the quality of life questionnaires; and to Amy Thommasen, Carol Thommasen, Julie Orlando, Bill Tallio, Rhonda Elliott, and Andy Bottomley for their help with various parts of this research. Special thanks to Pat Lenci for providing compliance ratings for diabetic people; and Liz Howard for piloting an initial Quality of Life Survey. We would also like to acknowledge the Community-Based Clinician-Investigator Program, the United Church Health Services, the University of Northern British Columbia, and the Rural and Remote Health Institute of UNBC for financial assistance with this project.

Appendix A

See Table A.3.

Table A.3 Morbidity scoring system

Eye disease	
1. None	None known
2. Minimal	Background retinopathy
3. Moderate	Proliferative retinopathy/laser Rx
4. Severe	Blindness
Cerebrovascular disease	
1. None	None known
2. Minimal	Carotid bruit
3. Moderate	hx of TIA's; thromboenderectomy
4. Severe	CVA's
Neuropathy	
1. None	None known
2. Minimal	Decreased touch/temp
3. Moderate	Neuropathic pain
4. Severe	Decreased touch/temp and pain
Coronary artery disease	
1. None	None known
2. Minimal	Angina (stable); ischemic ECG/Positive stress changes
3. Moderate	CABG; prior MI—now stable; angioplasty
4. Severe	*Post-MI; post-CABG, but still unstable e.g. CHF or persisting angina*

(continued)

Table A.3 (continued)

Peripheral vascular disease	
1. None	None known
2. Minimal	Decreased/absent pedal pulses; and/or femoral bruit
3. Moderate	Claudication pains
4. Severe	Bypass or amputation toes/foot/leg; ischemia of bowel
Nephropathy	
1. None	None known
2. Minimal	Proteinuria
3. Moderate	Peritoneal/hemodialysis
4. Severe	Transplant

Note Each person's *overall* morbidity score was calculated based on his or her individual morbidity ratings: (1.0) none were greater than 1.0; (2.0) one was 2.0, and all others were less than 2.0; (2.5) more than one was 2.0, and all others were less than 2.0; (3.0) one was 3.0, and all others were less than 3.0; (3.5) more than one was greater than three, and all others were less than three; (4.0) one was 4.0, and all other were less than 4.0; (4.5) more than one was 4.0, and all others were less than 4.0. For example, someone with proteinuria and no other known diabetes-related disease would have an overall morbidity score of 2.0

References

American Diabetes Association. (2001). Clinical practice recommendations 2001. *Diabetes Care, 24,* S80–S82.

Berger, M. (1999). Rationale for the use of insulin therapy alone as the pharmacological treatment of type II diabetes. *Diabetes Care, 22*(Suppl 3), C71–C75.

British Columbia Provincial Health Officer. (2002). A report on the health of British Columbians: Provincial health officer's annual report 2001. Feature report: The health and well-being of Aboriginal people in British Columbia. Victoria, BC: Ministry of Health and Ministry Responsible for Seniors.

British Columbia Vital Statistics Agency. (2003a, June). *P.E.O.P.L.E.* 27, BC Ministry of Management Services. Health Data Warehouse.

British Columbia Vital Statistics Agency. (2003b). *2001 British Columbia census.* Victoria, BC: Government of British Columbia.

Brown, S. A. (1996). Promoting weight loss in type II diabetes. *Diabetes Care, 19,* 613–621.

Camacho, F., Anderson, R. T., Bell, R. A., Goff, D. C., Duren-Winfield, V., Doss, D. D., et al. (2002). Investigating correlates of health related quality of life in a low-income sample of patients with diabetes. *Quality of Life Research, 11,* 783–796.

Canadian Diabetes Association. (2003). Clinical Practice Guidelines for the Prevention and Management of Diabetes in Canada. http://www.diabetes.ca/cpg2003/.

Diabetes Control and Complications Trial Research Group. (1993). The effect of intensive treatment of diabetes on the development and progression of long-term complications in insulin-dependent diabetes mellitus. *The New England Journal of Medicine, 329,* 977–986.

Expert Committee of the Canadian Advisory Board. (1998). Clinical practice guidelines for the management of diabetes in Canada. *CMAJ, 159*(Suppl 8), S1–S29.

Fugl-Meyer, A. R., Melin, R., & Fugl-Meyer, K. S. (2002). Life satisfaction in 18- to 64-year-old Swedes: In relation to gender, age, partner and immigrant status. *Journal of Rehabilitation Medicine, 34,* 239–246.

Gafvels, C., Lithner, F., & Borjeson, B. (1993). Living with diabetes: Relationship to gender, duration and complications. A survey in northern Sweden. *Diabetic Medicine, 10,* 768–773.

Harvey, G. (1994). *EXCEL for dummies* (2nd ed., p. 366). Foster City, CA: IDG Books.

Hu, F., & Stampfer, M. J. (2001). Physical activity and risk of cardiovascular events in diabetic women. *Annals of Internal Medicine, 134,* 96–103.

Hudson, W. W. (1982). *The clinical measurement package: A field manual.* Homewood, IL: Dorsey Press.

Ilkova, H. (1997). Induction of long term glycemic control in newly diagnosed type II diabetic patients by transient intensive insulin treatment. *Diabetes Care, 20,* 1353–1357.

Jacobson, A. M., Samson, J. A., & de Groot, M. (1994). The evaluation of two measures of quality of life in patients with type I and type II diabetes. *Diabetes Care, 17*(4), 267–274.

Johnson, J. A., Nowatzki, T. E., & Coons, S. J. (1996). Health-related quality of life in diabetic Pima Indians. *Medical Care, 34*(2), 97–102.

Lean, M. E., Han, T. S., & Seidell, J. C. (1999). Impairment of health and quality of life using new US federal guidelines for the identification of obesity. *Archives of Internal Medicine, 159,* 837–843.

Lindstorm, T. (1999). Sustained improvement of glycemic control by insulin treatment after 9 years in patients with type 2 diabetes and secondary failure. *Diabetes Care, 22,* 1373–1374.

Mercier, C., Peladeau, N., & Tempier, R. (1998). Age, gender and quality of life. *Community Mental Health Journal, 34*(5), 487–500.

Michalos, A. C., & Zumbo, B. D. (2000). *Quality of life in Quesnel.* British Columbia: Institute for Social Research and Evaluation, UNBC.

Michalos, A. C., & Zumbo, B. D. (2001). Ethnicity, modern prejudice and the quality of life. *Social Indicators Research, 53,* 189–222.

Michalos, A. C., Zumbo, B. D., & Hubley, A. (2000). Health and the quality of life. *Social Indicators Research, 51,* 245–286.

Michalos, A. C., Thommasen, H. V., Anderson, N., Read, R. & Zumbo, B. D. (2004). Determinants of health and the quality of life in the Bella Coola Valley. Social Indicators Research (In press).

Michalos, A. C. (1986). Job satisfaction, marital satisfaction and the quality of life: A review and a preview. In F. M. Andrews (Ed.), *Research on the quality of life* (pp. 57–83). Ann Arbour: Institute for Social Research, University of Michigan.

Michalos, A. C. (1991). *Global report on student well-being: vol. 1, life satisfaction and happiness.* New York: Springer.

Michalos, A. C. (2002, January). Prince George Papers on the Quality of Life. Institute for Social Research and Evaluation. Prince George, BC. Canada. V2N 4Z9, University of Northern British Columbia.

Michalos, A. C. (2003). Social indicators research and health-related quality of life research. *Social Indicators Research, 65*(1), 27–72.

Murphy, S. W. (2000). Deaths: Final data for 1998. *National Vital Statistics Report, 48*(11), 1–105.

Pan, X., & Li, G. (1997). Effects of diet and exercise in preventing NIDDM in people with impaired glucose tolerance. *Diabetes Care, 20,* 537–543.

Schneider, S. H. (1992). Ten year experience with an exercise-based outpatient lifestyle modification program in the treatment of diabetes mellitus. *Diabetes Care, 15,* 1800–1809.

Snedecor, G. W., & Cochran, W. G. (1980). *Statistical methods* (7th ed.). Ames, Iowa: Iowa State University Press.

Stewart, A. L., Greenfied, S., Hays, R. D., Wells, K., Rogers, W. H., Berry, S. D., et al. (1989). Functional status and well-being of patients with chronic conditions. *Journal of the American Medical Association, 262,* 907913.

Thompson, D. M. (1997). Diabetes. *BC Medical Journal, 39*(2), 76.

Tildesley, H. (1997). Diabetes teaching centres in BC. *BC Medical Journal, 39*(2), 77–79.

UK Prospective Diabetes Study (UKPDS) Group. (1998). Intensive blood glucose control with sulphonylurea or insulin compared with conventional treatment and risk of complications in patients with type II diabetes (UKPDS 33), Lancet 352 (pp. 837–853).

United Kingdom Prospective Diabetes Study Group. (2000). Association of glycaemia with macrovascular and microvascular complications of type 2 diabetes (UKPDS 35): Prospective observational study. *BMJ, 321,* 405–412.

Vaaler, S. (2000). Optimal glycemic control in type II diabetic patients. *Diabetes Care, 23*(Suppl 2), B30–B34.

Ware, J. E., Snow, K. K., Kosinski, M., & Gandek, B. (1993). *SF-36 health survey: Manual and interpretation guide.* Boston, MA: The Health Institute, New England Medical Center.

Watkins, K. W., Connell, C. M., Fitzgerald, J. T., Klem, L., Hickey, T., & Ingersoll-Dayton, B. (2000). Effect of adults' self-regulation of diabetes on quality-of-life outcomes. *Diabetes Care, 23*(10), 1511–1515.

Wilson, P. W., Cupples, L. A., & Kannel, W. B. (1991). Is hyperglycemia associated with cardiovascular disease? Framingham study. *American Heart Journal, 121,* 586–590.

Chapter 7
The Relationship Between Health Survey and Medical Chart Review Results in a Rural Population

Donald C. Voaklander, Harvey V. Thommasen and Alex C. Michalos

Introduction

Co-morbidity is an important dimension of health, particularly in older persons or persons with chronic conditions (Guralnik 1996). The importance of controlling for co-morbidity in outcome studies has been identified by others (Guralnik 1996; Iezzoni 1997) and various types of co-morbid measures have been used as covariates in research addressing mortality (Incalzi et al. 1997), health resource utilization (Librero et al. 1999; Rochon et al. 1996), re-admission to hospital (Librero et al. 1999), and health related quality of life (HRQL) (Jones et al. 2000, 2001). In addition, data on height, weight and obesity is often collected in clinical and survey research as the variable of interest or as an important covariate (Rowland 1989).

Voaklander, D.C., Thommasen, H.V., & Michalos, A.C.: 2006. The relationship between health survey and medical chart review results in a rural population. Social Indicators Research, 77, pp. 287–305. © Springer 2006.

D.C. Voaklander
BC Rural and Remote Health Research Institute, University of Northern British Columbia, 3333 Way, Prince George, BC V2N 4Z9, Canada
e-mail: voakland@unbc.ca

H.V. Thommasen
UBC Faculty of Medicine, University of Northern British Columbia, 4202 Davie Avenue, Prince George, BC V2M 4G7, Canada
e-mail: thommas@pgonline.com; thommash@unbc.ca

A.C. Michalos (✉)
University of Northern British Columbia, Prince George, BC, Canada
e-mail: michalos@brandonu.ca

A.C. Michalos, *Connecting the Quality of Life Theory to Health, Well-Being and Education*, DOI 10.1007/978-3-319-51161-0_7

An area of interest to health care researchers is how well health survey derived co-morbidity and height/weight information matches the clinical data of the same people as revealed by a review of their medical charts. In general height and weight information collected via survey has been reported to be reasonably valid and reliable (Palta et al. 1982; Pirie et al. 1981; Stewart 1982; Stunkard and Albaum 1981). However, others have commented that the reliability of selfreport measures of height and weight is compromised when composite measures of obesity such as body mass index (BMI) are calculated (Nieto-Garcia et al. 1990). It has also been reported that error is not uniform across subjects but can be mitigated by such things as gender, race, and upper or lower extremes of height and weight (Rowland 1989).

The accuracy of co-morbidity data from self-report has been shown to have generally good agreement with physician or medical records on serious diseases such as cancer, diabetes, liver disease and stroke but less agreement for conditions such as arthritis, back problems and depression (Bergmann et al. 1998; Bush et al. 1989; Haapanen et al. 1997; Harlow and Linet 1989; Kriegsman et al. 1996).

The object of this study is to understand the relationship between health survey and medical chart review results in a defined rural population.

Methods

Community Participation

This research project has been carried out in a participatory fashion, following the recommendations outlined in a recently published policy statement entitled "A Guide for Health Professionals Working with Aboriginal Peoples" and other guides to participatory action research (Brown et al. 1996; Cave and Ramsden 2002; Macaulay et al. 1999; Ramsden and Cave 2002; Redwood-Campbell et al. 1999; Smylie 2001). A goal of these recommendations is to make the relationship between Aboriginal people and non-Aboriginal Healthcare providers a fair and honorable one. There was extensive consultation with the Nuxalk Band Council, community members and local health care providers on our plans to study determinants of health and disease of people living in the Bella Coola valley. Prior to collecting data we obtained letters of support from the Nuxalk Band Council, from the Bella Coola Transitional Health Authority, and from Central Coast Regional District for a comprehensive study on determinants of health for people living in the Bella Coola valley. Last, but not least, we participated in potlatches asking for community support and explained the types of health projects we were planning to do.

Data Collection

A Health and Quality of Life Survey was offered to all adults (age 17 and up) living in the Bella Coola Valley between August 2001 and May 2002. Details of this survey methodology are reported elsewhere (Michalos et al. in press). Seven questions in this Health and Health Care Survey form the basis for this research paper. The first three questions are demographic questions—age, sex, and aboriginal status. Next, a question on the number of times a physician was seen in the past year. The next two were weight and height questions. Finally the question, "What is the major impairment(s) or health problem(s) that limits your activities" followed by 12 choices: (1) arthritis, (2) back or neck problem, (3) fractures, bone/joint injury, (4) lung/breathing problem, (5) hearing problem, (6) eye/vision problem, (7) heart problem, (8) stroke problem, (9) hypertension/high blood pressure, (10) diabetes, (11) cancer, and (12) depression/anxiety/emotional problem.

An identification number was given to each questionnaire sent out. A single investigator (HT) was the only one able to link this number to the 2001 clinic patient list. This information was used for the purposes of re-mailing, and for linking questionnaire responses to clinic charts. All recipients were asked to read an informed consent form or were read an informed consent form prior to completion of a questionnaire.

At the same time the Health and Quality of Life Survey was being offered to residents of the Bella Coola Valley, Dr. H. Thommasen did a detailed retrospective review of all clinic charts located in the Bella Coola Medical Clinic. Demographic information (age, sex, and aboriginal status), number of times a physician was seen in the past year, weight and height (if available), and the presence of 'health problems' was collected.

Definitions of health 'problems' were constructed prior to data collection and were designed to cover conditions listed in the Health and Quality of Life Survey (Michalos et al. in press).

(1) *Arthritis* (Edworthy and Arbillago 2001; Khraishi 2000; Wade and Watterson 1999). The term arthritis includes inflammatory arthritis (46%) and osteoarthritis (59%). Inflammatory arthritis refers to a collection of diseases in which the joint or joints are involved in a presumed autoimmune, inflammatory process. In this study, this includes rheumatoid arthritis, systemic lupus erythematosus, mixed connective tissue disease, polyarthralgia with positive rheumatoid factor or positive ANA, polymyalgia rheumatica, ankylosing spondylitis, psoriatic arthritis, and gout. The term arthritis does not include fibrositis/fibromyalgia syndrome (Edworthy and Arbillago 2001; Khraishi 2000; Wade and Watterson 1999). Osteoarthritis is a common degenerative joint disease characterized by progressive loss of articular cartilage and by formation of new bone at joint margins. These patients were identified here by X-ray confirmation of above, or clinic/consultant note that the patient had had joint replacement surgery because of debilitating osteoarthritis.

(2) *Back or neck problem* (Davis 1991; Gillies and Griesdale 1997). Patients were said to be suffering from back or neck problems if chart review revealed he or she had been seen more than once for a condition related to the neck or back that was causing pain or significant discomfort. Mechanical low back pain (64%), vertebral fractures (14%), discogenic nerve root pain (12%), spine degeneration (6%), followed by whiplash and other forms of musculo-ligamentous strain (4%) were the most commonly reported causes for a patient seeing a physician for back or neck problems. Vertebral fractures were mostly of the compression variety.

(3) *Bone/joint injury (includes fractures)* (Marx et al. 2001; Miller 2001). Patients said to be suffering from a bone/joint injury were those who presented to clinic with complaints of pain related to various musculoskeletal structures (66%); those who presented with pain associated with fractures (7%), trauma (8%), or amputation (3%); and those who presented with pain due to tendonitis (12%) or neuropathy (3%). The knee, shoulder, and hip were the most commonly mentioned joints causing pain and limitation.

(4) *Lung/breathing problem* (Baum et al. 1998). Clinic patients seen for asthma (72%), chronic obstructive pulmonary disease (27%), or other lung diseases (e.g. restrictive lung diseases) causing shortness of breath were said to have a lung/breathing problem. Asthma is an inflammatory respiratory condition characterized by increased responsiveness of the bronchi and bronchioles to various stimuli and manifested by widespread narrowing of the airways. Patients with asthma were identified by clinic notes recording wheezing or if they were being prescribed some sort of inhaled anti-asthmatic medication. Chronic Obstructive Pulmonary Disease includes emphysema and chronic bronchitis. Patients were identified as having COPD if there was a CXR report stating the person had COPD; if there was pulmonary function tests suggesting this person had COPD; or if there was a specialist report stating this person had probable COPD.

(5) *Hearing problem* (Ballenger and Snow 1996; Kennedy-Vosu and Brooks 1989). People noted to be wearing a hearing aid, and/or noted to be suffering from significant hearing loss were said to have a hearing problem. Details on causes of hearing loss were not collected.

(6) *Eye/vision problem* (Bains 1998). People said to have a significant eye/vision problem based on chart review were those who were said to have amblyopia (10%), retinal disease (45%), iritis/uveitis (15%), blindness due to trauma (7.5%), and chronic conjunctivitis, episcleritis, dry eye syndrome (17%). Examples of retinal disease include retinal vessel occlusion, detachment, and diabetic retinopathy.

(7) *Heart problem* (Braunwald et al. 2001; Gillis 2001). People said to have a heart problem based on chart review were those who had documented coronary artery disease (54%), cardiac dysrhythmias (35%) (including atrial fibrillation (27%)) which were felt significant enough to warrant medications (e.g. B-blockers, digoxin, amiodarone, calcium channel blockers) or

pacemaker treatment, valvular or congenital heart disease (9%), and/or congestive heart failure (25%).
Coronary Artery Disease refers to a condition characterized by narrowing of the lumen of coronary arteries due to accumulation of atherosclerotic plaque in the arterial wall. These changes result in possible compromising of the blood supply to the heart. Patients with coronary artery disease included those with: (1) Effort related chest pains responding to anti-angina medications (i.e. angina); myocardial infarction, (2) ECG changes consistent with recent or old myocardial infarction, (3) Clinical presentation consistent with recent myocardial infarction (e.g. elevated cardiac enzyme levels), (4) Consultant report confirming this person has probable coronary artery disease, (5) Angiographic changes consistent with coronary artery disease, and (6) If chart records this person had bypass surgery for their coronary artery disease. Congestive Heart Failure refers to a state of dysfunctional cardiac pumping that results in congestion of blood behind the dysfunctional cardiac pump. People were given this diagnosis if they were taking medications to treat congestive heart failure (CHF), if there was a cardiologist report stating this person had congestive heart failure, if there was an x-ray or other diagnostic test suggesting congestive heart failure, or if there was marked improvement of symptoms (e.g. ankle swelling, basal lung rales, and jugular venous distension) after being started on anti-CHF medications (e.g. ACE inhibitor, digoxin, diuretic, and B-blocker)

(8) *Stroke problem* (Copstead and Banasik 2000; Rowland 1995). People said to have a 'stroke problem' were those who had documentation in their chart indicating that they suffered from a major cerebrovascular accident (62.5%), or from recurring transient ischemic attacks (37.5%). Over 59% of people identified as suffering from a stroke problem were taking anti-platelet medications (e.g. ASA, clopidrogel).

(9) *Hypertension/high blood pressure* (Feldman 2003; Feldman et al. 1999). Hypertensive patients were identified as being patients who had elevated blood pressure (e.g. Systolic > 160 mm Hg or Diastolic > 95 mm Hg) documented on more than two clinic visits. The vast majority of these people (88%) were being prescribed antihypertensive medications (e.g. diuretics, B-blockers, Calcium channel blockers, ACE-inhibitors) and there is a note in chart that these medications are being prescribed for hypertension. The most commonly given reason for not taking medications is that the patient refused to take a prescription.

(10) *Diabetes* (Expert Comittee on the Diagnosis and Classification of Diabetes Mellitus 2002; Meltzer et al. 1998). Diabetes is a disorder of blood glucose metabolism. Diabetics were diagnosed on the basis of having repeatedly elevated blood glucose and/or elevated glycosylated hemoglobin (HGBA1c) values. Approximately 63% of diabetics in the chart review were taking oral hypoglycemic medications (e.g. glyburide, gliclazide, metformin); 15% were taking insulin; and 29% were 'controlled' by diet and exercise only.

(11) *Cancer* (DeVita et al. 1997; Fauci et al. 1998; Habif 1996). Cancer is a condition of disorderly cell division. Characteristics of cancer cells include lack of normal growth controls, decreased differentiation and function, ability to invade surrounding normal tissue and potential to travel to distant sites to produce secondary tumors (metastases). Cancer cells can arise from many different tissues in the body. The diagnosis of cancer is made by a pathologist based on observed changes to cell and tissue structure. Patients given the diagnosis of cancer had some sort of pathology report confirming malignancy; or had a specialist report stating this person had a pathology proven malignancy. The most common reported cancers in the clinic survey were breast (20%), gynecologic (20%), skin cancer (18%), urologic cancers (15%), gastrointestinal (14%), and others (12%). Gynecologic cancers include cervical, uterine, and ovarian cancers. Urologic cancers include prostate and testicular cancers. Skin cancers include squamous cell cancer, basal cell cancer, and malignant melanoma.

(12) *Depression/anxiety/emotional problem* (American Psychiatric Association 1997; Hutchison 2002; Reesal and Ewing 2001; Remick 2002). Patients presenting to family physician with affective depressive disorder (62%), situation depression (6%), anxiety disorder (12%), a mixture of debilitating depressive/anxiety symptoms (18%), and bipolar disorder (2%) were said to be suffering from depression/anxiety/emotional problem. Approximately 79% of people identified as suffering from depression/anxiety/emotional problem were taking an antidepressant medication. In this study it does not include patients with stress or anxiety symptoms alone. Antidepressant medications prescribed included tricyclic's (TCA), selective serotonin reuptake inhibitor's (SSRI), reversible monoamine oxidase inhibitor's (RIMA), norepinephrine and dopamine modulator's (NDM), serotonin antagonist and reuptake inhibitor's (SARI), and serotonin norepinephrine reuptake inhibitor's (SNRI).

After excluding clinic charts of people not living within the Bella Coola Valley and not currently living in the Bella Coola Valley, 2329 patients made up the September 2001 Clinic population list—approximately 102% of the May 2001 census estimate. A comparison of age distributions from May 2001 Canadian Census and a September 2001 chart review is shown in Table 7.1.

After completing the retrospective review of all clinic charts in the Bella Coola Medical Clinic, survey respondent answers were linked to the matching information retrieved from the chart review.

Analysis

Descriptive data are presented as means and frequencies. To determine the agreement between self-report versus clinically diagnosed morbidity intraclass

Table 7.1 Comparing census population to bcv clinic population

Age groups	May 2001 census Bella Coola Valley	September 2001 BCV clinic
0–4 years	155	181
5–14 years	365	371
15–19 years	195	197
20–24 years	120	122
25–44 years	695	696
45–54 years	355	371
55–64 years	210	190
65–74 years	120	131
75 years and over	70	70
Total	2285	2329

correlation (ICC) and kappa statistics were generated for continuous and dichotomous variables respectively. Excellent agreement was defined as kappa at 0.75 or greater, good agreement at kappa 0.40–0.74, and poor agreement for kappa below 0.40 (Landis and Koch 1977). For the ICC, excellent agreement occurred above 0.90, good when above 0.75, and poor when below 0.75 (Portney and Watkins 1993).

Results

Sample Characteristics

A total of 674 charts were successfully linked to the quality of life and disease prevalence surveys for a coverage rate of 39%. Table 7.2 describes the subject characteristics for those comprising the study group. For survey and clinic charts, 57% of the population was female. This rate is higher than that for the Bella Coola Valley (48%) reflecting the fact that more women than men completed the health questionnaire. According to survey results 36% of respondents were of aboriginal descent, which was slightly lower than the 37% calculated from reviewing respondent's clinic charts. These rates are lower than those that were calculated for the Bella Coola Valley (44%), reflecting the fact fewer aboriginal people completed the health questionnaire.

The average age (years) for the clinic population and survey populations was 48 years. The average number of times a survey respondent reported seeing a physician in the past year was 5.3. According to chart review the average number of times these survey respondents saw a physician (family physician and specialist) in 2001 was 5.4. In contrast, the entire Bella Coola Clinic population (aged 17 years and greater) averaged 4.2 physician visits in 2001. The lower number for the entire clinic population reflects the older population responding to the survey.

Table 7.2 Health survey and matched clinic population demographics and health conditions

	Health survey ($N = 674$)	Matched clinic population ($N = 674$)	Intraclass correlation co-efficient	Complete clinic population 17 years and older ($N = 1734$)
Age (years)	48.1 (16.1)	48.3 (16.5)	0.96^{***}	44 (16.7)
Height (cm)	168 (10.0)	168 (10.0)	0.93^{***}	168 (10.0)
Weight (kg)	78 (18.0)	80 (19.0)	0.92^{***}	81 (19.0)
BMI (kg/m^2)	27.6 (6.0)	29.7 (6.7)	0.87^{***}	29.4 (6.6)
Physician visits	5.3 (9.9)	5.4 (6.4)	0.56^{***}	4.2 (5.5)
			Kappa	
Sex (female)	384 (57)	385 (58)	0.97^{***}	877 (51)
Aboriginal ancestry	235 (36)	252 (37)	0.96^{***}	768 (44)
Diabetes	55 (8)	67 (10)	0.84^{***}	128 (7)
Cancer	13 (2)	31 (5)	0.53^{***}	65 (4)
Heart problems	32 (5)	45 (7)	0.49^{***}	107 (6)
Hypertension	64 (10)	118 (18)	0.47^{***}	223 (13)
Arthritis	115 (17)	113 (17)	0.45^{***}	163 (9)
Breathing problems	71 (10)	63 (9)	0.45^{***}	125 (7)
Depression	89 (13)	88 (13)	0.37^{***}	163 (9)
Back/neck problems	170 (25)	75 (11)	0.32^{***}	125 (7)
Eye problems	61 (9)	35 (5)	0.31^{***}	40 (2)
Stroke	10 (2)	8 (3)	$0\ 27^{***}$	34 (2)
Hearing problems	54 (8)	8 (1)	0.21^{***}	25 (1)
Bone/joint problems	62 (9)	55 (8)	0.13^{**}	156 (9)

***Significant at $P \leq 0.001$
**Significant at $P \leq 0.05$

Demographically there was excellent agreement between self-report and clinic data for age, sex, height, weight and Aboriginal ancestry.

Comparison of Health Problems: Survey Versus Clinic Data

Survey respondents were asked to circle from a list of 12 health problems ones which limited their activities. A summary of the prevalence rates calculated from the health survey information and from a review of medical charts is found in Table 7.2. Survey and chart prevalence rates for stroke (2% vs. 2%), arthritis (17% vs. 17%), and depression (13% vs. 13%) were identical. Survey prevalence rates were lower than chart prevalence rates for cancer (2% vs. 5%), heart problems (5% vs. 7%), diabetes (8% vs. 10%), and hypertension (9% vs. 18%). Survey prevalence rates were higher than chart prevalence rates for hearing problems (8% vs. 1%), vision problems (9% vs. 5%), lung/breathing problems (11% vs. 9%), and back/neck pain (25% and 11%).

For morbidity, there was excellent agreement between self-reported and clinically recorded diabetes. Good agreement was observed for diagnoses of cancer, heart problems, hypertension, arthritis and breathing problems. Poor agreement was observed for diagnoses of depression, back/neck problems, eye problems, walking problems, stroke, hearing problems and bone/joint problems. There was poor agreement between the number of self-reported and charted clinic visits. There were no significant differences in agreement between genders.

Height, Weight and Obesity

Excellent agreement was shown between self-reported height and weight and clinic height and weight. However when BMI was calculated only good agreement was achieved between self-report and chart data. In general subjects reported lower than actual weights. Figure 7.1 shows the difference between clinic BMI and self-report BMI. Fifty-two percent of subjects were at least one kg/m^2 great than their selfreported BMI. Figure 7.2 illustrates how this error can effect the classification of obesity in a survey population. Fourteen percent of subjects were classified in at least one lower obesity classification (normal, overweight, and obese) when self-report data is used. There was a small positive but significant correlation with weight and BMI error (r = 0.27; $p < 0.001$). Gender or age were not related to BMI error.

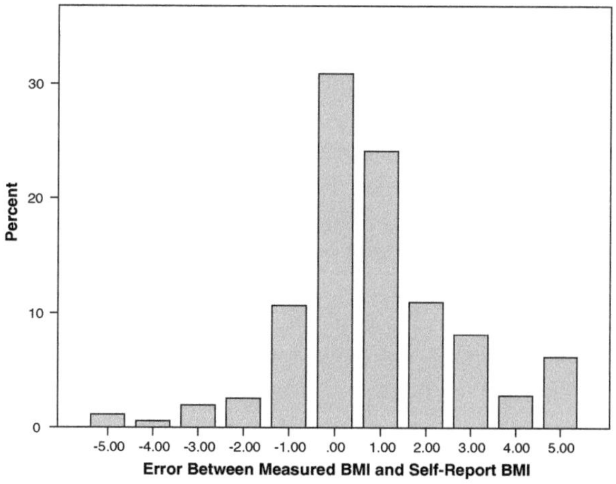

Fig. 7.1 Differences between self-report and clinic calculated BMI

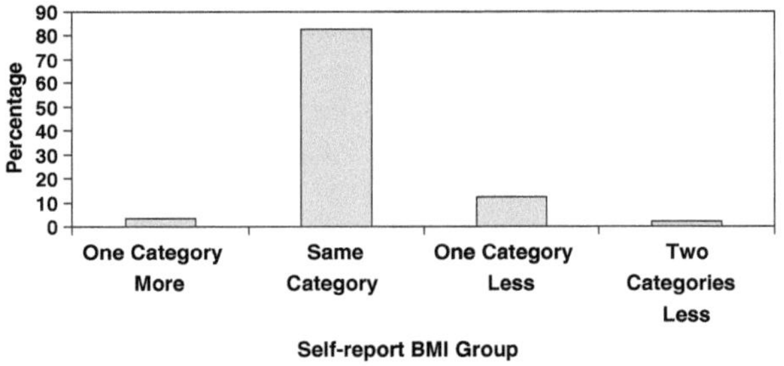

Fig. 7.2 Error in the classification of BMI category using self-report height and weight

Discussion

Demographics (age, sex, ethnicity, weight, and height), reported by Bella Coola residents on a Health and Quality of Life questionnaire matched up very well to the same information obtained from a review of respondents medical charts. However, the aggregate error when height and weight are converted to BMI is some cause for concern with a substantial number of persons categorized into lower obesity categories. As with other studies, increased weight was associated with greater error in reporting (Palta et al. 1982; Stunkard and Albaum 1981). Individuals have a tendency to aspire to their ideal weights, thus, the greater the deviation from that ideal weight, the greater the associated error in reporting (Stunkard and Albaum 1981).

For co-morbid conditions some health problems (diabetes, cancer, heart problems, hypertension, arthritis, and breathing problems) matched up well between self-report and chart. For other health problems there was a poor match (depression, back/neck problems, eye problems, walking problems, stroke, hearing problems, and bone/joint problems).

Comparison of self-reported health problem to chart health problem revealed discrepancies in health problem agreement which appears to reflect the degree to which a given health problem limits activity. For example, someone with hypertension could be taking medication for this problem and be identified from chart review as being hypertensive. That same person might have no signs or symptoms related to being hypertensive and so would not record on the health survey that he or she is limited by hypertension. For this reason, one would predict that hypertension would be a condition where chart review would reveal a higher health problem prevalence rate than that reported in the health survey. Cancer would be similar in that the chart review identifies people with cancer but does not take into account whether the cancer is limiting to one's activities. For example, cancers like squamous cell or basal cell skin cancers are readily cured by surgical excision. Conversely, hearing loss was reported much higher in the survey population, suggesting that clinic physicians rarely inquire about this problem. Presumably people suffering with this problem believe there is not much one can do about hearing loss so they rarely inquire or ask something be done about it. Alternatively, hearing loss may not be something which is clearly documented in the chart, and is easily missed when doing a chart review. Chronic back pain is something physicians can't cure as a general rule, and patients are generally told to cope with as best they can. Because of this, it makes sense that the survey population would report a higher prevalence rate for chronic neck/back pain than would the matched clinic chart review population. It has also been reported that persons self-report co-morbidity that is related to their quality of life rather than to their clinical profile (Voaklander et al. 2004).

There are some limitations in this study. First, not everyone living in the valley completed the health questionnaire. However we did calculate prevalence rates by reviewing all clinic charts so it is known how much the survey prevalence rates differ from the overall clinic recorded prevalence. The generalizability of the study is also an issue, as the Bella Coola Valley is a rural, remote community with over 40% of the residents being of aboriginal descent. Aboriginal people in British Columbia, across Canada, and across North America, have more health problems per capita—both physical and psychosocial—than non-native people. Looking at mortality rates for example; the infant death rate for aboriginals is over twice that for all of Canada; the death rate from injury and poisonings is four times the Canadian average; the suicide rate among 15–19 year old natives is six times the Canadian rate; and death from diabetes is six times the Canadian average (British Columbia Division of Vital Statistics 1989; British Columbia Provincial Health Officer 1997, 2002; Foster et al. 1995; Smylie 2001). One would predict that rates reported in our study would be higher than those reported for a community with a lower proportion of aboriginal people. However, as northern, rural and Aboriginal communities are generally under-sampled in the majority of national Canadian health surveys; this may be considered one of the few estimates of co-morbidity and obesity in these unique populations. Notwithstanding these limitations, the main objective of this study, to understand the relationship between health survey and medical chart review results in a defined rural population was still achieved.

In conclusion, the relationship between chart review and selfreport health information observed in this rural population is similar to findings from other populations. Researchers who use self-report data on co-morbidity and obesity measures as covariates should be aware of possible error in their estimates and how this would affect their findings.

Acknowledgements We would like to express thanks to the staff at the Bella Coola Medical Clinic for their assistance in distributing and collecting quality of life surveys. Thanks to Andy Bottomley for assistance with inputting survey data into electronic spreadsheets. We wish to thank the British Columbia Rural and Remote Research Institute for their financial support of this proposal. Dr. Thommasen would like to acknowledge the Community-Based-Clinical-Investigator Program for financial support.

References

American Psychiatric Association. (1997). *Diagnostic and statistical manual of mental disorders* (p. 317). Washington: American Psychiatric Association.

Bains, R. A. (1998). Managing the ten most common eye problems. *Canadian Journal of Diagnosis*, 68–79.

Ballenger, J. J., & Snow, J. B. (1996). *Otorhinolaryngology: Head and neck surgery* (p. 879). Philadelphia: Williams & Wilkins.

Baum, G. L., Crapo, J. D., Bartolome, R., & Karlinksy, J. B. (1998). *Textbook of pulmonary diseases* (Vols. 1–2, p. 341). Philadelphia: Lippincott-Raven.

Bergmann, M. M., Byers, T., Freedman, D. S., & Mokdad, A. (1998). Validity of selfreported diagnoses leading to hospitalization: A comparison of self-reports with hospital records in a prospective study of American adults. *American Journal of Epidemiology, 147,* 969–977.

Braunwald, E., Zipes, D. P., & Libby, P. (2001). *Heart disease: A textbook of cardiovascular disease* (p. 941). Toronto: WB Saunders Company.

British Columbia Division of Vital Statistics. (1989). Status Indians in British Columbia 1989, a vital statistics overview. *Division of Vital Statistics Quarterly Review,* 20–25.

British Columbia Provincial Health Officer. (1997). *A report on the health of British Columbians: Provincial health officer's annual report 1996* (p. 95). Ministry of Health and Ministry Responsible for Seniors: Victoria.

British Columbia Provincial Health Officer. (2002). A report on the health of British Columbians: Provincial health officer's annual report 2001 (p. xx). Victoria: Ministry of Health and Ministry Responsible for Seniors.

Brown, D., Calam, B., Grams, G. D., Grzybowski, S., Heffernan, C., Herbert, C. P., et al. (1996). The Haida Gwaii diabetes project: Non-insulin-dependent diabetes mellitus among the Haida. Summary Report to the British Columbia Health Research Foundation (p. 1). Vancouver: Department of Family Practice, University of British Columbia.

Bush, T. L., Miller, S. R., Golden, A. L., & Hale, W. E. (1989). Self-report and medical record report agreement of selected medical conditions in the elderly. *American Journal of Public Health, 79,* 1554–1556.

Cave, A. J., & Ramsden, V. R. (2002). Hypothesis: The research page-participatory action research. *Canadian Family Physician, 48,* 1671–1672.

Copstead, L. C., & Banasik, J. L. (2000). *Pathophysiology: Biological and behavioral perspectives* (2nd ed., p. 1023). Toronto: WB Saunders Company.

Davis, H. (1991). The cervical sprain syndrome: Psycho-organic aspects. *BC Medical Journal, 33,* 144–146.

DeVita, V. T., Jr., Hellman, S., & Rosenberg, S. A. (1997). *Cancer—Principles and practice of oncology* (Vols. 1–2, p. 79). Philadelphia: Lippincott-Raven Publishers.

Edworthy, S. M., & Arbillago, H. (2001). Osteoarthritis and degenerative joint disease. *Canadian Journal of Continuing Medical Education,* 93–109.

Expert Committee on the Diagnosis and Classification of Diabetes Mellitus. (2002). Report of the expert committee on the diagnosis and classification of diabetes mellitus. *Diabetes Care, 25,* S5–S20.

Fauci, A. S., Braunwald, E., Isselbacher, K. J., Wilson, J. D., Martin, J. B., Kasper, D. L., et al. (1998). *Harrison's principles of internal medicine* (Vols. 1–2, p. 491). Toronto: McGraw-Hill.

Feldman, R. (2003). The 2003 hypertension recommendations: What's new? *Canadian Journal of Diagnosis*, 81–84.

Feldman, R. D., Campbell, N., Larochelle, P., Bolli, P., Burgess, E. D., Carruthers, G., et al. (1999). Canadian recommendations for the management of hypertension. *Canadian Medical Association Journal, 161,* S1–S22.

Foster, L. T., Macdonald, J., Tuk, T. A., Uh, S. H., & Talbot, D. (1995). Native health in British Columbia. In P. H. Stephenson, S. J. Elliot, L. T. Foster, & J. Harris (Eds.), *A persistent spirit:*

Towards understanding aboriginal health in British Columbia (Vol. 31, pp. 43–94). Victoria: Western Geographic Press).

Gillies, J. H., & Griesdale, E. G. (1997). The mystery of low-back pain. *The Canadian Journal of Continuing Medical Education*, 55–68.

Gillis, A. M. (2001). Management of cardiac arhythmias. *Canadian Journal of Continuing Medical Education*, 167–179.

Guralnik, J. M. (1996). Assessing the impact of comorbidity in the older population. *Annals of Epidemiology, 6,* 376–380.

Haapanen, N., Miilunpalo, S., Pasanen, M., Oja, P., & Vuori, I. (1997). Agreement between questionnaire data and medical records of chronic diseases in middle-aged and elderly Finnish men and women. *American Journal of Epidemiology, 145,* 762–769.

Habif, T. P. (1996). *Clinical dermatology: A color guide to diagnosis and therapy* (p. 627). Toronto: Mosby.

Harlow, S. D., & Linet, M. S. (1989). Agreement between questionnaire data and medical records: The evidence for accuracy of recall. *American Journal of Epidemiology, 129,* 233–248.

Hutchison, R. (2002). Full remission: More likely with newer antidepressant drugs. *Patient Care Canada, 13,* 25–33.

Iezzoni, L. I. (1997). Dimensions of risk. In L. I. Iezzoni (Ed.), *Risk adjustment for measuring healthcare outcomes* (pp. 43–168). Chicago: Health Administration Press.

Incalzi, R. A., Capparella, O., Gemma, A., Landi, F., Bruno, E., Meo, F., et al. (1997). The interaction between age and comorbidity contributes to predicting the mortality of geriatric patients in the acute-care hospital. *Journal of Internal Medicine, 242,* 291–298.

Jones, C. A., Voaklander, D. C., Johnston, D. W. C., & Suarez-Almazor, M. E. (2000). Health-related quality of life outcomes after total hip and knee arthroplasties in a community-based sample. *Journal of Rheumatology, 27,* 1745–1752.

Jones, C. A., Voaklander, D. C., Johnston, D. W. C., & Suarez-Almazor, M. E. (2001). The effect of age on pain, function, and quality of life. *Archives of Internal Medicine, 161,* 454–460.

Kennedy-Vosu, L., & Brooks, C. (1989). Who is a candidate for a hearing aid? *Canadian Journal of Diagnosis*, 37–47.

Khraishi, M. M. (2000). Evaluation of fibromyalgia syndrome. *Canadian Journal of Continuing Medical Education*, 111–119.

Kriegsman, D. M., Penninx, B. W., van Eijk, J. T., Boeke, A. J., & Deeg, D. J. (1996). 'Self-reports and general practitioner information on the presence of chronic diseases in community dwelling elderly. A study on the accuracy of patients', selfreports and on determinants of inaccuracy. *Journal of Clinical Epidemiology, 49,* 1407–1417.

Landis, J. R., & Koch, C. G. (1977). The measurement of observer agreement for categorical data. *Biometrics, 33,* 159–174.

Librero, J., Peiro, S., & Ordinana, R. (1999). Chronic comorbidity and outcomes of hospital care: Length of stay, mortality, and readmission at 30 and 365 days. *Journal of Clinical Epidemiology, 52,* 171–179.

Macaulay, A. C., Gibson, N., Freeman, W., Commanda, L., McCabe, M., Robbins, C., et al. (1999). Participatory research maximizes community and lay involvement. *British Medical Journal, 319,* 774–778.

Marx, J. A., Hackberger, R. S., Walls, R. M., Adams, J., Barkin, R. M., Barsan, W. G., et al. (2001). *Rosen's emergency medicine: Concepts and clinical practice* (Vols. 1–2, p. 467). Toronto: Mosby.

Meltzer, S., Leiter, L. A., Daneman, D., Gerstein, H. C., Lau, D., Ludwig, S., et al. (1998). 1998 clinical practice guidelines for the management of diabetes in Canada. *Canadian Medical Association Journal, 159,* S1–S29.

Michalos, A. C., Thommasen, H. V., Anderson, N., Zumbo, B. D. (in press). Determinants of health and the quality of life in the Bella Coola valley. *Social Indicators Research.*

Miller, T. A. (2001). Repetitive-strain injuries: Description, not diagnosis. *Canadian Journal of Continuing Medical Education*, 201–214.

Nieto-Garcia, F. J., Bush, T. L., & Keyl, P. M. (1990). Body mass definitions of obesity: Sensitivity and specificity using self-reported weight and height. *Epidemiology, 1,* 146–152.

Palta, M., Prineaus, R. J., Berman, R., & Hannan, P. (1982). Comparison of selfreported and measured height and weight. *American Journal of Epidemiology, 115,* 223–230.

Pirie, P., Jacobs, D., Jeffery, R., & Hannan, P. (1981). Distortion in self-reported height and weight. *Journal of the American Dietetic Association, 78,* 601–606.

Portney, L. G., & Watkins, M. P. (1993). *Foundation of clinical research: Application to practice.* East Norwalk: Appleton and Lange.

Ramsden, V. R., & Cave, A. J. (2002). Hypothesis: The research page—Participatory methods to facilitate research. *Canadian Family Physician, 48,* 548–549.

Redwood-Campbell, L., MacDonald, W. A., & Moore, K. (1999). Residents' exposure to aboriginal health issues: Survey of family medicine programs in Canada. *Canadian Family Physician, 45,* 325–330.

Reesal, R. T., & Ewing, H. (2001). The art of managing depression in primary care. *Canadian Journal of Continuing Medical Education*, 209–220.

Remick, R. A. (2002). Diagnosis and management of depression in primary care: A clinical update and review. *Canadian Medical Association Journal, 167,* 1253–1260.

Rochon, P. A., Katz, J. N., Morrow, L. A., McGlinchey-Berroth, R., Ahlquist, M. M., Sakkarati, M., et al. (1996). Comorbid illness is associated with survival and length of hospital stay in patients with chronic disability: A prospective comparison of three comorbidity indices. *Medical Care, 34,* 1093–1101.

Rowland, M. L. (1989). Reporting bias in height and weight data. *Statistical Bulletin*, 3–9.

Rowland, L. P. (Ed.). (1995). *Merrit's textbook of neurology* (p. 227). Philadelphia: Williams & Wilkins.

Smylie, J. (2001). A guide for health professionals working with aboriginal peoples: Health issues affecting aboriginal peoples. *Journal of the Society Obstetrics and Gynaecology of Canada, 100,* 54–68.

Stewart, A. L. (1982). The reliability and validity of self-reported weight and height. *Journal of Chronic Disease, 35,* 295–309.

Stunkard, A. J., & Albaum, J. M. (1981). The accuracy of self-reported weights. *American Journal of Clinical Nutrition, 34,* 1593–1599.

Voaklander, D. C., Kelly, K. D., Jones, C. A., & Suarez-Almazor, M. E. (2004). Selfreport co-morbidity and health related quality of life—A comparison with record based co-morbidity measures. *Social Indicators Research, 66,* 213–228.

Wade, J. P., & Watterson, J. (1999). Keys to diagnosing inflammatory arthritis. *Canadian Journal of Continuing Medical Education*, 93–104.

Chapter 8
Health and Quality of Life of Older People, a Replication After Six Years

Alex C. Michalos, P. Maurine Hatch, Dawn Hemingway, Loraine Lavallee, Anne Hogan and Bev Christensen

Introduction

Celebrating the United Nations' International Year of Older Persons, in September 1999 a survey research project on people 55 years old or more was undertaken throughout an area of British Columbia designated as the Northern Interior Health Region (NIHR). The boundaries of all the health regions of the province have since been changed, but in September 2005 we undertook a replication of that survey in the same area. This report summarizes our main findings, including comparisons between the 2005 and 1999 samples wherever possible.

In section "Sampling Technique and Questionnaire" our sampling techniques and questionnaire are described, and following that some basic demographics of the two samples are provided (section "Sample Characteristics"). The health status of respondents in the two samples is reviewed in section "Health Status According to SF-36", followed by descriptive statistics regarding respondents' satisfaction with many specific domains of their lives (e.g., housing, friendships, sense of meaning in life) as well as with life as a whole and the overall quality of life, and happiness (section "Domain Satisfaction, Global Satisfaction and Happiness"). In section "Crime and Personal Safety" some descriptive statistics for the two samples are given concerning respondents' perceptions of criminal activity in the area,

Michalos, A.C., Hatch, P.M., Hemingway, D., Lavallee, L., Hogan, A., & Christensen, B.: 2007. Health and quality of life of older people: a replication after six years. Social Indicators Research, 84, pp. 127–158. © Springer Science+Business Media B.V. 2007.

A.C. Michalos (✉)
University of Northern British Columbia, Prince George, BC, Canada
e-mail: michalos@brandonu.ca

P.M. Hatch · D. Hemingway · L. Lavallee · A. Hogan · B. Christensen
Institute for Social Research and Evaluation, University of Northern British Columbia, Prince George, BC V2N 4Z9, Canada

A.C. Michalos, *Connecting the Quality of Life Theory to Health, Well-Being and Education*, DOI 10.1007/978-3-319-51161-0_8

criminal victimization, Crime-Related worries and defensive behaviours. Section "Issues and Troubles" contains a comparative review of respondents' views about some issues that our questionnaire-designing committee thought would have significance for the quality of people's lives, including an array of potential problems. In section "Social Support and Activities" we describe respondents' networks of social relations, social activities and social support. Section "Plan of the Following Seven Sections" provides an overview of the plan of analyses for sections "Explaining Health"–"Explaining SWB", which concerns only the 2005 sample. In these sections multiple regression analysis is applied in order to measure the impact (collectively and individually) that the great variety of aspects of life considered here actually have on respondents' perceived health, quality of life, happiness, life satisfaction, contentment with life and subjective wellbeing. Following these analyses, in section "Multiple Discrepancies Theory (MDT)" Multiple Discrepancies Theory (MDT) is used to explain the same set of dependent variables with an aim to comparing the relative explanatory power of the two types of explanatory models. Section "Conclusion" gives an overview of our most important results.

Sampling Technique and Questionnaire

In September 2005, 22-page questionnaires were distributed throughout the former NIHR of British Columbia with the aim of replicating a 1999 survey of the same region. Since there was no complete and authoritative list of older people for the region, we used a variety of means to assemble our sample. Questionnaires were given to all of the area's main seniors' organizations, recreation centres, local places of worship, the District Labour Council, native health centres, intermediate care homes, home care service providers, Meals on Wheels, commercial medical services providers, the local Advisory Council on Seniors, Alzheimer's Society, some independent seniors' housing units, friends, relatives and generally any eligible resident of the region. Arrangements were made for volunteers to help any respondents with visual or other types of problems filling out paper questionnaires.

The first four pages contained questions related to current housing accommodations and needs. These were followed by four pages dealing with a variety of problems regarding, for example, winter mobility in a northern community, older persons' stereotypes, activity centres and legal issues (e.g., wills and power-of-attorney). Then there were three and a half pages containing the 36-item Medical Outcomes Study Short Form (SF-36). Three pages of items concerning social relations, support and care-giving relationships came next. Then there were three pages of questions related to perceptions of criminal activity in the area, crime-related worries, defensive behaviour patterns and criminal victimization. There was a page of questions about respondents' satisfaction with particular domains or aspects of their lives (e.g., their family relations, housing and sense of meaning in life), their overall happiness, satisfaction with life as a whole and with the overall quality of their lives. Following the questions assessing various aspects of their lives, there were two pages of questions asking respondents to compare their lives to seven standards, e.g., to the lives of others their age and sex, and to the lives they think they deserve. Then there was another page of questions inviting respondents to reflect on their lives from various points of view. The questions concerning diverse standards and points of view about life were not in the 1999 questionnaire, but were added to this one in order to test some explanatory theories about people's health and quality of life. Finally, the questionnaire ended with some questions about public transit use and needs, and two pages of our standard demographic questions.

Sample Characteristics

By the end of October 656 useable questionnaires were returned, which formed the working data-set for the survey. The city of Prince George is the main urban settlement area in the region and its residents accounted for about 70% of the dataset. Of the 651 respondents who identified their gender, 417 (64%) were females. Their average age was 68, with a range running from 55 to 96 years. The average age of the 233 males was also 68, with a range running from 55 to 97 years. Forty-one percent of all respondents were aged 55–64 and within that group 67% were female. Sixty-two percent of respondents aged 65 years and older were female.

Fifty-six percent (364) of those who answered the marital status question were now married, including 65% (150) of the males and 51% (212) of the females. Another 3% (22) of respondents had live-in or common-law partners (3% (6) of the males and 4% (16) of the females). Twenty-two percent (143) of respondents were widowed, including 12% (27) of the males and 28% (115) of the females. Fourteen percent (92) of the sample were divorced or separated (14% (34) of the males and 14% (58) of the females). The remaining respondents were never married.

Ten percent (63) of the sample had some university education (8% (19) of the males and 11% (44) of the females) and 20% (129) held a university degree (20% (45) of the males and 20% (83) of the females). At the other end of the scale, 7% (48) of respondents had no education beyond elementary school (11% (26) of the males and 5% (21) of the females).

Ten percent (65) of respondents were employed full-time, including 12% (27) of the males and 9% (38) of the females. Another 6% (39) were employed part-time (4% (9) males and 7% (30) females).

For the 493 respondents who answered the income question, the median total household income was $38,000. For the 185 reporting males, the median household income was $45,000 and for the 308 reporting females, it was $35,000.

Compared to the 1999 sample, the 2005 sample was smaller (875 in 1999 vs. 656 in 2005), the average ages were nearly identical (69 vs. 68), the age ranges were identical (55–97), and the percentages of married respondents and respondents with some university education were identical, 56% and 10%, respectively. The percentages of females in each sample were close (68% in 1999 vs. 64% in 2005), as were the percentages of respondents employed full-time (9% vs. 10%) and part-time (7% vs. 6%). Apart from the total sample sizes, the biggest difference between the two samples was in the percentages of respondents holding university degrees, 8% in 1999 versus 20% in 2005. Considering all these figures, then, the 1999 sample provides a fairly good basis for comparing results from the 2005 sample.

Health Status According to SF-36

The 36-item Medical Outcomes Study Short Form (SF-36) was used in other studies of Prince George residents (Michalos and Zumbo 2003; Michalos et al. 2000, 2001) and has been shown to have good reliability and validity in several studies (Murray et al. 1998; Ware and Sherbourne 1992; McHorney et al. 1993, 1994; Ware et al. 1993, 1994). Table 8.1 summarizes its basic eight health status dimensions.

In the next two tables we summarize the eight SF-36 profile scores for males and females, aged 55–64 and 65 and over in the old NIHR, and compare the 1999 and 2005 sample scores. SF-36 profile scores are designed such that 0 represents the worst and 100 represents the best state of health.

Table 8.2 lists the scores for males in the four groups. The scores for the 2005 sample of male respondents aged 55–64 ranged from 85.4 for Social Functioning to 63.3 for General Health, with a mean of 76.1. This mean is a bit higher than the 74.4 mean of 1999. The scores for the 2005 male respondents aged 65 and older ranged from 83.2 for Social Functioning to 57.5 for Vitality, with a mean of 69.0. This mean is slightly higher than the 68.3 mean for the same age group in 1999, but considerably lower than the mean for the younger age group in 2005. Apparently age has its price. Based on these mean scores for the 8 dimensions, then, it is fair to say that the overall health status of males aged 55 years and older in the region was better in 2005 than in 1999.

Comparing the eight component scores for the 2005 and 1999 male respondents aged 55–64, we find that the 2005 scores are superior on 6 of the 8 dimensions. The only dimensions on which the 1999 sample scored better were General Health and Mental Health. Comparing the eight component scores for the 2005 and 1999 male respondents aged 65 and over, we find that the 2005 scores are again superior on 6 of the 8 dimensions, although a couple of the 6 are substantially the same. The two clear cases in which the 1999 sample in this age group was better off than the 2005 sample were Bodily Pain and Vitality, although the sample scores were very similar for the dimensions of General Health and Mental Health.

Table 8.3 lists the scores for females in the four groups. The scores for the 2005 sample of female respondents aged 55–64 ranged from 83.2 for Social Functioning to 61.3 for Vitality, with a mean of 73.1. This mean is practically identical to the

Table 8.1 Content of the SF-36 questionnaire

Concepts	Number of items	Meaning of low scores	Meaning of high scores
Physical functioning	10	Limited a lot in performing all physical activities including bathing or dressing due to health	Performs all types of physical activities including the most vigorous without limitations due to health
Role limitation physical	4	Problems with work or other daily activities as a result of physical health	No problems with work or other daily activities as a result of physical health
Bodily pain	2	Very severe and extremely limiting pain	No pain or limitations due to pain
General health	5	Evaluates personal health as poor and believes it is likely to get worse	Evaluates personal health as excellent
Vitality	4	Feels tired and worn out all of the time	Feels full of pep and energy all of the time
Social functioning	2	Extreme and frequent interference with normal social activities due to physical or emotional problems	Performs normal social activities without interference due to physical or emotional problems
Role limitation emotional	3	Problems with work or other daily activities as a result of emotional problems	No problems with work or other daily activities as a result of emotional problems
Mental health	5	Feelings of nervousness and depression all of the time	Feels peaceful, happy, and calm all of the time
Reported health transition	1	Believes general health is much worse now than one year ago	Believes general health is much better now than one year ago

Source Ware et al. (1993, p. 3:5)

Table 8.2 Comparisons of the 1999 and 2005 male scores on the 8 health dimensions of SF-36

Dimension	1999, 55–64, N = 90	1999, 65 and over N = 189	2005, 55–64, N = 86	2005, 65 and over, N = 147
PF	82.7	66.8	84.3	69.1
RP	74.4	55.7	79.0	57.9
BP	67.0	64.3	70.7	61.1
GH	65.8	62.2	63.3	62.8
VT	61.5	58.8	64.3	57.5
SF	82.4	79.5	85.4	83.2
RE	83.7	79.9	85.0	81.3
MH	77.9	79.0	76.9	79.2

mean of 73.0 for the same age group in 1999. The scores for the 2005 female respondents aged 65 and older ranged from 80.2 for Role Emotional to 55.0 for Role Physical, with a mean of 67.0. This mean is higher than the 65.4 mean for the

Table 8.3 Comparisons of the 1999 and 2005 female scores on the 8 health dimensions of SF-36

Dimension	1999, 55–64, *N* = 205	1999, 65 and over, *N* = 368	2005, 55–64, *N* = 179	2005, 65 and over, *N* = 235
PF	79.0	60.4	81.2	64.9
RP	70.1	54.7	70.5	55.0
BP	64.8	56.6	66.3	57.5
GH	68.1	63.9	63.6	63.4
VT	60.3	54.1	61.3	57.5
SF	81.7	78.7	83.2	79.8
RE	82.4	78.6	81.3	80.2
MH	77.2	76.4	77.6	77.5

same age group in 1999, but still lower than the mean for the younger age group in 2005. Age has its price for women too. Based on these mean scores for the 8 dimensions, then, it is fair to say that the overall health status of females aged 55 years and older in the region in 2005 was at least as good as (i.e., the same as or better than) that in 1999.

Comparing the eight component scores in turn for the 2005 and 1999 female respondents aged 55–64, we find that the 2005 scores are superior on 6 of the 8 dimensions. The only dimensions on which the 1999 sample scored better were General Health and Role Emotional. Comparing the eight component scores for the 2005 and 1999 female respondents aged 65 and over, we find that the 2005 scores are superior on all 8 dimensions, although the 1999 sample scores in this age group for Role Physical and General Health are fairly close to the 2005 scores.

Finally, comparing the mean scores for the eight dimensions for males with the mean scores for females for the two age groups, we find that males aged 55–64 were better off than females (76.1 vs. 73.1) and males aged 65 and over were also better off than females (69.0 vs. 67.0). Comparing the means of the eight dimensions taking each dimension in turn, we find that males aged 55–64 scored higher than females in 6 of 8 dimensions. For this age group, females scored slightly higher on General Health and Mental Health. For the 65 and over group, males again scored higher than females in 6 of 8 dimensions, with identical scores for Vitality and a higher female score for General Health.

Domain Satisfaction, Global Satisfaction and Happiness

Table 8.4 lists the mean scores for respondents' reported levels of satisfaction with several aspects of their lives and with life as a whole, including scores on the same items from the 1999 sample. The general format of the questions has been used in several studies (Michalos 2003), i.e., 'How satisfied are you with…?', with response categories running from 1 = very dissatisfied, through 4 = evenly

Table 8.4 Mean satisfaction and happiness levels, 2005/1999

How satisfied are you with your	Males 2005/1999	Females 2005/1999	Total 2005/1999
Housing	5.8/5.9	5.8/5.8	5.8/5.8
Neighbourhood	5.9/5.9	5.9/5.8	5.9/5.8
Family relations	5.8/6.0	5.9/6.0	5.9/6.0
Living partner	**6.4***/**6.5***	6.1/6.0	6.2/6.2
Job	5.6/5.4	5.7/5.3	5.7/5.3
Life as a whole	5.6/5.7	5.6/5.6	5.6/5.7
Friendships	5.5/5.7	5.7/5.9	5.6/5.8
Romantic relationships	5.2/5.5	5.1/5.0	5.1/5.2
Health	5.1/4.9	5.2/4.9	5.2/4.9
Access to health care	4.8/na	4.8/na	4.8/na
Religion or spiritual fulfilment	5.4/5.4	5.4/5.7	5.4/5.6
Financial security	5.0/4.9	5.0/4.7	5.0/4.8
Recreation activities	5.1/5.0	4.9/5.0	5.0/5.0
Level of physical activity	4.8/na	4.5/na	4.6/na
Level of social activity	4.9/na	4.9/na	4.9/na
Self-esteem	5.7/**5.5***	5.5/5.3	5.6/5.4
Air quality where you live	4.4/na	4.3/na	4.3/na
Quality of drinking water…live	5.3/na	5.2/na	5.3/na
Land pollution…live	5.0/na	4.8/na	4.9/na
Sense of meaning in life	5.6/na	5.7/na	5.7/na
Amount of free time	5.6/na	5.6/na	5.6/na
Personal safety around home	5.8/na	5.7/na	5.7/na
Federal gov. officials	3.3/3.1	3.3/3.0	3.3/3.1
Provincial gov. officials	3.2/2.8	3.1/2.5	3.1/2.6
Local gov. officials	3.8/3.8	3.8/3.7	3.8/3.8
Overall quality of life	5.6/5.4	5.6/5.5	5.6/5.5
Overall happiness	5.6/5.7	5.6/5.6	5.6/5.6
What you achieve in life	5.4/na	5.2/na	5.3/na
Future security	5.1/na	5.0/na	5.0/na
Feeling part of community	5.3/na	5.3/na	5.3/na
Caregiving role (N = 72/N = 136)	5.0/5.5	4.6/4.7	4.8/5.0

*Difference in the pair is significant at 0.05% level. Satisfaction scores range from 1 = very dissatisfied to 7 = very satisfied. Happiness scores range from 1 = very unhappy to 7 = very happy

balanced to 7 = very satisfied. Results for the two samples are remarkably similar. Generally speaking, for samples like these, pairs of scores are usually only statistically significant if the difference in their values are 0.3 or greater.

Regarding the 2005 sample as a whole, highest levels of satisfaction were reported for living partners (6.2), followed by family relations and neighbourhood, tied at (5.9). The first two of these domains registered the top two highest scores in 1999. Satisfaction with housing (5.8) followed in third place in both surveys. Satisfaction with jobs (5.7) in 2005 showed some significant improvement over 1999 (5.3). Two new items also had relatively high mean scores, namely, satisfaction with one's sense of meaning in life and personal safety around one's home (5.7 each).

In the previous section it was shown that self-reported health improved for men and women aged 55 and over in the 1999–2005 period. Reported satisfaction with health also revealed some improvement, from 4.9 to 5.2, largely based on improvement in women's reported satisfaction.

At the other end of the scale, highest levels of dissatisfaction were reported for provincial government officials (3.1), federal government officials (3.3) and local government officials (3.8). These were the domains registering lowest levels of satisfaction in 1999 in the same order, although there were some changes over the 6 years. Most notably, the Liberal provincial government of 2005 scored better than its New Democratic predecessor of 1999, 3.1 versus 2.6. Setting aside these government assessments, the domains registering the lowest mean satisfaction scores were air quality (4.3), level of physical activity (4.6) and access to health care (4.8). None of these domains were included in the 1999 survey. Of those included in both surveys, lowest scores were reported for financial security and recreation activities (5.0 each), followed by health (5.2). Apart from the government scores, these were also the lowest scores reported in 1999.

Regarding assessments of their lives as a whole for the total 2005 sample, all three global indicators (satisfaction with life as a whole and with the overall quality of life, and happiness) had the same mean score, 5.6. These were practically unchanged since 1999.

Examining the male and female scores for the 2005 sample, one finds only one pair of scores that are statistically significantly different. Males reported higher levels of satisfaction (6.4) than females (6.1) with their living partners. In 1999 that was one of only two cases in which there were statistically significant figures. We are not going to hazard a guess as to why men are apparently more satisfied than women with their living partners, most of whom are marriage partners.

Thus, considering the results summarized in this section, it seems fair to say that the perceived quality of life of older people in the former NIHR in 2005, so far as it is revealed in 28 domain and 3 global satisfaction and happiness scores, is at least as good as it was in 1999.

Crime and Personal Safety

Table 8.5 lists the percentage responses to the question 'Compared to 2 years ago would you say that crime has increased, remained the same or decreased in…?' for the 2005 and 1999 samples. For both samples, there was a striking difference between perceived local neighbourhood crime, which majorities of respondents thought stayed the same, and crime everywhere else, which majorities of respondents thought increased. Some of this difference is probably due to ego-centric bias.

In 2005, 68% of respondents thought local neighbourhood crime had stayed the same over the past two years, while 28% thought it increased and 4% thought it decreased. Over the same period, 59% of the same sample of respondents thought that crime in the city had increased, 71% thought that crime in British Columbia increased and 68% thought that crime in Canada increased. In each of the four cases, smaller percentages of respondents in the 2005 sample thought that crime had increased and larger percentages of respondents thought that crime had stayed the same. The percentages of respondents reporting decreases for the four cases were uniformly small, from 3 to 5%, and nearly the same for each time period for the four jurisdictions.

Objective statistics about levels of crime in the country, province and city are obtainable, but there are no neighbourhood statistics because we do not have a clearly defined set of neighbourhoods. According to a news release from Statistics Canada on July 21, 2005 (*The Daily*),

> Canada's crime rate, based on data reported by police services, fell a marginal 1% last year [2004]… Except for an increase in 2003, the crime rate has generally been falling since 1991 when it peaked. Police reported about 2.6 million offences in 2004, resulting in a crime rate [per 100,000 population] that was 12% lower than a decade ago.

Tables presented later in the story indicated that for British Columbia there was a slight increase of 0.2% in the 2003–2004 period. A *Municipal Crime Rate Report* dated July 2005 (Ministry of Public Safety and Solicitor General, B.C.) indicated that the Criminal Code total offence rate per 100, 000 for the municipality of Prince George was 176 in 2004 and 203 in 2003. It is likely, then, that there was in fact a decrease in crime in the region in the 2 years prior to our September 2005 survey.

Twenty-four percent of the respondents in 2005 reported that they never went out alone at night and another 24% said they rarely did so. In the 1999 survey, these figures were 36% and 26%, respectively. Forty-four percent of the 2005 sample

Table 8.5 Percentages of respondents saying that crime increased, remained the same or decreased compared to two years ago, 2005/1999

Area	Increased	Stayed same	Decreased
Your neighbourhood	28/39	68/56	4/5
This city	59/71	38/26	3/3
British Columbia	71/80	26/17	3/3
Canada	68/78	27/18	5/4

claimed they would feel reasonably safe going out alone in their neighbourhoods after dark and another 17% said they would feel very safe. The 1999 figures were 39% and 8%, respectively. Seventy-eight percent were very satisfied or satisfied with their personal safety around their homes, an item that was not included in the 1999 survey. As we found in our earlier surveys and as others have found (e.g., Braungart et al. 1980; Kennedy and Silverman 1984–1985), women reported higher levels of fear than men.

Table 8.6 lists the six items in our Index of Crime-Related Worries, with item mean and total mean scores for the 2005 and 1999 samples. The index was created by calculating each respondent's average score on the six items, finding the sum and dividing it by six. (The two negative items were recoded positively for the scale.) The average score for the 645 individuals who responded to the questions used in the construction of this index in 2005 was 2.8 (vs. 3.6 in 1999) and the range ran from 0 indicating 'never worry' to 10 indicating 'worry a great deal'. The Cronbach reliability coefficient alpha for the index was $\alpha = 0.90$. Respondents' biggest worry (4.2) was that someone would steal a personal item (e.g., coat or purse) when it was left somewhere unattended. That was the biggest worry for the 1999 sample too, but with a higher value of 4.9. The smallest worry in 2005 was that someone would cheat or con them out of a large amount of money (1.8), which was also the smallest worry in 1999, but more so (2.2). Compared to the 1999 survey, then, people responding to the 2005 survey tended to worry less about being victimized.

The relatively lower levels of worry about criminal victimization in 2005 were consistent with the lower levels of reported victimization. Only 7% of the 2005 sample reported being a victim of some crime, compared to 11% of the 1999 sample. Twenty-seven percent of the offences committed against the respondents were cases of breaking and entering a dwelling, house, outside building or business, and 28% of the offences involved theft of items costing less than $5,000. The 1999 figures were 46% and 40%, respectively. Ten percent of the offences in 2005 involved physical violence, e.g., spousal abuse (4%), assault, sexual assault and

Table 8.6 Mean scores of items in crime-related worries index, 2005/1999

Item [0 = never worry 10 = worry a great deal]	2005/1999
A thief will break into your home while you are away	3.4/4.3
Someone will use a weapon to take something from you by force	2.4/3.4
Someone will steal a personal item (e.g., coat, purse) when you have left it somewhere unattended	4.2/4.9
A thief will break into your home while you are home	2.3/3.4
Someone will cheat or con you out of a large amount of your money	1.8/2.2
Someone will assault you	2.5/3.2
Average score	2.8/3.6

elder abuse (2% each). The 1999 figure was 7%, with the increase mainly in spousal abuse.

Eighty-nine percent of the 2005 respondents reported that they locked the doors whenever they left home, compared to 95% in 1999. Fifty-two percent said they kept their doors locked when they were at home during the day, compared to 62% in 1999. Twelve percent said they avoided going downtown in their communities because of concern about crime, compared to 9% in 1999. Asked specifically about Prince George, 12% reported that they avoided going downtown during the day because of concerns about crime.

Considering all the crime-related material presented in this section, it appears to be the case that there was some decrease in the municipal overall crime rate from 1999 to 2005, which probably implies that the regional rate dropped too, given the relative size of the city population compared to that of the rest of the region. In spite of these actual decreases over the 6 year period, including the 2 years prior to the 2005 survey, a large majority of our respondents thought that crime had increased in the latter period. Notwithstanding the large majority perceiving increases in crime in the 2 year period prior to the survey, smaller percentages of the 2005 sample than of the 1999 sample thought that crime had increased over the past two years, avoided going out at night, feared for their safety, had crime-related worries, engaged in crime-related defensive behaviours and were actually the victims of any crimes. Therefore, it seems fair to say that, so far as crime-related issues are concerned for the two samples of seniors responding to our surveys, there is more evidence of improvement than of deterioration. The inconsistency between respondents' perceptions of changes in criminal activity and actual changes in objective crime rates is troublesome, but not unexplainable. Some years ago MacKuen (1984) showed that public concern with crime is much more a function of media reports than of actual crime rates.

Issues and Troubles

Table 8.7 lists the mean scores of 12 of 16 items that were of particular interest to members of the questionnaire-designing committee. For all of the 16 items respondents were asked to indicate their levels of agreement or disagreement on a five-point Likert scale running from 1 meaning 'strongly disagree' to 5 meaning 'strongly agree'. In the interest of some analyses undertaken later in this study, the 12 items in Table 8.7 were used to form an Index of Troubles, which was constructed by adding the means of these items and dividing by 12 for each respondent. The mean score of the index was 2.4 and its Cronbach alpha was 0.75. Examination of the mean scores in Table 8.7 reveals that by far the most troublesome item in the list (4.0) was the frustration respondents experienced with automated phone service that prevents them from speaking to a person. Following that, respondents were

Table 8.7 Mean scores on Index of Troubles items, 2005/1999

Item [1 = strongly disagree 5 = strongly agree]	Mean score
I worry about my ability to operate bank machines	1.8/2.5
Most people treat me like a stereotypical older person rather than like an individual	2.1/2.2
I have little opportunity to influence public policy	2.8/3.1
I have little opportunity to interact with young people	2.1/2.4
There are enough stores in my area so that shopping is convenient[a]	2.7/2.5
There are stores in my area but they are difficult to access	1.9/2.3
The stores in my area do not carry supplies that fit many of my needs	2.4/2.6
I am frustrated by automated phone service that prevents me from speaking to a person	4.0/na
I worry about stray dogs harming me when I go out in town or in local parks	2.4/2.8
In winter I try to avoid going out because there is too much ice on walkways in my area	2.7/3.3
If I could afford to leave the neighbourhood I am now living in, I would move	1.9/na
The neighbourhood in which I am now living is a good place to retire[a]	2.2/na

[a]Item reverse coded

most troubled by their inability to influence public policy (2.8), and the inconvenience of stores for shopping and ice on their walkways in winter (2.7 each). While the total array of scores indicates that respondents were not trouble-free, it is important to notice that only one of the 12 mean scores is above the mid-point (3.0) of the 5-point scale. Since a mean score of 1 would have been the best one could do and 5 would have been the worst, our respondents were generally closer to the former than to the latter. The sample of respondents in 2005 had better scores in 8 of the 9 items that were included in the 1999 survey.

Of the 632 respondents who replied to the item 'There should be only one main seniors activity centre in town', 38% strongly disagreed and 36% disagreed, compared to only 6% who strongly agreed and another 6% who agreed. In 1999, there were 79% disagreeing or disagreeing strongly and 9% agreeing or agreeing strongly. So, although there was some slippage in resistance in the 6 year period, the overwhelming majority still opposed the idea of a single seniors activity centre serving the whole community. There was strong support for local government being engaged in planning housing for its older population, with 91% of the sample agreeing or strongly agreeing. Eighty-six percent agreed or strongly agreed that local government should be setting aside land to build housing. In the 1999 survey, these figures were 91% and 93%, respectively. Fifty percent strongly agreed and 18% agreed that they would like to see specific courses at post secondary institutions for older people.

Social Support and Activities

Table 8.8 lists the percentages of respondents saying that they had someone who they could count on for four kinds of social support, for the 2005 and 1999 samples. The results for both surveys are practically the same and indicate very high levels of support. In 2005, from 86 to 92% of respondents indicated that they knew such a person, compared to from 86 to 93% in 1999. We constructed a Social Support Index by summing the number of yes responses on the four items, obtaining Cronbach alphas of 0.76 and 0.75, for 2005 and 1999, respectively.

In addition to the very direct questions about social support, our questionnaire contained several questions about social activities, which were designed to measure diverse ways in which people may be connected to others in their community. Sixty-five percent of respondents were members of some kind of voluntary organization, such as school groups, church social groups, community centres, ethnic associations or social clubs. Of the 417 people who said they belonged to such organizations, 42% reported that they participated in organization-sponsored meetings or activities once or twice a week over the past 12 months, and another 25% participated about once a month. Forty percent (265) of our respondents said that they served as a volunteer an average of 5 h per week, with a wide range from 0.5 to 72 h per week.

Sixty-nine percent reported that they were not members of a Seniors Centre. In response to a question about why they had not become members, 33% said that they did not feel old enough, 16% did not have time and 11% were already active in some other organization. Of the 215 respondents who belonged to Seniors Centres, 31% said they participated in Centre-sponsored activities once or twice a week over the past 12 months, 13% said three or more times a week and 20% said not at all.

In response to a question about how often respondents attended religious services in the past 12 months, apart from special occasions like weddings and funerals, 54% said not at all, 19% said once or twice a week and 3% said three or more times a week.

Fifty-four percent reported that they had a romantic relationship with someone, 12% said they would like to have a relationship and 34% said they would not. Of

Table 8.8 Percent answering 'yes' to Social Support Index items, 2005/1999

Items	% yes
Do you have someone you can confide in or talk to about your private feelings or concerns?	86/86
Do you have someone you can really count on to help you out in a crisis situation?	92/93
Do you have someone you can really count on to give you advice when you are making important personal decisions?	86/86
Do you have someone who makes you feel loved and cared for?	91/93

the 427 people who answered our question about how satisfied they were with their romantic relationship(s), 32% said they were very satisfied and another 19% were satisfied. Only 8% were very dissatisfied and another 3% were dissatisfied.

Plan of the Following Seven Sections

In the next seven sections we make similar analyses explaining in turn self-reported health measured by the SF-36 General Health scale and a single item scale, satisfaction with life as a whole measured with a single item, happiness measured with a single item, satisfaction with the overall quality of life measured with a single item, satisfaction with life measured with the Satisfaction with Life Scale (SWLS), contentment with life measured with the Contentment with Life Assessment Scale (CLAS) and subjective wellbeing measured with the Index of Subjective Wellbeing (SWB).

The SF-36 General Health scale is one of the 8 dimensions of the SF-36 set and it is formed from five items. The first item says 'In general, would you say your health is excellent, very good, good, fair or poor'. This single item is often used by itself as a general measure of self-reported health (Michalos 2004), and its Pearson correlation with the SF-36 General Health scale is $r = 0.50$. So we thought it would be worthwhile to compare results using the two measures. The other four items in the SF-36 General Health scale are 'I seem to get sick a little easier than other people. I am as healthy as anybody I know. I expect my health to get worse. My health is excellent.' Each of the latter has five response categories running from 'definitely true' to 'definitely false'.

The three single item global indicators regarding life as a whole, overall quality of life and happiness were described earlier. The SWLS came from Diener et al. (1985) and has five items with seven response categories running from 7 = strongly agree to 1 = strongly disagree. The items are 'The conditions of my life are excellent. So far I have gotten the important things I want in life. In most ways my life is close to my ideal. I am satisfied with my life. If I could live my life over, I would change almost nothing. For the 2005 sample SWLS has a Cronbach alpha of 0.92.

The CLAS came from Lavallee et al. (in press) and also has five items with the same response categories as SWLS. The items are 'I am very content with my life. I am living my life to the fullest. Nothing is currently lacking in my life. When I examine my life as a whole, I feel that I am not meeting my aspirations. I feel dissatisfied because I'm not doing everything that I want to be doing in my life'. (The two negative items were recoded positively for the scale.) For the 2005 sample, the CLAS has a Cronbach alpha of 0.86.

The SWB was developed by Michalos and Zumbo and has been used in several studies, e.g., Michalos et al. (2005). It has four global items, including the single items on happiness, satisfaction with life as a whole and satisfaction with the overall quality of life, plus satisfaction with one's standard of living. The SWB Cronbach alpha is 0.87.

In each of the next seven sections there are five stepwise regression analyses involving a different dependent variable, with mean replacement of missing values of predictor variables. Because the SF-36 General Health scale is being used as a dependent variable and we want to use the same set of predictors to explain all of our dependent variables, only the remaining 7 SF-36 dimensions of health are used as predictors in all of our analyses. In the first regression, a dependent variable is regressed on the 7 SF-36 health dimensions, with results reported in the column under 'Health'. Second, the same dependent variable is regressed on the Social Support Index, frequency of activity participation, satisfaction with family, living partner, friendships, romantic relationships and feeling part of the community, with results reported in the column under 'Social Relations'. Third, that dependent variable is regressed on the Index of Troubles, Crime-Related Worries Index, difficulty meeting housing costs and percent of income spent on housing, with results reported in the column under 'Problems'. Fourth, the dependent variable is regressed on 11 satisfaction measures involving housing, neighbourhoods, religion, financial security, recreation, self-esteem, environment (mean of air, water and land items), government officials (mean of federal, provincial and local items), sense of meaning in life, achievements in life and future security, with results reported in the column under 'Domain Satisfaction'. Finally, the dependent variable is regressed on all the statistically significant predictors from the first four regressions, with results reported in the column under 'All Predictors'. Following this plan, each of the five numerical columns of the next seven tables reveals the explanatory power of each of our predictors in combination with others. For every dependent variable, we will be able to assess the total explanatory power of each set of predictors, and the relative impact of particular predictors on particular dependent variables when the impact of all the others is held constant.

Explaining Health

For ease of comparison, results for the two measures of general health (i.e., the SF-36 General Health scale and the single item) are printed side by side (e.g., x/x) in Table 8.9. The results reported in the first column of this Table 8.9. The results reported in the first column of this table are based on regressing each health measure on the seven remaining dimensions of SF-36. Interestingly enough, the seven dimensions do a better job explaining the variation in the single item scores ($R^2 = 0.45$) than in the General Health scale scores ($R^2 = 0.32$). As well, 4 of the 7 dimensions have significant impacts on the single item, compared to 3 for the General Health scale. Nevertheless, in both cases the SF-36 Social Functioning scale was the strongest predictor, with standardized regression coefficients (Betas) of $\beta = 0.40$ for the General Health scale and $\beta = 0.33$ for the single item health measure. Figuratively speaking, one might say, for example, that with all variables

Table 8.9 Regressions of SF-36 General Health/single item health on other SF-36 health scales, social relations, problems and domain satisfaction (decimal points omitted)

Predictor clusters →	Health[a]	Soc. relat.[b]	Problems[c]	Domain sat.[d]	All pred.[e]
Percentage of variance explained	32/45	7/9	10/14	14/20	33/47
Predictors ↓	Betas	Betas	Betas	Betas	Betas
Physical functioning	10/25	f/f	f/f	f/f	10/23
Role limitation physical	g/13	f/f	f/f	f/f	f/13
Bodily pain	g/11	f/f	f/f	f/f	f/10
Vitality	40/33	f/f	f/f	f/f	39/28
Social functioning	14/g	f/f	f/f	f/f	12/f
Role limitation emotional	g/g	f/f	f/f	f/f	f/f
Mental health	g/g	f/f	f/f	f/f	f/f
Social support index	f/f	g/10	f/f	f/f	f/g
Frequency of activity participation	f/f	g/g	f/f	f/f	f/f
Satisfaction with family	f/f	g/g	f/f	f/f	f/f
Satisfaction with living partner	f/f	g/−8	f/f	f/f	f/−10
Satisfaction with friendships	f/f	11/g	f/f	f/f	g/f
Sat. with romantic relationships	f/f	g/g	f/f	f/f	f/f
Sat. with feeling part of community	f/f	20/28	f/f	f/f	g/g
Index of troubles	f/f	f/f	−21/−25	f/f	g/−9
Crime-related worries index	f/f	f/f	−8/g	f/f	g/f
Difficulty meeting housing costs	f/f	f/f	−14/−15	f/f	g/g
Percentage of income spent on housing costs	f/f	f/f	g/−10	f/f	f/g
Satisfaction with housing	f/f	f/f	f/f	g/g	f/f
Satisfaction with neighbourhood	f/f	f/f	f/f	10/g	10/f
Satisfaction with religion	f/f	f/f	f/f	g/g	f/f
Satisfaction with financial security	f/f	f/f	f/f	g/g	f/f
Satisfaction with recreation	f/f	f/f	f/f	25/36	g/g
Satisfaction with self-esteem	f/f	f/f	f/f	g/g	f/f
Satisfaction with environment	f/f	f/f	f/f	g/g	f/f
Sat. with government officials	f/f	f/f	f/f	g/g	f/f
Sat. with sense of meaning in life	f/f	f/f	f/f	g/g	f/f
Sat. with achievements in life	f/f	f/f	f/f	g/14	f/10
Satisfaction with future security	f/f	f/f	f/f	12/g	g/f

[a]Dimensions from SF-36
[b]Social Support Index, activity frequency, satisfaction with family, living partner, friendships, romantic relationships, feeling part of the community
[c]Index of Troubles, Crime-Related Worries Index, difficulty meeting housing costs, % of income spent on housing costs
[d]13 domain satisfaction scores
[e]a + b + c + d
[f]Variable not in equation
[g]Significance level too low for variable to enter equation

standardized to have means of zero and standard deviations of one, for every full step of increase in respondents' Social Functioning, there would be an increase of 40% of a full step in respondents' general health measured by the SF-36 scale and 33% of a full step measured by the single item, respectively, if the value of every other variable was held constant.

The second column of Table 8.9 reveals that our seven measures of social relations had relatively little influence on either of the two general health measures, explaining only 7 and 9% of the variance in the SF-36 scale and single item measure, respectively. In both cases, only 2 of the 7 measures had statistically significant influence and satisfaction with feeling part of the community was the strongest predictor, with $\beta = 0.20$ and $\beta = 0.28$ for the SF-36 scale and the single item measure, respectively.

The third column shows some improvement in explanatory power, with the four measures of problems explaining 10 and 14% of the variance in the SF-36 scale and the single item scale, respectively. In both cases, 3 of the 4 measures had statistically significant influence and the Index of Troubles was most influential and negatively so, with $\beta = -0.21$ and $\beta = -0.25$ for the SF-36 scale and the single item measure, respectively.

The fourth column indicates another increment in explanatory power, with only 3 and 2 of 11 domain satisfaction predictors accounting for 14% and 20% of the variance in the SF-36 scale and the single item scale, respectively.

Finally, the fifth column gives the results of regressing the two health measures on all the statistically significant predictors from the first four regressions for each measure. In the comprehensive set of 11 potential predictors, only 4 were significantly influential to the SF-36 General Health scale scores, explaining 33% of their variance. In the comprehensive set of 12 potential predictors, 7 were influential to the single item scores, explaining 47% of their variance. In both cases, the SF-36 Vitality scale was the strongest predictor, with $\beta = 0.39$ and $\beta = 0.28$ for the SF-36 scale and the single item measure, respectively.

Explaining Satisfaction with Life as a Whole

The first numerical column of Table 8.10 shows that 2 of the 7 SF-36 health dimensions explained 30% of the variation in Life Satisfaction scores. The most influential predictor was Mental Health ($\beta = 0.36$), followed by Social Functioning ($\beta = 0.25$). It should be noticed that the same set of predictors did a better job at explaining General Health (Table 8.9), and that the set of influential health-related predictors for Life Satisfaction was different from the set of influential predicators of General Health. Vitality was most influential for General Health, but had no significance for Life Satisfaction, while Mental Health was most influential for Life Satisfaction, but had no significance for General Health. Clearly, the idea of good health is different from the idea of a satisfying life.

Table 8.10 Regressions of life satisfaction on SF-36 health scales, social relations, problems and domain satisfaction (decimal points omitted)

Predictor clusters →	Health[a]	Soc. relat.[b]	Problems[c]	Domain sat.[d]	All pred.[e]
Percentage of variance explained	30	57	18	63	70
Predictors ↓	Betas	Betas	Betas	Betas	Betas
Physical functioning	g	f	f	f	f
Role limitation physical	g	f	f	f	f
Bodily pain	g	f	f	f	f
Vitality	g	f	f	f	f
Social functioning	25	f	f	f	g
Role limitation emotional	g	f	f	f	f
Mental health	36	f	f	f	5
Social support index	f	g	f	f	f
Frequency of activity participation	f	g	f	f	f
Satisfaction with family	f	11	f	f	g
Satisfaction with living partner	f	14	f	f	10
Satisfaction with friendships	f	51	f	f	31
Sat. with romantic relationships	f	g	f	f	f
Sat. with feeling part of community	f	19	f	f	g
Index of troubles	f	f	−22	f	g
Crime-related worries index	f	f	−18	f	−6
Difficulty meeting housing costs	f	f	−20	f	g
Percentage of income spent on housing costs	f	f	g	f	f
Satisfaction with housing	f	f	f	g	f
Satisfaction with neighbourhood	f	f	f	12	8
Satisfaction with health	f	f	f	35	24
Satisfaction with religion	f	f	f	g	f
Satisfaction with financial security	f	f	f	g	f
Satisfaction with recreation	f	f	f	g	f
Satisfaction with self-esteem	f	f	f	g	f
Satisfaction with environment	f	f	f	g	f
Sat. with government officials	f	f	f	−5	g
Sat. with sense of meaning in life	f	f	f	19	7
Sat. with achievements in life	f	f	f	16	12
Satisfaction with future security	f	f	f	17	11

[a]Dimensions from SF-36
[b]Social Support Index, activity frequency, satisfaction with family, living partner, friendships, romantic relationships, feeling part of the community
[c]Index of Troubles, Crime-Related Worries Index, difficulty meeting housing costs, % of income spent on housing costs
[d]13 domain satisfaction scores
[e]a + b + c + d
[f]Variable not in equation
[g]Significance level too low for variable to enter equation

The second column of Table 8.10 reveals that 4 of our 7 measures of social relations had a relatively powerful impact on Life Satisfaction, explaining 57% of the variance in Life Satisfaction scores. The most influential predictor was satisfaction with friendships ($\beta = 0.51$), followed at some distance by satisfaction with feeling part of the community ($\beta = 0.19$).

The third column shows that 3 of the 4 measures of problems explained 18% of the variance in Life Satisfaction scores, with the Index of Troubles most influential ($\beta = -0.22$), but relatively close to the other two predictors.

The fourth column indicates that 6 of the 11 domain satisfaction predictors accounted for 63% of the variance in Life Satisfaction scores, with satisfaction with one's own health most influential ($\beta = 0.35$), followed at some distance by satisfaction with a sense of meaning in life ($\beta = 0.19$).

The fifth column gives the results of regressing Life Satisfaction scores on all the statistically significant predictors from the first four regressions. In the comprehensive set of 15 potential predictors, 8 were significantly influential, explaining 70% of the variation. The most influential predictor was satisfaction with friendships ($\beta = 0.31$), followed by health satisfaction ($\beta = 0.24$).

People's assessments of their satisfaction with their health are not the same as their assessments of their health itself. For our respondents, health satisfaction correlated $r = 0.55$ with the SF-36 General Health scale and $r = 0.59$ with the single item general health measure. As we move through the set of non-health dependent variables, it should be noticed that in 5 of 6 cases health satisfaction has more influence than actual health measured by the SF-36 scales. In the present case, the only SF-36 scale that remained statistically significant in the final regression was Mental Health, and its explanatory power was greatly reduced to $\beta = 0.05$.

Explaining Happiness with Life as a Whole

The first numerical column of Table 8.11 shows that 4 of the 7 SF-36 health dimensions explained 34% of the variation in Happiness scores, with Mental Health most influential ($\beta = 0.37$), followed by Social Functioning ($\beta = 0.20$).

The second column of Table 8.11 reveals that 5 of our 7 measures of social relations explained 41% of the variance in Happiness scores, with satisfaction with friendships ($\beta = 0.25$) and satisfaction with feeling part of the community ($\beta = 0.24$) most influential.

The third column shows that 3 of the 4 measures of problems explained 15% of the variance in Happiness scores, with the Index of Troubles most influential ($\beta = -0.22$), followed by difficulty meeting housing costs ($\beta = -0.18$).

The fourth column indicates that 5 of the 11 domain satisfaction predictors accounted for 45% of the variance in Happiness scores, with satisfaction with one's

Table 8.11 Regressions of happiness on SF-36 health scales, social relations, problems and domain satisfaction (decimal points omitted)

Predictor clusters →	Health[a]	Soc. relat.[b]	Problems[c]	Domain sat.[d]	All pred.[e]
Percentage of variance explained	34	41	15	45	53
Predictors ↓	Betas	Betas	Betas	Betas	Betas
Physical functioning	g	f	f	f	f
Role limitation physical	−11	f	f	f	g
Bodily pain	g	f	f	f	f
Vitality	15	f	f	f	g
Social functioning	20	f	f	f	g
Role limitation emotional	g	f	f	f	f
Mental health	37	f	f	f	24
Social support index	f	9	f	f	6
Frequency of activity participation	f	g	f	f	f
Satisfaction with family	f	13	f	f	g
Satisfaction with living partner	f	g	f	f	f
Satisfaction with friendships	f	25	f	f	9
Sat. with romantic relationships	f	20	f	f	17
Sat. with feeling part of community	f	24	f	f	7
Index of troubles	f	f	−22	f	g
Crime-related worries index	f	f	−15	f	g
Difficulty meeting housing costs	f	f	−18	f	g
Percentage of income spent on housing costs	f	f	g	f	f
Satisfaction with housing	f	f	f	12	11
Satisfaction with neighbourhood	f	f	f	g	f
Satisfaction with health	f	f	f	27	16
Satisfaction with religion	f	f	f	g	f
Satisfaction with financial security	f	f	f	g	f
Satisfaction with recreation	f	f	f	g	f
Satisfaction with self-esteem	f	f	f	g	f
Satisfaction with environment	f	f	f	g	f
Sat. with government officials	f	f	f	g	f
Sat. with sense of meaning in life	f	f	f	20	11
Sat. with achievements in life	f	f	f	11	g
Satisfaction with future security	f	f	f	14	8

[a]Dimensions from SF-36
[b]Social Support Index, activity frequency, satisfaction with family, living partner, friendships, romantic relationships, feeling part of the community
[c]Index of Troubles, Crime-Related Worries Index, difficulty meeting housing costs, % of income spent on housing costs
[d]13 domain satisfaction scores
[e]a + b + c + d
[f]Variable not in equation
[g]Significance level too low for variable to enter equation

own health most influential ($\beta = 0.27$), followed by satisfaction with a sense of meaning in life ($\beta = 0.20$).

The fifth column gives the results of regressing Happiness scores on all the statistically significant predictors from the first four regressions. In the comprehensive set of 17 potential predictors, 9 were significantly influential, explaining 53% of the variation. The most influential predictor was the SF-36 scale of Mental Health ($\beta = 0.24$), followed by satisfaction with romantic relationships ($\beta = 0.17$) and health satisfaction ($\beta = 0.16$). Clearly, the idea of a happy life is not the same as the idea of a satisfying life.

Explaining Satisfaction with the Overall Quality of Life

The first numerical column of Table 8.12 shows that 3 of the 7 SF-36 health dimensions explained 28% of the variation in Satisfaction with the overall Quality of Life scores, with Mental Health and Social Functioning most influential ($\beta = 0.22$ each).

The second column reveals that 5 of our 7 measures of social relations explained 41% of the variance in Quality of Life Satisfaction scores, with satisfaction with feeling part of the community most influential ($\beta = 0.34$), followed by satisfaction with friendships ($\beta = 0.30$).

The third column shows that the four measures of problems explained 23% of the variance in Quality of Life Satisfaction scores, with the Index of Troubles most influential ($\beta = -0.26$), followed by difficulty meeting housing costs ($\beta = -0.21$).

The fourth column indicates that 8 of the 11 domain satisfaction predictors accounted for 63% of the variance in scores for Satisfaction with the overall Quality of Life, with satisfaction with a sense of meaning in life most influential ($\beta = 0.21$), followed by satisfaction with health ($\beta = 0.17$) and financial security ($\beta = 0.15$).

The fifth column gives the results of regressing overall Quality of Life Satisfaction scores on all the statistically significant predictors from the first four regressions. In the comprehensive set of 20 potential predictors, 11 were significantly influential, explaining 64% of the variation. The most influential predictor was satisfaction with a sense of meaning in life ($\beta = 0.19$), followed by satisfaction with health ($\beta = 0.16$) and financial security ($\beta = 0.14$). The fact that respondents' assessments of their satisfaction with the overall quality of their lives (perceived quality of life) drew significantly on more aspects of their lives apparently shows that the idea of the quality of life is more comprehensive or inclusive than the ideas of life satisfaction and happiness, and of course much more so than the idea of general health.

Table 8.12 Regressions of satisfaction with the overall quality of life on SF-36 health scales, social relations, problems and domain satisfaction (decimal points omitted)

Predictor clusters →	Health[a]	Soc. relat.[b]	Problems[c]	Domain sat.[d]	All pred.[e]
Percentage of variance explained	28	46	23	63	64
Predictors ↓	Betas	Betas	Betas	Betas	Betas
Physical functioning	g	f	f	f	f
Role limitation physical	g	f	f	f	f
Bodily pain	g	f	f	f	f
Vitality	19	f	f	f	g
Social functioning	22	f	f	f	g
Role limitation emotional	g	f	f	f	f
Mental health	22	f	f	f	g
Social support index	f	g	f	f	f
Frequency of activity participation	f	6	f	f	5
Satisfaction with family	f	8	f	f	g
Satisfaction with living partner	f	g	f	f	f
Satisfaction with friendships	f	30	f	f	7
Sat. with romantic relationships	f	14	f	f	8
Sat. with feeling part of community	f	34	f	f	8
Index of troubles	f	f	−26	f	g
Crime-related worries index	f	f	−8	f	g
Difficulty meeting housing costs	f	f	−21	f	g
Percentage of income spent on housing costs	f	f	−12	f	g
Satisfaction with housing	f	f	f	11	10
Satisfaction with neighbourhood	f	f	f	g	f
Satisfaction with health	f	f	f	17	16
Satisfaction with religion	f	f	f	g	f
Satisfaction with financial security	f	f	f	15	14
Satisfaction with recreation	f	f	f	14	12
Satisfaction with self-esteem	f	f	f	13	12
Satisfaction with environment	f	f	f	g	f
Sat. with government officials	f	f	f	8	8
Sat. with sense of meaning in life	f	f	f	21	19
Sat. with achievements in life	f	f	f	9	g
Satisfaction with future security	f	f	f	g	f

[a]Dimensions from SF-36
[b]Social Support Index, activity frequency, satisfaction with family, living partner, friendships, romantic relationships, feeling part of the community
[c]Index of Troubles, Crime-Related Worries Index, difficulty meeting housing costs, % of income spent on housing costs
[d]13 domain satisfaction scores
[e]a + b + c + d
[f]Variable not in equation
[g]Significance level too low for variable to enter equation

Explaining SWLS Scores

The first numerical column of Table 8.13 shows that 4 of the 7 SF-36 health dimensions explained 33% of the variation in SWLS scores, with Mental Health most influential ($\beta = 0.28$), followed by Social Functioning ($\beta = 0.20$).

The second column reveals that 5 of our 7 measures of social relations explained 40% of the variance in SWLS scores, with satisfaction with feeling part of the community most influential ($\beta = 0.31$), followed by satisfaction with friendships ($\beta = 0.23$).

The third column shows that the four measures of problems explained 24% of the variance in SWLS scores, with the Index of Troubles most influential ($\beta = -0.23$), followed by the Crime-Related Worries Index ($\beta = -0.19$).

The fourth column indicates that 5 of the 11 domain satisfaction predictors accounted for 53% of the variance in SWLS scores, with satisfaction with financial security most influential ($\beta = 0.24$), followed by satisfaction with health ($\beta = 0.22$) and achievements in life ($\beta = 0.21$).

The fifth column gives the results of regressing SWLS scores on all the statistically significant predictors from the first four regressions. In the comprehensive set of 18 potential predictors, 10 were significantly influential, explaining 58% of the variation. The most influential predictor was satisfaction with financial security ($\beta = 0.22$), followed by satisfaction with achievements in life ($\beta = 0.18$) and health satisfaction ($\beta = 0.14$).

Explaining CLAS Scores

The first numerical column of Table 8.14 shows that 3 of the 7 SF-36 health dimensions explained 30% of the variation in CLAS scores, with Mental Health most influential ($\beta = 0.25$), followed by Social Functioning ($\beta = 0.22$).

The second column reveals that 3 of our 7 measures of social relations explained 34% of the variance in CLAS scores, with satisfaction with feeling part of the community most influential ($\beta = 0.33$), followed by satisfaction with friendships ($\beta = 0.25$).

The third column shows that the four measures of problems explained 18% of the variance in CLAS scores, with the Index of Troubles most influential ($\beta = -0.20$), followed by the cluster of percent of income spent on housing costs ($\beta = -0.15$), Crime-Related Worries ($\beta = -0.14$) and difficulty meeting housing costs ($\beta = -0.13$).

The fourth column indicates that 4 of the 11 domain satisfaction predictors accounted for 45% of the variance in CLAS scores, with satisfaction with health most influential ($\beta = 0.28$), followed by satisfaction with future security ($\beta = 0.23$).

The fifth column gives the results of regressing CLAS scores on all the statistically significant predictors from the first four regressions. In the comprehensive set

Table 8.13 Regressions of SWLS on SF-36 health scales, social relations, problems and domain satisfaction (decimal points omitted)

Predictor clusters →	Health[a]	Soc. relat.[b]	Problems[c]	Domain sat.[d]	All pred.[e]
Percentage of variance explained	33	40	24	53	58
Predictors ↓	Betas	Betas	Betas	Betas	Betas
Physical functioning	10	f	f	f	8
Role limitation physical	g	f	f	f	f
Bodily pain	g	f	f	f	f
Vitality	12	f	f	f	g
Social functioning	20	f	f	f	g
Role limitation emotional	g	f	f	f	f
Mental health	28	f	f	f	12
Social support index	f	g	f	f	f
Frequency of activity participation	f	g	f	f	f
Satisfaction with family	f	9	f	f	g
Satisfaction with living partner	f	8	f	f	8
Satisfaction with friendships	f	23	f	f	g
Sat. with romantic relationships	f	17	f	f	11
Sat. with feeling part of community	f	31	f	f	8
Index of troubles	f	f	−23	f	g
Crime-related worries index	f	f	−19	f	−13
Difficulty meeting housing costs	f	f	−15	f	8
Percentage of income spent on housing costs	f	f	−14	f	g
Satisfaction with housing	f	f	f	g	f
Satisfaction with neighbourhood	f	f	f	g	f
Satisfaction with health	f	f	f	22	14
Satisfaction with religion	f	f	f	g	f
Satisfaction with financial security	f	f	f	24	22
Satisfaction with recreation	f	f	f	10	9
Satisfaction with self-esteem	f	f	f	13	g
Satisfaction with environment	f	f	f	g	f
Sat. with government officials	f	f	f	g	f
Sat. with sense of meaning in life	f	f	f	g	f
Sat. with achievements in life	f	f	f	21	18
Satisfaction with future security	f	f	f	g	f

[a]Dimensions from SF-36
[b]Social Support Index, activity frequency, satisfaction with family, living partner, friendships, romantic relationships, feeling part of the community
[c]Index of Troubles, Crime-Related Worries Index, difficulty meeting housing costs, Percentage of income spent on housing costs
[d]13 domain satisfaction scores
[e]a + b + c + d
[f]Variable not in equation
[g]Significance level too low for variable to enter equation

Table 8.14 Regressions of CLAS on SF-36 health scales, social relations, problems and domain satisfaction (decimal points omitted)

Predictor clusters →	Health[a]	Soc. relat.[b]	Problems[c]	Domain sat.[d]	All pred.[e]
Percentage of variance explained	30	34	18	45	48
Predictors ↓	Betas	Betas	Betas	Betas	Betas
Physical functioning	g	f	f	f	f
Role limitation physical	g	f	f	f	f
Bodily pain	g	f	f	f	f
Vitality	17	f	f	f	g
Social functioning	22	f	f	f	g
Role limitation emotional	g	f	f	f	f
Mental health	25	f	f	f	15
Social support index	f	g	f	f	f
Frequency of activity participation	f	g	f	f	f
Satisfaction with family	f	g	f	f	f
Satisfaction with living partner	f	g	f	f	f
Satisfaction with friendships	f	25	f	f	g
Sat. with romantic relationships	f	18	f	f	13
Sat. with feeling part of community	f	33	f	f	12
Index of troubles	f	f	−20	f	g
Crime-related worries index	f	f	−14	f	g
Difficulty meeting housing costs	f	f	−13	f	g
Percentage of income spent on housing costs	f	f	−15	f	g
Satisfaction with housing	f	f	f	g	f
Satisfaction with neighbourhood	f	f	f	g	f
Satisfaction with health	f	f	f	28	24
Satisfaction with religion	f	f	f	g	f
Satisfaction with financial security	f	f	f	g	f
Satisfaction with recreation	f	f	f	13	11
Satisfaction with self-esteem	f	f	f	g	f
Satisfaction with environment	f	f	f	g	f
Sat. with government officials	f	f	f	g	f
Sat. with sense of meaning in life	f	f	f	g	f
Sat. with achievements in life	f	f	f	16	g
Satisfaction with future security	f	f	f	23	20

[a]Dimensions from SF-36
[b]Social Support Index, activity frequency, satisfaction with family, living partner, friendships, romantic relationships, feeling part of the community
[c]Index of Troubles, Crime-Related Worries Index, difficulty meeting housing costs, % of income spent on housing costs
[d]13 domain satisfaction scores
[e]a + b + c + d
[f]Variable not in equation
[g]Significance level too low for variable to enter equation

of 14 potential predictors, 6 were significantly influential, explaining 48% of the variation. The most influential predictor was satisfaction with health ($\beta = 0.24$), followed by satisfaction with future security ($\beta = 0.20$).

Explaining SWB

The first numerical column of Table 8.15 shows that 3 of the 7 SF-36 health dimensions explained 33% of the variation in SWB scores, with Mental Health most influential ($\beta = 0.31$), followed by Social Functioning ($\beta = 0.18$).

The second column reveals that 4 of our 7 measures of social relations explained 51% of the variance in SWB scores, with satisfaction with friendships most influential ($\beta = 0.36$), followed by satisfaction with feeling part of the community ($\beta = 0.29$).

The third column shows that the 4 measures of problems explained 21% of the variance in SWB scores, with difficulty meeting housing costs most influential ($\beta = -0.21$), followed by the Index of Troubles ($\beta = -0.18$).

The fourth column indicates that 6 of the 11 domain satisfaction predictors accounted for 64% of the variance in SWB scores, with satisfaction with health most influential ($\beta = 0.28$), followed by satisfaction with financial security ($\beta = 0.21$) and with a sense of meaning in life ($\beta = 0.19$).

The fifth column gives the results of regressing SWB scores on all the statistically significant predictors from the first four regressions. In the comprehensive set of 18 potential predictors, nine were significantly influential, explaining 68% of the variation. The most influential predictors were satisfaction with friendships ($\beta = 0.19$) and financial security ($\beta = 0.18$), followed by satisfaction health ($\beta = 0.17$).

Examination of the results displayed in the final columns of Tables 8.9, 8.10, 8.11, 8.12, 8.13, 8.14 and 8.15 suggests a few general comments. We have not reported any percent changes attached to successive steps in the stepwise regressions presented here. Generally, the stepwise procedure begins by formulating an equation with the most influential predictor, then with the two most influential, and so on until additional predictors fail to make a significant contribution to the total variance explained in the dependent variable. Usually, there is a substantial jump in the percent of variance explained from the first to the second step, with even more modest percent changes with each additional predictor added to the explanatory equation. So, examination of only the first two predictors for every dependent variable can be very illuminating.

First, then, it should be noticed that the pair of most influential predictors of each of the eight dependent variables is different in every case. Some of the same predictors occur several times, but there are no cases in which exactly the same pair appears.

Second, for the SF-36 General Health and the single item general health measure, only SF-36 scales were included in the top two predictors, with Vitality most influential in both cases.

Third, for the remaining six dependent variables, the only predictor that appeared as most influential in more than one case was satisfaction with friendships, which was first for Life Satisfaction and for SWB. Each of the remaining four dependent variables had a different predictor in first place, namely, the SF-36 Mental Health scale for Happiness, satisfaction with a sense of meaning in life for Satisfaction with the overall Quality of Life, satisfaction with financial security for SWLS and satisfaction with health for CLAS.

Fourth, satisfaction with health was the second most influential predictor for 3 of the 6 dependent variables, Life Satisfaction, Happiness and Satisfaction with the overall Quality of Life. For the remaining three dependent variables, second place went to satisfaction with achievements in life for SWLS, satisfaction with future security for CLAS and satisfaction with financial security for SWB.

Taken together, these comments pretty clearly show that all these important dependent variables capture whole-life assessments that have distinct core connotations with some overlapping meaning. At a minimum, that should alert researchers to be careful about the claims made about determinants of such things as general health, happiness and the quality of life.

Multiple Discrepancies Theory (MDT)

MDT was initially described in detail and tested in Michalos (1985). After that, it was applied to a group of seniors in Ontario (Michalos 1986) and to 18,000 undergraduates in 39 countries (Michalos 1991a, b, 1993a, b). The 1985 paper was the third most frequently cited paper in *Social Indicators Research* in the first 30 years of that journal's life (Michalos 2005), but the theory has been rarely examined in its entirety. A review paper of the complete citation history of the article is in preparation, including an examination of the theory's strengths, weaknesses, necessary revisions and future prospects. In the present investigation, we only look at the explanatory power of the seven core discrepancies used in the theory, plus income. The primary aims here are to (1) compare the relative power of MDT to the more primitive linear models of explanation used for the results described in Tables 8.9, 8.10, 8.11, 8.12, 8.13, 8.14 and 8.15, (2) identify some discrepancies that might be dropped from the theory, and (3) demonstrate again the fact that income is not as important as other predictors in MDT for the set of dependent variables considered in this study.

Here are the postulates as stated in Michalos (1985, pp. 347–413).

H1 Reported net satisfaction is a function of perceived discrepancies between what one has and wants, relevant others have, the best one has had in the past,

Table 8.15 Regressions of SWB on SF-36 health scales, social relations, problems and domain satisfaction (decimal points omitted)

Predictor clusters →	Health[a]	Soc. relat.[b]	Problems[c]	Domain sat.[d]	All pred.[e]
Percentage of variance explained	33	51	21	64	68
Predictors ↓	Betas	Betas	Betas	Betas	Betas
Physical functioning	8	f	f	f	7
Role limitation physical	g	f	f	f	f
Bodily pain	g	f	f	f	f
Vitality	13	f	f	f	g
Social functioning	18	f	f	f	g
Role limitation emotional	g	f	f	f	f
Mental health	31	f	f	f	9
Social support index	f	g	f	f	f
Frequency of activity participation	f	g	f	f	f
Satisfaction with family	f	11	f	f	f
Satisfaction with living partner	f	g	f	f	f
Satisfaction with friendships	f	36	f	f	19
Sat. with romantic relationships	f	18	f	f	12
Sat. with feeling part of community	f	29	f	f	g
Index of troubles	f	f	−18	f	g
Crime-related worries index	f	f	−13	f	g
Difficulty meeting housing costs	f	f	−21	f	g
Percentage of income spent on housing costs	f	f	−15	f	g
Satisfaction with housing	f	f	f	14	14
Satisfaction with neighbourhood	f	f	f	g	f
Satisfaction with health	f	f	f	28	17
Satisfaction with religion	f	f	f	g	f
Satisfaction with financial security	f	f	f	21	18
Satisfaction with recreation	f	f	f	g	f
Satisfaction with self-esteem	f	f	f	g	f
Satisfaction with environment	f	f	f	g	f
Sat. with government officials	f	f	f	g	f
Sat. with sense of meaning in life	f	f	f	19	15
Sat. with achievements in life	f	f	f	12	g
Satisfaction with future security	f	f	f	8	8

[a]Dimensions from SF-36
[b]Social Support Index, activity frequency, satisfaction with family, living partner, friendships, romantic relationships, feeling part of the community
[c]Index of Troubles, Crime-Related Worries Index, difficulty meeting housing costs, % of income spent on housing costs
[d]13 domain satisfaction scores
[e]a + b + c + d
[f]Variable not in equation
[g]Significance level too low for variable to enter equation

expected to have 3 years ago, expects to have after 5 years, deserves and needs

H2 All perceived discrepancies, except that between what one has and wants, are functions of objectively measurable discrepancies, which also have direct effects on satisfaction and actions

H3 The perceived discrepancy between what one has and wants is a mediating variable between all other perceived discrepancies and reported net satisfaction

H4 The pursuit and maintenance of net satisfaction motivates human action in direct proportion to the perceived expected levels of net satisfaction

H5 All discrepancies, satisfaction and actions are directly and indirectly affected by age, sex, education, ethnicity, income, self-esteem and social support

H6 Objectively measurable discrepancies are functions of human action and conditioners

In the questionnaire, discrepancies were measured with items like 'Considering your life as a whole, how does it measure up to your general aspirations or what you want out of life? Generally, does life provide what you want fairly poorly, fairly well, etc.?' Response categories ran from 1 = provides nothing that you want, through 4 = provides half of what you want, to 7 = provides all that you want.

In Michalos (1991a), '(happiness or subjective well-being)' was inserted after 'satisfaction' in H1 to emphasize the point that MDT was intended to be a theory sufficient to explain all three notions. Based on the different relationships among these three concepts and a diverse array of other variables that have been revealed in many empirical studies, including the present one, it is clear that these three concepts have somewhat distinct cores with overlapping connotations. Also, as indicated in Michalos (1991a, pp. 3–4),

> ...a fully developed scientific theory of subjective well-being would...be applicable to satisfaction or happiness with life as a whole (i.e., global satisfaction or happiness) as well as to satisfaction or happiness with specific domains of life (i.e., domain satisfaction) such as marital satisfaction and job satisfaction.

Thus, a general theory like MDT could be used on its own to explain global and domain satisfaction (happiness or subjective well-being) or it could be used in combination with the familiar simple linear, bottom-up model in which, say, Life Satisfaction is explained by aggregated domain satisfaction and satisfaction in each of the domains is explained by MDT. The main virtue of MDT is that it provides explanations of satisfaction in terms of something else. It is, therefore, a conceptually deeper sort of explanatory theory than the standard simple linear model that, for example, explains Life Satisfaction in terms of satisfaction with friends, recreation and so on.

It is probably worthwhile to notice that the phrase 'quality of life' does not appear in the postulates because it was assumed that the quality of one's life is a function of the objective features of one's life and one's subjective assessment of those features. MDT is supposed to provide an explanation of the subjective assessment. This view of a good quality of life or a good life in general is very similar to Aristotle's notion of *eudaimonia* in his *Nicomachean Ethics* and his earlier *Eudemian Ethics,* understood as "living well and doing well" in his longer phrase or as "wellbeing" in a shorter phrase. Unfortunately, because of the linguistic flexibility of 'happiness' compared to the other phrases, for years translators have used 'happiness' more often than any other word or phrase as a translation of *eudaimonia* (Jost 2002). Since current usage tends to treat happiness as a purely subjective, experienced matter, it is a poor substitute for a good quality of life, good life or well-being for those of us following the Aristotelian tradition.

Tables 8.16, 8.17, 8.18, 8.19, 8.20, 8.21 and 8.22 give the results of Path Analyses constructed from two regressions for each of our eight dependent variables, mainly involving only postulates H1 and H3 of MDT. The basic idea is that the eight predictors listed in the first columns of these tables have both direct and indirect effects on the dependent variables. The sum of these effects is called the Total Effects, and these are listed in the final column of each table. The direct effects of each of the eight predictors are simply the beta values obtained by regressing each dependent variable on the predictors, with results listed in the column under the name of each dependent variable. The indirect effects are obtained in two steps. First, Self-Wants scores are regressed on the remaining seven predictors, with results listed in the column under 'Self-Wants' in each table. Second, the beta value for each predictor in the Self-Wants column is multiplied times the beta value of Self-Wants in the dependent variable column. This product is a measure of the indirect effect of a predictor. The Total Effects of a predictor, then, equal the sum of this product and the direct effect. Most importantly, the square of the total effect of a predictor on a dependent variable equals the percent of the variance of that variable explained by that predictor (Pedhazur 1982, p. 183).

For example, in the last column of Table 8.17, under 'Total Effect' for the Self-Others predictor, the 30 (decimal points omitted in the tables) was obtained by multiplying 0.26 (the beta value of Self-Others in the Self-Wants regression) times 0.36 (the beta value of Self-Wants in the Life Satisfaction regression) to get 0.09 (the indirect effect of Self-Others scores on Life Satisfaction scores), and adding 0.21 (the beta value of Self-Others in the Life Satisfaction regression = the direct effect of Self-Others scores on Life Satisfaction scores). Squaring 0.30, one gets the percent of variance in Life Satisfaction scores accounted for by Self-Others scores, i.e., 9% of the variance in Life Satisfaction scores may be explained by Self-Others scores. All other total effects in the other tables are obtained in a similar fashion.

Table 8.16 shows that 5 of the 7 core discrepancy predictors explained 13% and 25% of the variance in SF-36 General Health scores and single item general health scores, respectively. These results are less impressive than those shown in Table 8.9. Examining the Total Effects column, one finds that the most influential predictors of the SF-36 scale scores were Self-Best and Self-Others scores, with Total Effects tied at 0.18. For the single item measure, the most influential predictor based on Total Effects was Self-Others (TE = 0.27). Income had no direct effects on the two dependent variables, but had a tiny 0.01 Total Effect.

Table 8.16 Regressions of SF-36 General Health/single item health scores on MDT core discrepancies and income (decimal points omitted)

Predictors ↓	Gen. health/sing. item betas/betas	Self-wants betas	Total effects
Income	0/0	8	1/0
Self-others	14/27	26	18/27
Self-deserved	−13/−13	18	−10/−13
Self-needs	0/16	13	2/16
Self-progress	0/0	0	0/0
Self-future	13/11	8	14/11
Self-best	15/18	21	18/18
Self-wants	16/0		16/0
Percentage of variance expl.	13/25	49	

Table 8.17 Regression of life Satisfaction scores on MDT core discrepancies and income (decimal points omitted)

Predictors ↓	Life satisfaction betas	Self-wants betas	Total effects
Income	0	8	3
Self-others	21	26	30
Self-deserved	0	18	7
Self-needs	14	13	19
Self-progress	0	0	0
Self-future	0	8	3
Self-best	0	21	8
Self-wants	36		36
Percentage of variance expl.	38	49	

Table 8.18 Regression of happiness scores on MDT core discrepancies and income (decimal points omitted)

Predictors ↓	Life satisfaction betas	Self-wants betas	Total effects
Income	0	8	3
Self-others	15	26	24
Self-deserved	0	18	6
Self-needs	19	13	23
Self-progress	0	0	0
Self-future	0	8	3
Self-best	9	21	16
Self-wants	33		33
Percentage of variance expl.	41	49	

Table 8.19 Regression of satisfaction with overall quality of life scores on MDT core discrepancies and income (decimal points omitted)

Predictors ↓	Life satisfaction betas	Self-wants betas	Total effects
Income	6	8	9
Self-others	14	26	23
Self-deserved	0	18	6
Self-needs	20	13	24
Self-progress	0	0	0
Self-future	0	8	3
Self-best	10	21	17
Self-wants	34		34
Percentage of variance expl.	44	49	

Table 8.20 Regression of SWLS scores on MDT core discrepancies and income (decimal points omitted)

Predictors ↓	Life satisfaction betas	Self-wants betas	Total effects
Income	0	8	3
Self-others	13	26	22
Self-deserved	0	18	6
Self-needs	16	13	20
Self-progress	8	0	8
Self-future	0	8	3
Self-best	20	21	27
Self-wants	34		34
Percentage of variance expl.	57	49	

Table 8.21 Regression of CLAS scores on MDT core discrepancies and income (decimal points omitted)

Predictors ↓	Life satisfaction betas	Self-wants betas	Total effects
Income	0	8	2
Self-others	14	26	21
Self-deserved	0	18	5
Self-needs	15	13	19
Self-progress	10	0	10
Self-future	−7	8	−5
Self-best	22	21	28
Self-wants	28		28
Percentage of variance expl.	47	49	

Table 8.22 Regression of SWB scores on MDT core discrepancies and income (decimal points omitted)

Predictors ↓	Life satisfaction betas	Self-wants betas	Total effects
Income	0	8	3
Self-others	14	26	24
Self-deserved	0	18	7
Self-needs	24	13	29
Self-progress	0	0	0
Self-future	0	8	3
Self-best	8	21	16
Self-wants	39		39
Percentage of variance expl.	52	49	

Table 8.17 shows that 3 of the 7 core discrepancy predictors explained 38% of the variance in Life Satisfaction scores, with the Self-Wants predictor having the greatest total effect (TE = 0.36), followed by the Self-Others predictor (TE = 0.30). Income had a Total Effect of 0.03.

Table 8.18 shows that 4 of the 7 core discrepancy predictors explained 41% of the variance in Happiness scores, with the Self-Wants predictor having the greatest total effect (TE = 0.33), followed by the Self-Others (TE = 0.24) and Self-Needs (TE = 0.23) predictors. Income had a Total Effect of 0.03.

Table 8.19 shows that 5 of the 7 core predictors explained 44% of the variance in Satisfaction with the overall Quality of Life scores, with the Self-Wants predictor having the greatest total effect (TE = 0.34), followed by the Self-Needs (TE = 0.24) and Self-Others (TE = 0.23) predictors. Income had a Total Effect of 0.09.

Table 8.20 shows that 5 of the 7 core discrepancy predictors explained 57% of the variance in SWLS scores, with the Self-Wants predictor having the greatest total effect (TE = 0.34), followed by the Self-Best (TE = 0.27) and Self-Others (TE = 0.22) predictors. Income had a Total Effect of 0.03.

Table 8.21 shows that 6 of the 7 core discrepancy predictors explained 47% of the variance in CLAS scores, with the Self-Wants and Self-Best predictors having the greatest total effects (TE = 0.28 each), followed by the Self-Others (TE = 0.21) and Self-Needs (TE = 0.19) predictors. Income had a Total Effect of 0.02.

Table 8.22 shows that 4 of the 7 core discrepancy predictors explained 52% of the variance in SWB scores, with Self-Wants having the greatest Total Effects (TE = 0.39), followed by the Self-Needs (TE = 0.29) and Self-Others (TE = 0.24) predictors. Income had a Total Effect of 0.03.

Examining the last seven tables to answer the three basic questions concerning MDT versus the simpler linear explanatory models, we find that (1) MDT displayed relatively less explanatory power than the simpler models for every dependent variable, although it was only 1% point below the mark for SWLS (57% vs. 58% of the variance explained) and CLAS (47% vs. 48%). This is fairly promising considering the fact that only the central core of predictors from MDT were employed.

(2) The Self-Progress predictor was ineffective for 6 of the 8 dependent variables. (3) Income had a relatively weak impact on every dependent variable, but in 6 out of 8 cases its impact was the result of indirect effects. In an application of the full MDT model, income has many more opportunities for influencing the dependent variables. So, income still has a role to play, though pretty clearly a relatively modest one judging from this and earlier research with MDT.

Conclusion

Replicating a survey of 875 people 55 years old or more undertaken in September 1999 throughout the former NIHR of British Columbia, in September 2005 a sample of 656 people completed a 22-page questionnaire. The average age of the respondents was 68, with a range running from 55 to 96 years, and 64% were women. Responses to the SF-36 questionnaire indicated that for male respondents aged 55–64, the mean score for the 8 dimensions was 76.1. This mean was a bit higher than the 74.4 mean of 1999. For male respondents aged 65 and older the mean was 69.0, which was also higher than the 68.3 mean of 1999. For females aged 55–64, the mean score for 8 dimensions was 73.1, versus 73.0 in 1999. For female respondents aged 65 and older, the mean score was 67.0, versus 65.4 in 1999. Based on these mean scores for the 8 dimensions, then, it is fair to say that the overall health status of males and females aged 55 years and older in the region in 2005 was at least as good as (i.e., the same as or better than) that in 1999.

Comparing 28 average figures for the 2005 respondents on satisfaction with specific domains of life (e.g., financial security, health, sense of meaning) and three global indicators (satisfaction with life as a whole and with the overall quality of life, and happiness) with those of the 1999 respondents, we found that the scores for the 2005 sample were at least as high as those of the other sample. Thus, it seems fair to say that the perceived quality of life of older people in the former NIHR, so far as it is revealed in domain and global satisfaction and happiness scores, is at least as good as the perceived quality of life of a similar sample in 1999.

Although a large majority perceived increases in crime in the 2 year periods prior to both surveys, smaller percentages of the 2005 sample than of the 1999 sample thought that crime had increased over the past two years, avoided going out at night, feared for their safety, had crime-related worries, engaged in crime-related defensive behaviours and were actually the victims of any crimes. Therefore, it seems fair to say that, so far as crime-related issues are concerned for the two samples of seniors responding to our surveys, there is more evidence of improvement than of deterioration.

In both surveys there was strong support for local government to be planning housing for its older population, including setting aside land to build housing. Most respondents did not believe that most people treated them like stereotypical older persons and most would not leave the neighbourhood they now live in if they could afford it. In general, over 86% of respondents in both samples indicated that they knew someone who really cared about them and who could be counted upon in a crisis situation.

Applying stepwise multiple regression, each of the eight dependent variables was explained on the basis of four clusters of predictors separately and then a final regression was run using only the statistically significant predictors from the four clusters. Broadly speaking, 7 SF-36 health status scales explained from 28% to 45% of the variance in the eight dependent variables, running from satisfaction with the overall quality of life (28%) to the single item measure of general health (45%). The seven predictors in the Social Relations cluster explained from 7% of the variance in the SF-36 General Health scale scores to 57% of the variance in the Life Satisfaction scores. The four predictors in the Problems cluster explained from 10% of the variance in the SF-36 General Health scale scores to 24% of the variance in the SWLS scores. The 11 predictors in the Domain Satisfaction cluster explained from 14% of the variance in the SF-36 General Health scale scores to 64% of the variance in the SWB scores. Putting all the significant predictors together for each dependent variable, in the weakest case, 4 of 11 potential predictors explained 33% of the variance in the SF-36 General Health scale scores and in the strongest case, 9 of 15 potential predictors explained 70% of the variance in Life Satisfaction scores. Among other things, these results clearly show that respondents' ideas about a generally healthy life are different from, but not independent of, their ideas about a happy, satisfying or contented life, or about the perceived quality of their lives or their subjective wellbeing.

Finally, the 7 core discrepancy predictors of MDT plus incomes were used to explain the eight dependent variables. From 13% of the variance in the SF-36 General Health scale scores to 57% of the variance in SWLS scores were explained using those predictors. Based on an examination of the Total Effects scores for the predictors of the eight dependent variables, the most influential predictors were Self-Wants, followed by Self-Others and then Self-Best. In other words, the most influential discrepancy predictors of respondents' overall life assessments were those between what respondents have versus what they want, followed by what they have versus what others of the same age and sex have, and then by what they have versus the best they ever had in the past.

References

Braungart, M., Braungart, R., & Hoyt, W. (1980). Age, sex and social factors in fear of crime. *Sociological Focus, 13*(1), 55–66.

Diener, E., Emmons, R. A., Larsen, R. J., & Griffin, S. (1985). The satisfaction with life scale. *Journal of Personality Assessment, 49*(1), 71–75.

Jost, L. J. (2002). Introduction. In L. J. Jost & R. A. Shiner (Eds.), *Eudaimonia and well-being: Ancient and modern conceptions* (pp. ix–xxxiii). Kelowna, BC: Academic Printing and Publishing.

Kennedy, L. W., & Silverman, R. A. (1984–1985). Significant others and fear of crime among the elderly. *International Journal of Aging and Human Development, 20*(4), 241–256.

Lavallee, L. F., Hatch P. M., Michalos, A. C., & McKinley, T. (in press). Development of the contentment with life assessment scale (CLAS): Using daily life experiences to verify levels of self-reported life satisfaction. *Social Indicators Research.*

MacKuen, M. B. (1984). Reality, the press and citizens' political agendas. In C. F. Turner & E. Martin (Eds.), *Surveying subjective phenomena* (Vol. 2, pp. 443–474). New York: Russell Sage Foundation.

McHorney, C. A., Ware, J. E., Lu, J. F. R., & Donald Sherbourne, C. (1994). The MOS 36-item short-form health survey (SF-36): III tests of data quality, scaling assumptions, and reliability across diverse patient groups. *Medical Care, 32*(1), 40–66.

McHorney, C. A., Ware, J. E., & Raczek, A. E. (1993). The MOS 36-item short-form health survey (SF-36): II. Psychometric and clinical tests of validity in measuring physical and mental health constructs. *Medical Care, 31*(3), 247–263.

Michalos, A. C. (1985). Multiple discrepancies theory (MDT). *Social Indicators Research, 16,* 347–413.

Michalos, A. C. (1986). An application of multiple discrepancies theory to seniors. *Social Indicators Research, 18,* 349–373.

Michalos, A. C. (1991a). *Global report on student well-being: Vol. 1, Life satisfaction and happiness.* New York: Springer.

Michalos, A. C. (1991b). *Global report on student well-being: Vol. 2, Family, friends, living partner and self-esteem.* New York: Springer.

Michalos, A. C. (1993a). *Global report on student well-being: Vol. 3, Employment, finances, housing and transportation.* New York: Springer.

Michalos, A. C. (1993b). *Global report on student well-being: Vol. 4, Religion, education, recreation and health.* New York: Springer-Verlag.

Michalos, A. C. (2003). *Essays on the quality of life.* Dordrecht: Kluwer Academic Publishers.

Michalos, A. C. (2004). Social indicators research and health-related quality of life research. *Social Indicators Research, 65,* 27–72.

Michalos, A. C. (Ed.). (2005). *Citation classics from social indicators research.* Dordrecht: Springer Publishers.

Michalos, A. C., Hubley, A., Zumbo, B. D., & Hemingway, D. (2001). Health and other aspects of the quality of life of older people. *Social Indicators Research, 54*(3), 239–274.

Michalos, A. C., Thommasen, H. V., Read, R., Anderson, N., & Zumbo, B. D. (2005). Determinants of health and the quality of life in the Bella Coola valley. *Social Indicators Research, 72,* 1–50.

Michalos, A. C., & Zumbo, B. D. (2003). Leisure activities, health and the quality of life. In A. C. Michalos (Ed.), *Essays on the quality of life* (pp. 217–238). Dordrecht: Kluwer Academic Publishing.

Michalos, A. C., Zumbo, B. D., & Hubley, A. (2000). Health and the quality of life. *Social Indicators Research, 51,* 245–286.

Murray, M., Lefort, S., & Ribeiro, V. (1998). The SF-36: Reliable and valid for the institutionalized elderly? *Aging & Mental Health, 2*(1), 24–27.

Pedhazur, E. J. (1982). *Multiple regression in behavioral research: Explanation and prediction.* New York: Holt, Rinehart and Winston.

Ware, J. E., & Donald Sherbourne, C. (1992). The MOS 36-item short-form health survey (SF-36): I. Conceptual framework and item selection. *Medical Care, 30*(6), 473–483.

Ware, J. E., Kosinsky, M., & Keller, S. D. (1994). *SF-36 physical and mental health summary scales: A user's manual.* Boston, MA: The Health Institute, New England Medical Center.

Ware, J. E., Snow, K. K., Kosinski, M., & Gandek, B. (1993). *SF-36 health survey: Manual and interpretation guide.* Boston, MA: The Health Institute, New England Medical Center.

Chapter 9
Good Health is Not the Same as a Good Life: Survey Results from Brandon, Manitoba

Alex C. Michalos, Douglas Ramsey, Derrek Eberts and P. Maurine Kahlke

Introduction

The aim of this investigation is to obtain some baseline self-reported data on the health status and overall quality of life of a sample of residents of the city of Brandon, Manitoba (pop. approx. 42,000) aged 18 years or older, and to measure the impact of a set of designated health determinants, comparison standards and satisfaction with diverse domains or aspects of life on their health and quality of life measured with 7 different indicators. The paper begins with a description of the sampling technique, questionnaire, demographic composition of the sample and a descriptive analysis of measures of health status, health-related behaviour, health care and (domain specific and overall) quality of life. Multivariate explorations, including an overview of the variance explained and the most influential explanatory measures for 7 dependent variables, form the central analytic findings

Michalos, A.C., Ramsey, D., Eberts, D., & Kahlke, P.M.: 2011, Good health is not the same as a good life: survey results from Brandon, Manitoba. Social Indicators Research, 107(2), pp. 201–234.

A.C. Michalos (✉)
University of Northern British Columbia, Prince George, BC, Canada
e-mail: michalos@brandonu.ca

D. Ramsey
Department of Rural Development, Brandon University, Brandon, MB, Canada
e-mail: ramsey@brandonu.ca

D. Eberts
Department of Geography, Brandon University, Brandon, MB, Canada
e-mail: Ebertsd@brandonu.ca

P. Maurine Kahlke
9005 College Drive, Coldstream, BC V1B 2P7, Canada
e-mail: pmhatch@shaw.ca

A.C. Michalos, *Connecting the Quality of Life Theory to Health, Well-Being and Education*, DOI 10.1007/978-3-319-51161-0_9

of the paper. In the conclusion, key highlights are summarized which outline the importance of the research in better understanding health and quality of life, and differentiating the two.

Sampling Technique, Questionnaire and Sample Demographics

In May and June 2010, 2,500 households from the city of Brandon, Manitoba were randomly selected and mailed a 16-page questionnaire that could be completed by any (one) resident in the household 18 years of age or older. The first three and a half pages contained the 36-item Medical Outcomes Study Short Form (SF-36) profile (Ware et al. 1993) and 13 items from the United States Centers for Disease Control and Prevention, Behavioral Risk Factor Surveillance System (BRFSS) (CDC 2000). There are 14 items in the BRFSS, the first of which is a general health question that is also the first question in SF-36. Seven items measuring socializing activities and social support came next, followed by 6 items forming a Community Health Index and an item measuring free-time exercise levels. This was followed by 9 questions about health-related behaviours, e.g., tobacco smoking, drinking alcoholic beverages, eating and sleeping routines, and use of over-the-counter and prescription drugs. Ten items were devoted to health care issues, e.g., rating personal and most people's health care, frequency of seeking medical and dental care in the past year, types of health problems requiring care, and distances travelled to receive care. After these, there were 3 items concerning housing needs and problems, followed by a standard set of 41 quality of life items, e.g., happiness and satisfaction with life as a whole, and satisfaction with specific domains of life like one's housing, friendships and financial security. Seven items were included concerning the fundamental postulates of Multiple Discrepancies Theory (Michalos 1985), and 11 more to craft 2 additional dependent variables, i.e., the Satisfaction with Life Scale (SWLS from Diener et al. 1985) and Contentment With Life Assessment Scale (CLAS from Lavallee et al. 2007). Ten items focused on neighbourhood issues and 13 on growth in the city over the past 10 years which were followed by two pages of items concerning crime, personal safety, worries about and behaviours concerning criminal victimization and actual victimization. The last two pages had basic demographic questions, including age, gender and education.

By the end of June we had received 518 (21%) useable, completed questionnaires. A simple random sample of this size provides sampling error margins of about plus or minus 4% points on responses, 19 times out of 20. Additional non-sampling errors may occur as a result of questions being poorly expressed or understood, respondent fatigue, mood or bias, the weather and other things that are often difficult to measure and beyond the researchers' control.

Of the 503 respondents who identified their gender, 53% (267) were females. Sixty percent (308) of those who answered the marital status question were married. The average age was 60, and the range ran from 18 to 94. Twenty-nine percent of the 482 respondents answering the question had a university degree at the bachelor's level or higher. Forty-eight percent reported their employment status as retired, 33% were employed full-time and 8% part-time. The total household income question had 399 respondents, providing an average income of $72,978. Regarding cultural or ethnic background, 77% simply reported being Canadian and 3% reported being First Nations or Métis. Using standard measures of Body Mass Index, 4.9% of our sample would be classed as having insufficient weight, 31.4% having acceptable weight, 25.9% with some excess weight and 37.9% overweight.

According to the 2006 census for the City of Brandon, there were 31,495 residents aged 20 or older, with 16,804 (53%) women, 51% were legally married and 14% had a "university certificate, diploma or degree" (Statistics Canada 2006). Although the sample size and range is not clear, according to the Brandon Regional Health Authority (2009, pp. 4–10), about 38% of the adult population of Brandon would be classed as overweight and 21% as obese. Therefore, it is fair to say that our sample is representative of the Brandon population regarding percentages of women and men, but married people, older people and people who have some excess weight or are overweight are over-represented. Given the over-representation of older people, it may safely be assumed that any average measures of health status would be improved somewhat if younger people were appropriately represented. It may also be assumed that the average level of awareness of and attention to health status would be higher in our sample than in a more representative sample.

Health Status Measures

The 36-item Medical Outcomes Study Short Form (SF-36) profile is sometimes referred to as the 'gold standard' for health status measurement and its norms for several populations provide useful benchmarks for other developed countries (Ware and Sherbourne 1992; McHorney et al. 1993, 1994; Ware et al. 1993, 1994). Table 9.1 summarizes its basic elements.

The SF-36 scale works best as a health profile measure with eight dimensions, rather than as a single summative measure. SF-36 profile scores are designed such that 0 represents the worst and 100 represents the best state of health. Using a panel study of 3,445 patients McHorney et al. (1994), found that the internal-consistency reliability (Cronbach's alpha) for each of the eight concepts measured in the SF-36 with this panel ranged from 0.78 to 0.93, with a mean of 0.85.

Tables 9.2, 9.3, and 9.4 summarize the eight SF-36 profile scores for the respondents in Brandon taken all together and for males and females. The most useful comparisons that can be made with surveys like this one are usually those involving the same population at different times, and those tracking the very same

Table 9.1 Content of the SF-36 questionnaire

Concepts	Number of items	Meaning of low scores	Meaning of high scores
Physical functioning	10	Limited a lot in performing all physical activities including bathing or dressing due to health	Performs all types of physical activities including the most vigorous without limitations due to health
Role physical	4	Problems with work or other daily activities as a result of physical health	No problems with work or other daily activities as a result of physical health
Bodily pain	2	Very severe and extremely limiting pain	No pain or limitations due to pain
General health	5	Evaluates personal health as poor and believes it is likely to get worse	Evaluates personal health as excellent
Vitality	4	Feels tired and worn out all of the time	Feels tired and worn out all of the time
Social functioning	2	Extreme and frequent interference with normal social activities due to physical or emotional problems	Performs normal social activities without interference due to physical or emotional problems
Role emotional	3	Problems with work or other daily activities as a result of emotional problems	No problems with work or other daily activities as a result of emotional problems
Mental health	5	Feelings of nervousness and depression all of the time	Feels peaceful, happy, and calm all of the time
Reported health transition	1	Believes general health is much worse now than one year ago	Believes general health is much better now than one year ago

Source Ware et al. (1993, pp. 3:5)

people over time (longitudinal panel studies) are even better because they allow examination of changes at the level of individuals (versus aggregate changes) over time. In the absence of both kinds of comparisons for this study, we thought it would provide some context for considering results obtained from the Brandon sample if we included results obtained from other samples taken from earlier surveys. Accordingly, we included scores from samples from the Bella Coola Valley (pop. approx. 2300) and Prince George (pop. approx. 71,000), British Columbia;

Aberdeen, Scotland (pop. approx. 210,400) and the United States. While the age range of the respondents for each of the 6 samples is fairly similar, the composition may be somewhat different.

Table 9.2 lists the scores for our Brandon respondent group as a whole. The scores range from 83.5 for Social Functioning to 59.3 for Vitality, with a mean of 73.9. This mean score is similar to that for Aberdeen (73.7), higher than that of the Bella Coola Valley sample (62.7) and lower than the scores for the two Prince George samples and the USA sample. The latter is the highest of the lot (76.6).

Table 9.2 SF-36 comparisons of country and city scores

Health dimension	Brandon 2010	Bella C. Valley 2002	P.G 1998	P.G. 1999	Aberdeen 1993	USA 1993
PF	78.5	82.3	87.2	87.7	79.2	84.2
RP	70.4	67.5	81.8	76.6	76.5	81.0
BP	68.5	54.6	60.9	72.2	76.9	75.2
GH	69.6	55.5	73.7	71.7	68.7	72.0
VT	59.3	54.0	58.4	58.4	61.2	60.9
SF	83.5	50.0	83.5	81.8	78.6	83.3
RE	82.9	75.1	80.7	78.1	75.0	81.3
MH	78.2	62.4	74.5	75.2	73.7	74.7
Average	73.9	62.7	75.1	75.2	73.7	76.6

Brandon, May 2010, N = 494, ages 18–94: Bella Coola Valley, March 2002, N = 687, ages 17–90; Prince George, November 1998, N = 719, ages 17–92; Prince George, November 1999, N = 438, ages 17–86; Aberdeen, N = 542, ages 18 and older; USA, N = 2,474, ages 18 and older
Sources Ware et al. (1993), Garratt et al. (1993), Michalos et al. (2000, 2005), and Michalos and Zumbo (2003)

Using these means of the eight scores as broad and relatively rough indicators of the health of the 6 samples listed in Table 9.2, the Brandon sample would rank fourth.

Because the first question in the SF-36 list of questions was used in the Brandon RHA survey, an approximate comparison can be made between our two samples. For our sample, 47.6% reported being in excellent or very good health, compared to about 61% for the Brandon RHA sample (pp. 4–4). According to Statistics Canada's National Population Health Surveys and Canadian Community Health Survey, the national figures for this question ran from 63.1% in 1994 to 59.6% in 2007 (Michalos et al. 2010). Presumably, our sample score is lower because of the over-representation of older people.

Table 9.3 lists the scores for males in the 5 groups for which we had data. The scores for Brandon male respondents range from 85.0 for Social Functioning to 61.9 for Vitality, with a mean of 75.0. This mean puts the sample of Brandon males in third place among the 5.

Table 9.4 lists the scores for females in the 5 groups. The scores for Brandon female respondents range from 82.1 for Social Functioning to 57.1 for Vitality, with a mean of 73.1. So, on average our female respondents are not as healthy as our males. The Brandon female scores put them in fourth place among the 5 samples.

Because older people are relatively over-represented in the Brandon sample, we thought it might be worthwhile to make somewhat more precise comparisons using male and female groups aged 55–64 (younger old), and 65 and older (older old). Considering the relatively small sample sizes involved, one should exercise extra caution about the figures obtained. Tables 9.5 and 9.6 display our results.

Examining the Brandon figures for younger old males versus older old males (Table 9.5), one finds that the average value of the former is as expected, higher than that of the latter, namely, 81.3 versus 68.3, respectively. That is the case for the

Table 9.3 SF-36 comparisons of city and country male scores

Health dimensions	Brandon 2010	Bella C. Valley 2002	P.G. 1998	P.G. 1999	USA 1993
PF	80.9	82.4	87.1	88.3	87.2
RP	69.4	66.7	83.6	80.0	86.6
BP	68.7	53.4	61.9	74.5	76.9
GH	69.0	54.7	74.0	72.4	73.5
VT	61.9	54.1	60.2	59.6	63.6
SF	85.0	50.8	85.3	82.5	85.2
RE	84.9	76.2	81.5	78.4	83.3
MH	80.0	63.0	75.5	76.0	76.4
Average	75.0	62.7	76.1	76.5	79.1

Brandon, May 2010, N = 227, ages 20–94; Bella Coola Valley, N = 292, ages 17–90; Prince George, November 1998, N = 365, ages 17–82; Prince George, November 1999, N = 202, ages 17–86: USA, N = 1055, ages 18 and older

Source Ware et al. (1993), Michalos et al. (2000, 2005), and Michalos and Zumbo (2003)

Table 9.4 SF-36 comparisons of city and country female scores

Health dimensions	Brandon 2010	Bella C. Valley 2002	P.G. 1998	P.G. 1999	USA 1993
PF	76.8	82.1	87.3	87.1	81.5
RP	72.0	68.1	79.8	73.8	77.8
BP	68.2	55.5	59.7	70.2	73.6
GH	70.0	56.1	73.4	71.2	70.6
VT	57.1	54.0	56.5	57.3	58.4
SF	82.1	49.4	81.7	81.1	81.5
RE	81.8	74.3	79.8	77.8	79.5
MH	76.8	61.9	73.5	74.5	73.3
Average	73.1	62.7	74.0	74.1	74.5

Brandon, May 2010, N = 265, ages 18–93; Bella Coola Valley, N = 394, ages 17–88; Prince George, November 1998, N = 352, ages 17–92; Prince George, November 1999, N = 236, ages 20–86; USA, N = 1,412, ages 18 and older

Sources Ware et al. (1993), Michalos et al. (2000, 2001, 2005), and Michalos and Zumbo (2003)

samples from Prince George in 1999 and 2005, and for the USA in 1993. The 13% point difference in average scores for the Brandon samples of younger old and older old is larger than the differences for the other 3 samples. What drives the older old figures down are the scores for Role Physical (49.4) and Vitality (59.2). In fact, the same thing happens for the 2 Prince George samples. For the USA sample, while the Vitality score is the lowest of the 8, the General Health score is second lowest.

Examining the Brandon figures for younger old females versus older old females (Table 9.6), one finds that the average value of the former is again as expected, higher than that of the latter, namely, 70.5 versus 67.7, respectively. The female average for younger old people (70.5) is quite a bit lower than that for younger old

Table 9.5 Comparisons of older males' scores on the 8 health dimensions of SF-36

Dimension	Brandon 55–64 N = 67	Brandon 65 and over N = 81	PG 1999 55–64 N = 90	PG 1999 65 and over N = 189	PG 2005 55–64 N = 86	PG 2005 65 and over N = 147	USA 1993 55–64 N = 105	USA 1993 65 and over N = 293
PF	86.7	69.1	82.7	66.8	84.3	69.1	79.9	65.8
RP	83.3	49.4	74.4	55.7	79.0	57.9	76.0	59.7
BP	73.6	64.1	67.0	64.3	70.7	61.1	68.5	68.8
GH	70.8	64.5	65.8	62.2	63.3	62.8	66.6	58.6
VT	66.3	59.2	61.5	58.8	64.3	57.5	63.0	57.8
SF	91.3	81.6	82.4	79.5	85.4	83.2	83.6	79.7
RE	96.0	77.9	83.7	79.9	85.0	81.3	81.1	76.9
MH	82.1	80.5	77.9	79.0	76.9	79.2	76.9	77.4
Average	81.3	68.3	74.4	68.3	76.1	69.0	74.5	68.1

Sources Michalos et al. (2007), and Ware et al. (1993)

Table 9.6 Comparisons of older females' scores on the 8 health dimensions of SF-36

Dimension	Brandon 55–64 N = 58	Brandon 65 and over N = 88	PG 1999 55–64 N = 205	PG 1999 65 and over N = 368	PG 2005 55–64 N = 179	PG 2005 65 and over N = 235	USA 1993 55–64 N = 164	USA 1993 65 and over N = 413
PF	76.5	62.2	79.0	60.4	81.2	64.9	73.1	61.9
RP	70.3	55.1	70.1	54.7	70.5	55.0	71.6	56.1
BP	63.1	63.0	64.8	56.6	66.3	57.5	66.6	63.4
GH	67.9	64.5	68.1	63.9	63.6	63.4	62.9	61.6
VT	55.5	57.5	60.3	54.1	61.3	57.5	58.1	55.5
SF	79.7	78.0	81.7	78.7	83.2	79.8	79.4	77.0
RE	75.9	82.1	82.4	78.6	81.3	80.2	79.5	73.4
MH	75.1	79.3	77.2	76.4	77.6	77.5	73.4	74.7
Average	70.5	67.7	73.0	65.4	73.1	67.0	70.6	65.5

Sources Michalos et al. (2007), and Ware et al. (1993)

males (81.3). For the samples from Prince George in 1999 and 2005, and the USA in 1993, the younger old average scores for females are also higher than those of the older old. The differences among the female pairs of younger old versus older old samples is not as great as the differences for the males. While the Brandon difference was 13% points for males, it was only 2.8% points for females. The largest difference occurs with the Prince George 1999 sample (7.6). The 7.6% point difference in average scores for the Prince George 1999 samples of younger old and older old is larger than the differences for the other 3 samples. What drives the female older old figures down is a bit more complicated than the male picture. For the Brandon female older old sample, the lowest scores are for Role Physical (55.1) and Vitality (57.5). For the Prince George 1999 sample and the USA samples, the lowest scores are for Vitality, followed by that for Role Physical. For the Prince George 2005 sample, Role Physical is lowest, followed by a tie between Bodily Pain and Vitality.

The question we started with concerning the relative ranking of the Brandon sample of younger old and older old compared to the 2 samples from Prince George and the USA sample has been clearly answered. The Brandon sample of male younger old people had the highest average among the 4 samples and the Brandon sample of male older old people had the second highest average. In both cases the Brandon male sample for this age group moved up from last place. The Brandon sample of female younger old people ranked 3 out of 4 and the sample of female older old people ranked first. So, in both cases there was improvement, with the female older old sample moving from fourth place to first and the younger old sample moving from fourth place to third. Probably, then, Brandon's relatively low overall ranking (Table 9.2) was not the result of its having over-representation of older people, because our sample of older people generally compared well with samples of older people in other studies.

Since 1993 the United States Centers for Disease Control and Prevention (CDC) have been using a set of indicators to track the population health status of residents of all 50 States (CDC 2000). The whole system is known as the Behavioral Risk Factor Surveillance System (BRFSS). There were 4 items in the original core of the system and 10 were added to it in January 1995. Table 9.7 lists results from 6 surveys for 3 of the original items from the BRFSS that provide good summaries of people's health from different perspectives. Specifically, the items measure the number of days in the past 30 in which respondents experienced "not good health" physically, the number of days that were mentally "not good" and the number on which "not good" physical or mental health prevented respondents from engaging in their usual activities. All of the surveys were based on mailout questionnaires to adults 18 years of age or older in Brandon and Bella Coola Valley, Quesnel (pop. approx. 10,000) and Prince George, British Columbia.

The first two columns of the table reveal that on average the Brandon sample ran second behind the Bella Coola Valley sample for "not good" physical health days, with scores of 5.0 and 6.5, respectively. Brandon (3.3) was fourth behind Bella Coola Valley (5.5), Quesnel (4.2) and Prince George 2000 (3.5) for "not good"

Table 9.7 Mean scores for physical and mental not good health days, limited activity days, general health; 6 surveys

Indicator	Brandon 2010	Bella C. Valley 2002	Quesnel May 2000	P.G. April 2000	P.G. November 2000	P.G. May 2001
Sample size	505	687	642	607	437	695
P. H. not good days	5.0	6.5	3.7	3.4	4.1	3.2
M. H. not good days	3.3	5.5	4.2	3.5	3.2	3.1
Limited activity days	3.0	4.1	2.8	2.1	1.5	2.2

Sources Michalos and Zumbo (2000, 2003) Institute for Social Research and Evaluation surveys, 2000–2001, Michalos et al. (2005)

Table 9.8 Mean scores for additional five CDC items

Indicator: days in the past 30 in which you felt	Brandon 2010 (N = 497)	Bella C. Valley 2002 (N = 687)
Sad, blue or depressed	2.9	5
Worried, tense or anxious	3.7	6.7
You did not get enough sleep	7.3	9.5
Pain limited your usual activities	3.9	5
Very healthy and full of energy	17.6	16.4

Source Michalos et al. (2005)

mental health days. For limited activity days, Bella Coola Valley (4.1) was first and Brandon (3.0) second among the 6 samples.

Table 9.8 lists 5 other items from the CDC collection that were included in our questionnaire. The formats are the same as above, with respondents being asked to indicate the number of days in the past 30 in which they felt one way or another. The first four are negative and the last is positive. On average, the Brandon sample scores are better than the Bella Coola Valley sample scores on all 5 items. Brandon respondents felt sad on 2.9 of the past 30 days, worried on 3.7 days, did not get enough sleep on 7.3 days and had their usual activities limited by pain on 3.9 days. In general, they felt “very happy and full of energy” on 17.6 of the past 30 days.

Health-Related Behaviour and Exposure

Tables 9.9, 9.10, and 9.11 review health-related behaviour and exposure issues, including some comparisons with the Bella Coola Valley survey and the 1998 Prince George survey. Table 9.9 lists the percentages of respondents who were tobacco smokers and/or were exposed to second-hand smoke. Eighty-four percent

Table 9.9 Smoking behaviour and exposure

Behaviour and exposure	Brandon 2010 (N = 510)	Bella C. Valley 2002 (N = 685)	P.G. 1998 (N = 352)
Frequency of smoking tobacco (%)			
Never	84.3	66.5	77.1
Occasionally	4.5	10.2	6
Daily	7.3	13.1	8
Hourly	3.9	10.2	8.9
Frequency of exposure to second-hand smoke at home			
Never	84.7	68.7	68.5
Occasionally	8.0	13.7	15.8
Daily	4.9	11.6	10.1
Hourly	2.3	6.0	5.6
Frequency of exposure to second-hand smoke outside home			
Never	36.7	20.4	8.6
Occasionally	57.1	64.4	74.4
Daily	5.5	12.1	15.2
Hourly	0.8	3.1	1.8

Source Michalos et al. (2000, 2005)

Table 9.10 Drinking alcoholic beverages behaviour

Place →	Brandon 2010 (N = 510)	Bella C. Valley 2002 (N = 677)	P.G. 1998 (N = 352)
Frequency of drinking	%	%	%
Never	19.4	33.8	12.3
Less than once a month	18.4	17.1	22.5
Once a month	8.8	5	7.7
2–3 times a month	15.7	13	16.6
Once a week	10.0	6.4	9.4
2–3 times a week	13.3	12.4	16.1
4–6 times a week	7.8	6.9	10.5
Every day	6.5	5.4	5
Average # drinks per sitting	(N = 404)	(N = 448)	NA
1 or 2 drinks	80.2	63.6	71.3
3 or 4 drinks	16.1	21	21.7
5 or more drinks	3.7	15.4	7

'Drink' means one bottle or can of beer or a glass of draft, one glass of wine or a wine cooler, or one straight or mixed drink with one and a half ounces of hard liquor
Source Michalos et al. (2000, 2005)

Table 9.11 Mean number of times per week in the past month that respondents engaged in various kinds of physical activities in their leisure time for 15 min or more

Free time activities	Brandon 2010	Bella C. Valley 2002
Strenuous exercise (e.g., running, jogging, long distance cycling, singles tennis)	0.75 (N = 457)	1.0 (N = 567)
Moderate exercise (e.g., easy cycling, volleyball, easy swimming, folk dancing)	2.4 (N = 473)	2.3 (N = 585)
Mild exercise (e.g., yoga, golf, gardening, easy walking)	4.7 (N = 496)	5.5 (N = 616)

Source Michalos et al. (2005)

of the Brandon sample reported that they never smoked, compared to 66.5% of the Bella Coola Valley sample and 77.1% of the Prince George sample. In Brandon, 84.7% said they were never exposed to second-hand smoke at home, compared to 68.7% in Bella Coola Valley and 68.5% in Prince George. Thirty-seven percent of Brandon respondents reported that they were never exposed to second-hand smoke outside the home, compared to 20.4% of respondents in Bella Coola Valley and only 8.6% of the Prince George respondents. According to the Brandon RHA survey (pp. 4–9), about 25% of their sample were current smokers, compared to 15.7% of our sample.

Table 9.10 lists the percentages of respondents who drank alcoholic beverages with diverse frequencies and drinks per sitting. Nineteen percent of Brandon respondents reported that they never drank and 6.5% reported that they drank alcoholic beverages every day. Thirty-four percent of respondents in the Bella Coola Valley said they never drank and 5.4% drank every day, compared to 12.3% total abstainers and 5.0% daily drinkers in Prince George. Of those who drank, 80.2% of Brandon respondents reported that they drank an average of 1 or 2 drinks per sitting, compared to 63.6% of Bella Coola Valley respondents and 71.3% of Prince George respondents. At the other end of the scale, 15.4% of Bella Coola Valley respondents said that they drank 5 or more drinks per sitting on average, compared to 3.7% of Brandon respondents and 7.0% of Prince George respondents. Thus, Brandon respondents tended to be lighter drinkers in a given sitting.

Table 9.11 shows that on average, in their leisure time, Brandon respondents engaged in strenuous physical exercise for 15 min or more less than once per week (0.75) in the past month, moderate exercise about 2.4 times per week and mild exercise about 4.7 times per week. Bella Coola Valley respondents had more mild and strenuous exercise per week (5.5 and 1.0, respectively) and less moderate exercise (2.3 times per week).

Health Care

Table 9.12 lists results of several questions related to respondents' views about health care and aspects of their own care, including a column of scores from the Bella Coola Valley survey for comparison. For the Brandon sample, on a 5-point scale from 1 = poor to 5 = excellent, the mean respondent rating for their own health care services was 3.5, slightly better than their mean rating (3.3) for the health care services of most people. The Bella Coola Valley scores for the same questions were 3.4 for their own versus 3.3 for others.

In Brandon, 91.6% of respondents said they had a family physician, compared to 59.9% in the Bella Coola Valley. Nevertheless, Brandon respondents reported seeing a physician on average 4.9 times in the past year, compared to 5.6 times per year for Bella Coola Valley respondents. The former respondents had also been in hospital less often than the latter respondents, 0.3 times compared to 1.4 times per year. On average, Brandon respondents reported traveling 6.5 km the last time they needed routine medical care, compared to 67.9 km for Bella Coola Valley respondents. For specialist care, Brandon respondents traveled on average 84.3 km, compared to 579.0 km for Bella Coola Valley respondents.

Eighty-five percent of Brandon respondents had a dentist and had seen their dentist on average 1.5 times in the past year, compared to 61.4% of Bella Coola Valley respondents who had a dentist and had seen their dentist 1.6 times in the past year.

Table 9.12 Views about and aspects of health care

Health care issue	Brandon 2010 (N = 516)	Bella C. Valley 2002 (N = 663)
Mean rating of respondents' own health care services[a]	3.5	3.4
Mean rating of health care services for most people[a]	3.3	3.3
Percent having a family physician	91.6	59.9
Number of times seen a physician in the past year	4.9	5.6
Number of times been in hospital in the past year	0.3	1.4
Distance traveled for routine medical care last time it was needed (km)	6.5	67.9
Distance traveled for specialist care last time it was needed (km)	84.3	579

[a]Ratings on 5 point scale with 1 = poor, 2 = fair, 3 = average, 4 = good and 5 = excellent
Source Michalos et al. (2005)

Quality of Life Measures

Table 9.13 lists results for 19 measures of the quality of people's lives, including 15 measures of specific domains or aspects of life (e.g., housing, job, family relations) and 4 overall measures (e.g., overall happiness, satisfaction with life as a whole). All of the items were formatted in 7-point scales running from 1 = very dissatisfied (or very unhappy), through 4 = evenly balanced, to 7 = very satisfied (or very happy). Besides the Brandon sample, the table includes samples from the Bella Coola Valley and Prince George in May 2001, Quesnel in May 2000 and Jasper,

Table 9.13 Mean satisfaction and happiness levels

How satisfied are you with	Brandon 2010	Bella C. Valley 2002	P.G. May 2001	Quesnel May 2000	Jasper July 1997
Your house, apartment	6.0	5.4	5.6	5.6	5.7
Your neighborhood	6.0	5.7	5.5	5.4	5.7
Your family relations	6.0	5.7	5.9	5.9	5.8
Your living partner	6.4	5.8	6.2	6.3	5.4
Your job	5.5	5.1	5.2	5.4	4.6
Your life as a whole	5.7	5.5	5.7	na	5.9
Your friendships	5.7	5.7	5.8	5.8	6.0
Your health	5.4	4.9	5.4	5.5	5.8
Your religion/spiritual fulfilment	5.3	5.2	5.2	5.4	4.5
Your overall standard of living	5.8	5.4	5.4	5.3	5.7
Your financial security	5.3	4.4	4.6	4.7	4.9
Your recreation activities	4.9	4.6	5.1	4.8	na
Your self-esteem	5.6	5.2	5.5	5.7	5.8
Your personal safety around home	5.7	5.8	5.6	na	na
Federal government officials	4.0	3.3	2.9	3.6	3.0
Provincial government officials	4.1	3.3	2.6	3.7	3.0
Local government officials	4.4	3.6	3.4	4.1	na
Your overall quality of life	5.8	5.5	5.7	5.5	5.9
Your overall happiness	5.8	5.5	5.8	5.6	5.8
Average	5.4	5.0	5.1	5.2	5.2
N	512	687	695	642	447

Sources Michalos and Zumbo (2000), Zumbo and Michalos (2000), Michalos (2002), and Michalos et al. (2005)

Alberta (pop. approx. 4,300) in July 1997. The average score for the Brandon respondents was 5.4, ranging from 4.0 for satisfaction with federal government officials to 6.4 for satisfaction with living partners. Each of the average scores for the other 4 samples are lower than the Brandon average, i.e., Quesnel and Jasper (5.2 each), Prince George (5.1) and Bella Coola Valley (5.0). While the Brandon sample had 4 scores of 6.0 or above, there was only one such score in the other 4 samples. For these quality of life measures, with sample sizes of about 500, usually there must be a difference of 0.3 between any two scores to be statistically significant.

Considering only the rank ordering of only the domain satisfaction scores for the 5 samples, one finds some interesting similarities and differences at both ends of the satisfaction scales. For the samples from Brandon, Bella Coola Valley, Prince George and Quesnel, living partner satisfaction scores were ranked highest, while for the Jasper sample, it was friendship satisfaction. Curiously, the Bella Coola Valley personal safety satisfaction score was the same as the living partner satisfaction score. Family relations satisfaction scores ranked second for all 5 samples, although these scores were tied with several different scores in different samples, e.g., tied with housing and neighbourhood satisfaction scores in Brandon. At the other end of the scale, in every sample government officials at all 3 levels had the lowest satisfaction ratings, although the Brandon sample scores were higher than those for every other sample for every level of government. Local officials always faired a bit better than federal and provincial officials. Apart from government officials, which routinely serve as a sort of public punching bag in most surveys, lowest levels of satisfaction scores are reported for recreation activities in Brandon (4.9), and financial security in Bella Coola Valley (4.4), Prince George (4.6) and Quesnel (4.7). In Jasper, apart from government officials, the lowest scores are reported for religion or spiritual fulfillment (4.5).

In comparison, the Brandon Regional Health Authority (2009, pp. 1–22) reported that about 43% of their sample said that they were very satisfied with their life as a whole, while 33.9% of our sample gave that response.

Independent and Dependent Measures

Broadly speaking, we classified variables as independent if they belonged to the British Columbia Provincial Health Officer's (1994) list of determinants of health and dependent if they had been validated as relatively general measures of health status or overall quality of life. In some analyses in other studies we use health status indicators as predictors of overall quality of life, because the concept of the 'quality of life' is more comprehensive than the concept of 'health' (Michalos 2004). Table 9.14 provides an overview of how we view the most important ones. It should be noted that 3 of the items listed among the predictor variables in this table are most likely consequences rather than antecedents of ill health, namely, number of pain killers taken, number of visits to doctors, and number of times in

Table 9.14 Independent and dependent variables

Independent (predictors, determinants)	Dependent variables
Biological influences	Average of 8 SF-36 dimensions = general health
Age, gender, body mass index	Happiness
Social/economic environment	Satisfaction with life as a whole
Income, education level, social support index, good neighbourhood	Satisfaction with life scale
Index, crime worries index, community health index, frequency at religious services	Satisfaction with life scale Satisfaction with quality of life Subjective well-being index Contentment with life assessment scale
Health behaviours	
Smoking frequency, drinking frequency, drinking amount, eating breakfast, skipping meals, # pain killers taken, hrs sleep per night, frequency of moderate exercise	
Health services	
Personal health care rating, most people's health care rating, # times seeing doctor, # times in hospital, # times seeing dentist, distance to doctor, distance to specialist	
Comparison standards	
Self status compared to wants, others of same age and gender, deserves, needs, expected 3 years ago, expect in 5 years, best ever had	
Satisfaction with domains/aspects of life	
Home, neighbourhood, city, quality of air, land, water, personal safety, local government, Brandon programs for recreation, police/fire protection, social programs, shops/services, religious activities, public transportation, parks, treatment by locals, feel part of community, access to health care, family, living partner, friendships, spiritual fulfillment, financial security, recreation activities, self-esteem, sense of meaning in life, life achievements, future security	

hospital. Hours of sleep per night can be a determinant and a consequence of ill health.

Most of the measures listed in Table 9.14 have been explained with data presented in earlier tables, but some require additional explanations. One- and two-year test-retest reliabilities and sensitivity measures may be found for most of the domain satisfaction measures and all of the overall quality of life measures except Average Health in Michalos and Kahke (2010). Beginning with the dependent variables, we took the average of the 8 SF-36 dimension scores as a measure of Average Health. The measures of happiness, satisfaction with life as a whole and satisfaction with the overall quality of life were described earlier. Diener et al.'s (1985) 5-item Satisfaction with Life Scale (SWLS) Lavallee et al. (2007), 5-item Contentment with Life Assessment Scale (CLAS) and Michalos and Zumbo's (2000) 4-item Subjective Wellbeing (SWB) have been used and described in previous studies, e.g., Michalos (2003), Michalos et al. (2005), Michalos and Kahke (2010). Four new indexes were constructed for this investigation, and their basic features are given in Tables 9.15, 9.16, 9.17, and 9.18. Each scale was constructed by taking the average score of its constituent items.

Table 9.15 Good neighbourhood index (∝ = 0.87, N = 451)

Item	Item mean	Item-total correlation
I feel like I belong in my neighbourhood	5.4	0.67
I participate in neighbourhood activities	4.1	0.52
I feel comfortable reaching out to neighbours when I need help	4.7	0.59
My neighbourhood is clean	5.6	0.69
My neighbourhood is friendly	5.5	0.77
I am satisfied with the roads in my neighbourhood	4.6	0.53
I am satisfied with the sidewalks in my neighbourhood	4.6	0.48
I am satisfied with the parks/green spaces in my neighbourhood	5.0	0.55
The houses in my neighbourhood are in good condition	5.6	0.61
My neighbourhood is a good place to raise children	5.5	0.55

Table 9.16 Crime worries index (∝ = 0.99, N = 518)

Item: how much do you worry about the possibility that…	Item mean	Item-total correlation
A thief will break into your home while you are away	6.8	0.98
Someone will use a weapon to take something from you by force	6.5	0.94
Someone will steal a personal item (e.g., coat, purse, etc.) when you have left it somewhere unattended	8.0	0.98
A thief will break into your home while you are home	6.3	0.98
Someone will cheat or con you out of a large amount of money	5.7	0.99
Someone will assault you	6.4	0.96

Table 9.17 Community health index (∝ = 0.93, N = 482)

Item: considering the city of Brandon	Item mean	Item-total correlation
Alcohol abuse is a problem here	3.5	0.82
Drug abuse is a problem here	3.6	0.85
Family violence is a problem here	3.3	0.86
Unemployment is a problem here	2.9	0.69
Sexual abuse is a problem here	3.1	0.85
Racial discrimination is a problem here	3.1	0.68

Table 9.15 lists the 10 items of our Good Neighbourhood Index, with its Cronbach Alpha value ($\alpha = 0.87$) and item-total score correlations (averaging $r = 0.60$). Generally speaking, alpha coefficients above 0.70 are regarded as acceptable and those above 0.80 as relatively high. Alpha coefficients measure the inter-correlations (i.e., internal coherence or consistency) among the items in the set based on pairwise correlations.

Table 9.18 Social support index (∝ = 0.77, N = 508)

Item: considering the city of Brandon	Item mean	Item-total correlation
Do you have someone to confide in, or talk to about your private feelings/concerns?	1.2	0.56
Do you have someone you can really count on to help you out in a crisis situation?	1.1	0.62
Do you have someone you can really count on to give you advice when you are making important personal decisions?	1.1	0.67
Do you have someone that makes you feel loved and cared for?	1.1	0.47

Table 9.16 lists the 6 items of our Crime Worries Index, with its Cronbach Alpha value ($\alpha = 0.99$) and item-total score correlations (averaging $r = 0.97$). Table 9.17 lists the 6 items of our Community Health Index, with its Cronbach Alpha value ($\alpha = 0.93$) and item-total score correlations (averaging $r = 0.79$). Table 9.18 lists the 4 items of our Social Support Index, with its Cronbach Alpha value ($\alpha = 0.77$) and item-total score correlations (averaging $r = 0.58$).

Explaining Health and the Quality of Life: Multivariate Relationships

Tables 9.19, 9.20, 9.21, 9.22, 9.23, 9.24, and 9.25 summarize results of systematically regressing each of our 7 dependent variables (i.e., Average Health, Happiness, single item Satisfaction with Life, single item Satisfaction with the Quality of Life, and 3 indexes, SWLS, CLAS and SWB) on the set of 63 determinants listed in Table 9.14. Of all the potential predictors, the only ones that appear in any particular table are those that had at least one significant relationship to the dependent variable considered in that table.

The strategy of the analysis for each dependent variable was the same and the structure of each table is the same. Each of the numerical columns gives results of applying stepwise regression using the following sets of potential determinants: (1) columns 1–4 = biological, social/economic, health behaviour, health services; (2) all significant health variables from columns 1–4, (3) 7 comparison standards; (4) satisfaction in diverse domains or aspects of life (without health satisfaction), and (5) all statistically significant variables from the previous regressions indicated in the columns for all statistically significant health variables, comparison standards and satisfaction in diverse domains of life. The results in this final column may be compared to those in the column for all statistically significant health variables to estimate the relative strength of health determinants as quality-of-life determinants. We are interested in measuring:

Table 9.19 Explaining average of 8 SF-36 dimensions by health determinants, comparison standards and domain satisfaction, N = 411

	Biological determinants	Social/economic determinants	Health behaviour det.	Health services determinants	All health determinants	Comparison standard determinant	Domain Sat. determinants	All significant determinants
% Variance expl.	11	18	23	13	44	28	25	46
Predictors ↓	$\beta\downarrow$	$\beta\downarrow$	$\beta\downarrow$	$\beta\downarrow$	$\beta\downarrow$	$\beta\downarrow$	$\beta\downarrow$	$\beta\downarrow$
BMI	−0.16	a	a	a	b	a	a	b
Age	−0.32	a	a	a	−0.17	a	a	−0.19
Gender	−0.11	a	a	a	b	a	a	b
Income	a	0.26	a	a	0.14	a	a	b
G. neighbourhood index	a	0.22	a	a	0.20	a	a	b
Crime worries index	a	−0.12	a	a	−0.15	a	a	b
Social support index	a	0.14	a	a	0.18	a	a	b
Freq. moderate exercise	a	a	0.16	a	0.10	a	a	b
Hours sleep/night	a	a	0.11	a	b	a	a	b
# pain killers taken	a	a	−0.41	a	−0.34	a	a	−0.26
# times seeing doctor	a	a	a	−0.25	−0.22	a	a	−0.17
# times in hospital	a	a	a	−0.18	b	a	a	b

(continued)

Table 9.19 (continued)

	Biological determinants	Social/economic determinants	Health behaviour det.	Health services determinants	All health determinants	Comparison standard determinant	Domain Sat. determinants	All significant determinants
Self-wants	a	a	a	a	a	0.20	a	b
Self-best	a	a	a	a	a	0.34	a	0.21
Self-future	a	a	a	a	a	0.11	a	b
Recreation sat.	a	a	a	a	a	a	0.42	0.33
Self-esteem sat.	a	a	a	a	a	a	0.15	b
Life achievements sat.	a	a	a	a	a	a	0.14	b
Feel part community sat.	a	a	a	a	a	a	−0.19	b

a not in equation, *b* significance level too low to enter equation

Table 9.20 Explaining happiness by health determinants, comparison standards and domain satisfaction, N = 491

	Social/economic determinants	Health behaviour det.	Health services determinants	All health determinants	Comparison standard determinant	Domain sat. determinants	All significant determinants
% Variance expl.	23	12	5	20	40	43	45
Predictors↓	$\beta\downarrow$	$\beta\downarrow$	$\beta\downarrow$	$\beta\downarrow$	$\beta\downarrow$	$\beta\downarrow$	$\beta\downarrow$
G. neighbourhood index	0.27	a	a	0.19	a	a	b
Social support ind.	0.37	a	a	0.21	a	a	0.16
Hours sleep/night	a	0.20	a	0.21	a	a	b
# Pain killers taken	a	−0.14	a	b	a	a	b
Drink frequency	a	0.17	a	0.12	a	a	b
Drink amount	a	−0.12	a	b	a	a	b
Skipping meals	a	−0.11	a	b	a	a	b
Own health care rating	a	a	0.21	0.11	a	a	b
# Times in hospital	a	a	−0.10	b	a	a	b
Self-wants	a	a	a	a	0.43	a	0.31
Self-best	a	a	a	a	0.10	a	b
Self-others	a	a	a	a	0.21	a	0.19

(continued)

Table 9.20 (continued)

	Social/economic determinants	Health behaviour det.	Health services determinants	All health determinants	Comparison standard determinant	Domain sat. determinants	All significant determinants
Living partner sat.	a	a	a	a	a	0.21	b
Financial security sat.	a	a	a	a	a	0.16	b
Meaning in life sat.	a	a	a	a	a	0.28	0.23
Life achievements sat.	a	a	a	a	a	0.19	b

a not in equation, *b* significance level too low to enter equation

Table 9.21 Explaining satisfaction with life as a whole (single item) by health determinants, comparison standards and domain satisfaction, N = 332

	Biological determinants	Social/economic determinants	Health behaviour det.	Health services determinants	All health determinants	Comparison standard determinant	Domain sat. determinants	All significant determinants
% Variance expl.	1	29	8	10	34	39	65	66
Predictors↓	$\beta\downarrow$	$\beta\downarrow$	$\beta\downarrow$	$\beta\downarrow$	$\beta\downarrow$	$\beta\downarrow$	$\beta\downarrow$	$\beta\downarrow$
Gender	0.11	a	a	a	b	a	a	b
Income	a	0.11	a	a	b	a	a	b
G. neighbourhood index	a	0.35	a	a	0.25	a	a	b
Crime worries index	a	−0.12	a	a	b	a	a	b
Social support index	a	0.30	a	a	0.29	a	a	b
Hours sleep/night	a	a	0.14	a	0.12	a	a	b
# Pain killers taken	a	a	−0.14	a	−0.12	a	a	b
Drink frequency	a	a	0.17	a	0.18	a	a	b
Skipping meals	a	a	−0.12	a	b	a	a	b
Own health care rating	a	a	a	0.28	0.17	a	a	0.08
# Times seeing dentist	a	a	a	0.15	b	a	a	b
Self-wants	a	a	a	a	a	0.39	a	b

(continued)

Table 9.21 (continued)

	Biological determinants	Social/economic determinants	Health behaviour det.	Health services determinants	All health determinants	Comparison standard determinant	Domain sat. determinants	All significant determinants
Self-best	a	a	a	a	a	0.17	a	0.16
Self-other	a	a	a	a	a	0.12	a	b
Self-progress	a	a	a	a	a	0.11	a	b
Family sat.	a	a	a	a	a	a	0.12	b
Living partner sat.	a	a	a	a	a	a	0.26	0.18
Friendships sat.	a	a	a	a	a	a	0.29	0.29
Meaning in life sat.	a	a	a	a	a	a	0.22	0.21
Life achievements sat.	a	a	a	a	a	a	0.25	0.23

a not in equation, *b* significance level too low to enter equation

Table 9.22 Explaining satisfaction with the overall quality of life by health determinants, comparison standards and domain satisfaction, N = 392

	Social/economic determinants	Health behaviour det.	Health services determinants	All health determinants	Comparison standard determinant	Domain sat. determinants	All significant determinants
% Variance expl.	24	9	9	31	37	60	67
Predictors↓	β↓	β↓	β↓	β↓	β↓	β↓	β↓
Education	0.13	a	a	0.12	a	a	0.06
Income	0.11	a	a	b	a	a	b
G. neighbourhood index	0.33	a	a	0.25	a	a	b
Social support index	0.23	a	a	0.21	a	a	b
Hours sleep/night	a	0.14	a	b	a	a	b
# pain killers taken	a	−0.16	a	−0.14	a	a	−0.07
Drink frequency	a	0.15	a	0.14	a	a	b
Eating breakfast	a	0.14	a	0.16	a	a	b
Own health care rating	a	a	0.22	0.12	a	a	b
# Times seeing doctor	a	a	−0.19	b	a	a	b
Distance to doctor	a	a	−0.10	b	a	a	b

(continued)

Table 9.22 (continued)

	Social/economic determinants	Health behaviour det.	Health services determinants	All health determinants	Comparison standard determinant	Domain sat. determinants	All significant determinants
Self-wants	a	a	a	a	0.41	a	0.14
Self-other	a	a	a	a	0.17	a	0.14
Self-progress	a	a	a	a	0.14	a	b
Financial security Sat.	a	a	a	a	a	0.15	b
Meaning in life Sat.	a	a	a	a	a	0.30	0.34
Home sat.	a	a	a	a	a	0.18	0.14
Treatment by locals Sat.	a	a	a	a	a	0.35	0.26

a not in equation, *b* significance level too low to enter equation

Table 9.23 Explaining satisfaction with life scale (SWLS) by health determinants, comparison standards and domain satisfaction, N = 329

	Social/economic determinants	Health behaviour det.	Health services determinants	All health determinants	Comparison standard determinant	Domain sat. determinants	All significant determinants
% Variance expl.	33	14	9	39	68	56	74
Predictors↓	β↓	β↓	β↓	β↓	β↓	β↓	β↓
Income	0.16	a	a	0.12	a	a	b
G. neighbourhood index	0.41	a	a	0.33	a	a	b
Crime worries index	−0.09	a	a	b	a	a	b
Social support index	0.28	a	a	0.20	a	a	b
Hours sleep/night	a	0.19	a	0.17	a	a	b
# Pain killers taken	a	−0.13	a	b	a	a	b
Drink frequency	a	0.13	a	0.10	a	a	b
Skipping meals	a	−0.24	a	−0.16	a	a	b
Own health care rating	a	a	0.27	0.15	a	a	b
# Times in hospital	a	a	−0.14	b	a	a	b
Self-wants	a	a	a	a	0.47	a	0.30
Self-best	a	a	a	a	0.24	a	0.22

(continued)

Table 9.23 (continued)

	Social/economic determinants	Health behaviour det.	Health services determinants	All health determinants	Comparison standard determinant	Domain sat. determinants	All significant determinants
Self-other	a	a	a	a	0.14	a	0.17
Self-progress	a	a	a	a	0.12	a	b
Self-deserves	a	a	a	a	0.08	a	b
Living partner sat.	a	a	a	a	a	0.16	0.09
Self-esteem sat.	a	a	a	a	a	0.22	0.18
Life achievements sat.	a	a	a	a	a	0.27	0.12
Future security sat.	a	a	a	a	a	0.17	b
Treatment by locals sat.	a	a	a	a	a	0.13	0.09

a not in equation, *b* significance level too low to enter equation

Table 9.24 Explaining contentment with life assessment scale (CLAS) by health determinants, comparison standards and domain satisfaction, N = 458

	Social/economic determinants	Health behaviour det.	Health services determinants	All health determinants	Comparison standard determinant	Domain sat. determinants	All significant determinants
% Variance expl.	29	10	8	36	52	54	60
Predictors↓	$\beta\downarrow$	$\beta\downarrow$	$\beta\downarrow$	$\beta\downarrow$	$\beta\downarrow$	$\beta\downarrow$	$\beta\downarrow$
Income	0.15	a	a	0.11	a	a	b
G. neighbourhood index	0.35	a	a	0.27	a	a	b
# Relig. meetings	0.12	a	a	0.12	a	a	b
Social support index	0.29	a	a	0.23	a	a	b
Hours sleep/night	a	0.21	a	0.21	a	a	b
Drink frequency	a	0.12	a	0.09	a	a	b
Skipping meals	a	−0.18	a	−0.10	a	a	b
Own health care rating	a	a	0.24	0.09	a	a	b
# times seeing doctor	a	a	−0.11	−0.10	a	a	b
# times in hospital	a	a	−0.10	b	a	a	b
Self-wants	a	a	a	a	0.39	a	0.30
Self-best	a	a	a	a	0.16	a	0.25

(continued)

Table 9.24 (continued)

	Social/economic determinants	Health behaviour det.	Health services determinants	All health determinants	Comparison standard determinant	Domain sat. determinants	All significant determinants
Self-other	a	a	a	a	0.16	a	b
Self-progress	a	a	a	a	0.13	a	b
Self-future	a	a	a	a	0.10	a	b
Living partner sat.	a	a	a	a	a	0.12	b
Friendships sat.	a	a	a	a	a	0.14	0.13
Recreation activities sat.	a	a	a	a	a	0.16	b
Self-esteem sat.	a	a	a	a	a	0.23	0.15
Life achievements sat.	a	a	a	a	a	0.30	0.18

a not in equation, *b* significance level too low to enter equation

Table 9.25 Explaining subjective wellbeing (SWB) by health determinants, comparison standards and domain satisfaction, N = 325

	Social/economic determinants	Health behaviour det.	Health services determinants	All health determinants	Comparison standard determinant	Domain sat. determinants	All significant determinants
% Variance expl.	35	13	10	42	53	76	75
Predictors↓	β↓	β↓	β↓	β↓	β↓	β↓	β↓
Income	0.18	a	a	0.12	a	a	b
G. neighbourhood index	0.39	a	a	0.31	a	a	b
Crime worries index	−0.09	a	a	b	a	a	b
# Relig. meetings	0.11	a	a	b	a	a	b
Social support index	0.30	a	a	0.25	a	a	b
Hours sleep/night	a	0.19	a	0.16	a	a	b
# pain killers taken	a	−0.17	a	−0.10	a	a	b
Drink frequency	a	0.19	a	0.16	a	a	0.08
Skipping meals	a	−0.13	a	−0.11	a	a	b
Own health care rating	a	a	0.26	0.15	a	a	b
# times seeing doctor	a	a	−0.14	b	a	a	b

(continued)

Table 9.25 (continued)

	Social/economic determinants	Health behaviour det.	Health services determinants	All health determinants	Comparison standard determinant	Domain sat. determinants	All significant determinants
# times seeing dentist	a	a	0.13	b	a	a	b
Self-wants	a	a	a	a	0.45	a	0.14
Self-best	a	a	a	a	0.11	a	0.12
Self-other	a	a	a	a	0.21	a	b
Self-progress	a	a	a	a	0.12	a	b
Family sat.	a	a	a	a	a	0.09	b
Living partner sat.	a	a	a	a	a	0.13	b
Financial security sat.	a	a	a	a	a	0.26	0.25
Meaning in life sat.	a	a	a	a	a	0.26	0.28
Life achievements sat.	a	a	a	a	a	0.13	0.14
Home sat.	a	a	a	a	a	0.13	0.18
Treatment by locals sat.	a	a	a	a	a	0.17	b

a not in equation, *b* significance level too low to enter equation

1. the total explanatory power (R^2) of each set of determinants for each dependent variable;
2. the relative explanatory power (standardized regression coefficient or β value) of each determinant in the context of each set of predictors for each dependent variable;
3. the similarities and differences obtained in all the explanations of the measures of Average Health and the broader measures of overall quality of life.

We will comment on the results of each exhibit in turn and then provide some overview remarks in the next section.

Average of SF-36 Dimensions

Table 9.19 (column 1) shows that our 3 biological determinants explain 11% of the variation in the scores of Average Health. In the context of these determinants, respondents' age was most influential and negative ($\beta = -0.32$). Figuratively speaking, this β-value may be understood as indicating that when all predictors are standardized to have means of zero and standard deviations of one unit step, for every increase of one full unit step in respondents' age, the dependent variable (Average Health) decreases 32% of a step, with the values of the other predictors held constant (i.e., controlled).

Column 2 shows that 4 social/economic determinants could account for 18% of the variance in Average Health scores, with respondents' income most influential and positive ($\beta = 0.26$). As one might have expected, scores on the Good Neighbourhood Index ($\beta = 0.22$) and Social Support Index ($\beta = 0.14$) had a positive influence on Average Health, and scores on the Crime Worries Index had a negative influence ($\beta = -0.12$).

Three health behaviours accounted for 23% of the variance in Average Health scores (column 3), with respondents' average numbers of pain killers taken per week most influential and negative ($\beta = -0.41$).

Two health services determinants explained 13% of the variance in Average Health scores (column 4) and both influences were negative, namely, respondents' average number of times seeing a physician ($\beta = -0.25$) and being in hospital ($\beta = -0.18$) in the past year.

Using the 10 statistically significant health determinants, we found a narrower set of 8 significant predictors could account for 44% of the variance in Average Health scores. Of these 8, the most influential 2 are negative, i.e., respondents' average number of pain killers taken per week ($\beta = -0.34$) and average number of times in the past year seeing a doctor ($\beta = -0.22$), and the third most influential is positive, i.e., Good Neighbourhood Index scores ($\beta = 0.20$).

Of the 7 different comparison standards that might influence respondents' judgment of their Average Health, 3 were statistically significant (column 6). Most influential were comparisons made between respondents' current life as a whole and the best they had ever experienced ($\beta = 0.34$). The closer the gap became between their current status and the best they had ever experienced, the greater its influence. Comparisons made between their current status and what they wanted out of life ($\beta = 0.20$) were next most influential, and comparisons between their current status and what they thought they would have in the future came last ($\beta = 0.20$).

Levels of satisfaction in 4 of the 28 distinct domains of life explained 25% of the variance in Average Health scores (column 7), with respondents' satisfaction with their recreation activities most influential ($\beta = 0.42$). Given the relatively small sample size (N = 411), regressions involving 28 predictors would have been somewhat inaccurate. "Even when R^2 in the population is zero, the expectation of the sample R^2 is $k/(N - 1)$, where k is the number of predictors, and N is the sample size" (Pedhazur 1982, p. 148). For our sample and number of predictors, the expectation of our sample R^2 would have been 7% though the population R^2 might be zero. To reduce the risk of such inaccuracy, we undertook several regressions with about 5 predictors at a time, deleting statistically insignificant predictors until we reached a set with only significant predictors.

Finally, using the 15 significant health determinants, comparison standards and domain satisfaction scores together, we were able to explain 46% of the variation in Average Health scores (column 8). In the final regression, there were 5 statistically significant predictors, with recreation satisfaction ($\beta = 0.33$) and average number of pain killers taken per week ($\beta = -0.26$) most influential, the first positive and the second negative. It should be noted that our exploration of the influence of 7 comparison standards and 28 domain satisfaction scores allowed us to increase our power to explain the variation in Average Health scores beyond the power of health determinants alone from 44% to only 46%. This distribution of the explanatory power of health determinants versus other kinds will be radically different for all of our overall quality of life assessment variables, indicating quite clearly that respondents distinguish having good health from having a good quality of life, all things considered.

Happiness

Table 9.20 begins with a column listing social/economic determinants because none of our biological determinants had statistically significant relations to our measure of happiness. Column (1) shows that 2 social/economic determinants explain 23% of the variation in happiness scores, with respondents' Social Support Index scores most influential ($\beta = 0.37$), followed by Good Neighbourhood Index scores ($\beta = 0.27$).

Five health behaviour determinants accounted for 12% of the variance in happiness scores (column 2), with respondents' number of hours of sleep per night most influential ($\beta = 0.20$), followed by the frequency of drinking alcoholic beverages ($\beta = 0.17$). Number of pain killers taken ($\beta = -0.14$), average amount of alcoholic drinks taken at one sitting ($\beta = -0.12$) and average number of meals skipped per week ($\beta = -0.11$) were negative as expected.

Two health services determinants explained 5% of the variance in happiness scores (column 3), with respondents' ratings of their own health care weighing in first ($\beta = 0.21$) and average number of times being in hospital in the past year second ($\beta = -0.10$). It is curious that respondents' reported happiness with life as a whole increased with increases in their health care ratings, since the latter had no influence on their Average Health assessments.

Using the 9 statistically significant health determinants, we found a narrower set of 5 significant predictors accounted for 20% of the variance in happiness scores, with respondents' Social Support Index and average number of hours of sleep per night equally influential ($\beta = 0.21$).

Three comparison standards were statistically significant (column 5). Most influential were comparisons made between respondents' current life as a whole and what they wanted out of life ($\beta = 0.43$). Comparisons made between their current status and that of others of the same sex and age in their areas were second ($\beta = 0.21$), followed by comparisons between their current status and the best they had ever experienced ($\beta = 0.10$).

Levels of satisfaction in 4 distinct domains of life explained 43% of the variance in happiness scores (column 6), with respondents' satisfaction with their sense of meaning in life most influential ($\beta = 0.28$), followed by satisfaction with their living partner ($\beta = 0.21$).

Finally, using the 12 statistically significant health determinants, comparison standards and domain satisfaction scores, we were able to explain 45% of the variation in happiness scores (column 7). In the final regression, there were 4 statistically significant predictors, with the gap between respondents' current status and what they wanted being most influential ($\beta = 0.31$), followed by their satisfaction with their sense of meaning in life ($\beta = 0.23$). As suggested earlier, the explanatory power of our predictors more than doubled from 20 to 45% as we added comparison standards and domain satisfaction scores to our set of health determinants. Besides explaining a greater amount of variance in happiness scores than in Average Health scores, none of the statistically significant predictors in the final regression equations for happiness and Average Health were the same.

Satisfaction with Life as a Whole

Table 9.21 (column 1) shows that one biological determinant explained 1% of the variation in the single item satisfaction with life as a whole scores ($\beta = 0.11$), i.e., as we saw earlier, in our Brandon sample, male respondents had higher average scores than female respondents for the 8 SF-36 health dimensions.

Four social/economic determinants accounted for 29% of the variance in the single item satisfaction with life as a whole scores (column 2), led by the Good Neighbourhood Index ($\beta = 0.35$) and followed by the Social Support Index ($\beta = 0.30$). The Crime Worries Index had a negative impact ($\beta = -0.12$).

Four health behaviours accounted for 8% of the variance in the single item satisfaction with life as a whole scores (column 3), with respondents' frequency of drinking alcoholic beverages leading ($\beta = 0.17$), followed by their average number of hours of sleep per night ($\beta = 0.14$) and their average number of pain killers taken per week ($\beta = -0.14$).

Two health services determinants explained 10% of the variance in the single item satisfaction with life as a whole scores (column 4), with respondents' ratings of their own health care being most influential ($\beta = 0.28$), followed by their average numbers of times seeing a dentist in the past year ($\beta = 0.15$). No doubt the latter information will come as a pleasant surprise to dentists. Presumably, the frequency of dentists visits indicated successful prevention.

Using the 11 statistically significant health determinants, we found a narrower set of 6 significant predictors accounted for 34% of the variance in the single item satisfaction with life as a whole scores (column 5), with respondents' Social Support Index ($\beta = 0.29$) and Good Neighbourhood Index ($\beta = 0.25$) most influential.

Four comparison standards were statistically significant (column 6). Most influential were comparisons made between respondents' current life as a whole and what they wanted out of life ($\beta = 0.39$). Comparisons made between their current status and the best they had ever experienced ($\beta = 0.17$) came next at some distance.

Levels of satisfaction in 4 of the distinct domains of life explained 65% of the variance in the single item satisfaction with life as a whole scores (column 7), with respondents' satisfaction with their friendships most influential ($\beta = 0.29$), followed by satisfaction with their living partner ($\beta = 0.26$) and what they had achieved in life ($\beta = 0.25$). Part of the reason for the relatively big increase in the explanatory power of our predictors in this column lies in the fact that here we are explaining one sort of satisfaction (overall life satisfaction) by other sorts (satisfaction with specific domains and aspects of life).

Finally, using all the significant health, comparison standards and domain satisfaction determinants, we were able to explain 66% of the variation in the single item satisfaction with life as a whole scores (column 8). In that regression, 6 predictors remained statistically significant, with respondents' satisfaction with their friendships dominating the lot ($\beta = 0.29$), followed by their satisfaction with what they had achieved in life ($\beta = 0.23$) and satisfaction with their sense of meaning in life ($\beta = 0.21$).

Satisfaction with the Overall Quality of Life

Table 9.22 shows, first, that our biological determinants had no statistically significant influence on respondents' satisfaction with the overall quality of their lives. Four social/economic determinants accounted for 24% of the variance in their satisfaction with the overall quality of their lives (column 1), with respondents' Good Neighbourhood Index most influential ($\beta = 0.33$), followed by their Social Support Index ($\beta = 0.23$).

Four health behaviours accounted for 9% of the variance in respondents' scores for satisfaction with the overall quality of their lives (column 2), with respondents' average number of pain killers taken per week most influential and negative ($\beta = -0.16$), followed closely by their frequency of drinking alcoholic beverages ($\beta = 0.15$), and their average number of hours of sleep per night and average number of times per week that they eat breakfast ($\beta = 0.14$ for each variable).

Three health services determinants also explained 9% of the variance in respondents' scores for satisfaction with the overall quality of their lives (column 3). Respondents' ratings of their own health care were most influential ($\beta = 0.22$), followed negatively by their average number of times seeing a doctor in the past year ($\beta = -0.19$) and the average distance they had to travel to get routine medical care ($\beta = -0.10$).

Using the 11 statistically significant health determinants, we found that a narrower set of 7 significant predictors accounted for 31% of the variance in respondents' scores for satisfaction with the overall quality of their lives (column 4), with the Good Neighbourhood Index most influential ($\beta = 0.25$), followed by the Social Support Index ($\beta = 0.21$).

Three comparison standards were statistically significant in accounting for the variance in respondents' scores for satisfaction with the overall quality of their lives (column 5). Most influential were comparisons made between respondents' current life as a whole and what they wanted out of life ($\beta = 0.41$). Comparisons made between their current status and that of others of the same sex and age in their areas were a distant second ($\beta = 0.17$).

Levels of satisfaction in 4 of the distinct domains of life explained 60% of the variance in respondents' scores for satisfaction with the overall quality of their lives (column 6). Respondents' satisfaction with how local people treat them was most influential ($\beta = 0.35$), followed by satisfaction with their sense of meaning in life ($\beta = 0.30$).

Finally, using all the significant health, comparison standards and domain satisfaction determinants, we were able to explain 67% of the variation in respondents' scores for satisfaction with the overall quality of their lives (column 7), with satisfaction with their sense of meaning in life most influential ($\beta = 0.34$), followed by their satisfaction with how local people treat them ($\beta = 0.26$).

Satisfaction with Life Scale (SWLS)

Table 9.23 reveals, first, that our biological determinants did not explain any of the variation in Satisfaction With Life Scale (SWLS) scores. Four social/economic determinants accounted for 33% of the variance in SWLS scores (column 1), with respondents' Good Neighbourhood Index most influential ($\beta = 0.41$), followed by the Social Support Index ($\beta = 0.28$).

Four health behaviours accounted for 14% of the variance in SWLS scores (column 2), with respondents' average number of meals skipped per week most influential and negative ($\beta = -0.24$), followed by their average number of hours of sleep per night ($\beta = 0.19$). There was a tie between the positive influence of their frequency of drinking alcoholic beverages ($\beta = 0.13$) and the negative influence of their average number of pain killers taken per week ($\beta = -0.13$).

Two health services determinants explained 9% of the variance in SWLS scores (column 3), with respondents' ratings of their own health care being most influential positively ($\beta = 0.27$), followed negatively by the average number of times they had been in hospital in the past year ($\beta = -0.14$).

Using the 10 statistically significant health determinants, we found a narrower set of 7 significant predictors accounted for 39% of the variance in SWLS scores (column 4), with respondents' Good Neighbourhood Index most influential ($\beta = 0.33$), followed by the Social Support Index ($\beta = 0.20$).

Five comparison standards were statistically significant in accounting for 68% of the variance in respondents' SWLS scores (column 5). Most influential were comparisons made between respondents' current life as a whole and what they wanted out of life ($\beta = 0.47$). Comparisons made between their current status and the best they had ever experienced were a somewhat distant second ($\beta = 0.24$).

Levels of satisfaction in 5 of the distinct domains of life explained 56% of the variance in SWLS scores (column 6), with respondents' satisfaction with what they had achieved in life most influential ($\beta = 0.27$), followed by satisfaction with their own self-esteem ($\beta = 0.22$)

Finally, using all the significant health, comparison standards and domain satisfaction determinants, we were able to explain 74% of the variation in SWLS scores (column 7), with comparisons made between respondents' current life as a whole and what they wanted out of life most influential ($\beta = 0.30$), followed by comparisons between their current status and the best they had ever experienced ($\beta = 0.22$), and satisfaction with their own self-esteem ($\beta = 0.18$).

Contentment with Life Assessment Scale (CLAS)

Table 9.24 reveals, first, that our biological determinants did not explain any of the variation in Contentment with Life Assessment Scale (CLAS) scores. Four social/economic determinants could account for 29% of the variance in CLAS scores (column 1), with respondents' Good Neighbourhood Index most influential ($\beta = 0.35$), followed by their Social Support Index ($\beta = 0.29$).

Three health behaviours accounted for 10% of the variance in CLAS scores (column 2), with respondents' average number of hours of sleep per night most influential positively ($\beta = 0.21$), followed by their average number of meals skipped per week negatively ($\beta = -0.18$).

Three health services determinants explained 8% of the variance in CLAS scores (column 3), led by respondents' ratings of their own health care positively ($\beta = 0.24$), followed negatively by the average number of times they had seen a doctor in the past year ($\beta = -0.11$) and been in hospital ($\beta = -0.10$).

Using the 10 statistically significant health determinants, we found that a narrower set of 9 significant predictors accounted for 36% of the variance in CLAS scores, with respondents' Good Neighbourhood Index leading the set ($\beta = 0.27$), followed somewhat closely by their Social Support Index ($\beta = 0.23$) and their number of hours of sleep per night ($\beta = 0.21$).

Five comparison standards were statistically significant in accounting for 52% of the variance in respondents' CLAS scores (column 5). Most influential were comparisons made between respondents' current life as a whole and what they wanted out of life ($\beta = 0.39$). Comparisons made between their current status and the best they had ever experienced were tied with comparisons between their current status and that of others of the same sex and age in their areas ($\beta = 0.16$).

Levels of satisfaction in 5 of the distinct domains of life explained 54% of the variance in CLAS scores (column 6), with respondents' satisfaction with what they had achieved in life most influential ($\beta = 0.30$), followed by satisfaction with their own self-esteem ($\beta = 0.23$).

Finally, using all the significant health, comparison standards and domain satisfaction determinants, we were able to explain 60% of the variation in CLAS scores (column 7). In that regression, 5 predictors remained statistically significant, with comparisons made between respondents' current life as a whole and what they wanted out of life most influential ($\beta = 0.30$), followed by comparisons made between their current status and the best they had ever experienced in the past ($\beta = 0.25$).

Subjective Wellbeing (SWB)

Table 9.25 reveals again that our biological determinants did not explain any of the variation in Subjective Wellbeing Index (SWB) scores. Five social/economic determinants accounted for 35% of the variance in SWB scores (column 1), with respondents' Good Neighbourhood Index most influential ($\beta = 0.39$). The Social Support Index followed relatively closely ($\beta = 0.30$) compared to the third placed total household income ($\beta = 0.18$).

Four health behaviours accounted for 13% of the variance in SWB scores (column 2), with respondents' number of hours of sleep per night tied for most influential predictor with respondents' frequency of drinking alcoholic beverages ($\beta = 0.19$). Respondents' average number of pain killers taken per week had a negative influence ($\beta = -0.17$) as did their average number of meals skipped per week ($\beta = -0.13$).

Three health services determinants explained 10% of the variance in SWB scores (column 3), beginning with respondents' ratings of their own health care ($\beta = 0.26$), followed negatively by the average number of times they had seen a doctor in the past year ($\beta = -0.14$).

Using the 12 statistically significant health determinants, we found that a narrower set of 8 significant predictors accounted for 42% of the variance in SWB scores (column 4), with respondents' Good Neighbourhood Index dominating the set ($\beta = 0.31$), followed by the Social Support Index ($\beta = 0.25$). After these two predictors, there was a tie between respondents' average number of hours of sleep per night and their frequency of drinking alcoholic beverages ($\beta = 0.16$).

Four comparison standards were statistically significant in accounting for 53% of the variance in respondents' SWB scores (column 5). Most influential by a wide margin were comparisons made between respondents' current life as a whole and what they wanted out of life ($\beta = 0.45$). Comparisons made between their current status and that of others of the same sex and age in their areas came in a somewhat distant second ($\beta = 0.21$).

Levels of satisfaction in 7 of the distinct domains of life explained 76% of the variance in SWB scores (column 6), with a tie between respondents' satisfaction with their financial security and their sense of meaning in life ($\beta = 0.26$). Following these two, satisfaction with how local residents treat respondents' was most influential ($\beta = 0.17$).

Finally, using all the significant health, comparison standards and domain satisfaction determinants, we were able to explain 75% of the variation in SWB scores (column 7). In that regression, 7 predictors remained statistically significant, led by respondents' satisfaction with their sense of meaning in life ($\beta = 0.28$), followed closely by their satisfaction with their financial security ($\beta = 0.25$). The fact that we lost a percentage point of explanatory power as we moved from the penultimate to the final regression equation is probably the result of having a different set of predictors (rather than a suppressing variable) in the two equations.

Overview of Variance Explained and Most Influential Determinants

Table 9.26 lists the percent of variance explained in the scores for each of the 7 dependent variables by each cluster of health determinants, comparison standards and domain satisfaction scores. Taking all predictors together, we were able to explain as much as 75% of the variance in SWB scores and as little as 45% in happiness scores. The difference in the levels of explanation for both of these

Table 9.26 Percent of variance explained by health determinants, comparison standards and domain satisfaction

	8 SF-36 dim.	Happiness	Life sat.	QOL sat.	SWLS	CLAS	SWB
Biological determinants	11	0	1	0	0	0	0
Social/economic determinants	18	23	29	24	33	29	35
Health behaviour determinants	23	12	8	9	14	10	13
Health service determinants	13	5	10	9	9	8	10
All health determinants	44	20	34	31	39	36	42
Comparison standards	28	40	39	37	68	52	53
Domain satisfaction determinants	25	43	65	60	56	54	76
All significant determinants	46	45	66	67	74	60	75

overall life assessment variables is fairly typical (Michalos 2003). The relatively large percentage of variance explained for SWB and SWLS scores (74%) is a bit unusual. Usually these figures are in the 60% range.

The four clusters of health determinants explained from 20% (Happiness) to 44% (Average Health) of the variance in the dependent variables (row 5). Adding comparison standards and domain satisfaction scores to the set of health determinants increased our total explanatory power by only 2% points for Average Health (from 44 to 46%), but by 36% points for satisfaction with the overall quality of life (from 31 to 67%) and 35% points for SWLS (from 39 to 74%). In fact, the relative contribution of comparison standards and domain satisfaction scores to health determinants in terms of explanatory power for Average Health versus quality of life measured in 6 different ways provides additional clear evidence that there is more to a good life than good health. These results are quite similar to those reported in Michalos et al. (2005, 2007). To understand and appreciate the differences between good health and a good life, one must cast one's net of determinants beyond health determinants and one's net of dependent variables beyond health status measures, as argued in Michalos (2004). Unfortunately, many researchers are still using SF-36 scores to measure quality of life. See, for example, any issue of the journal *Quality of Life Research* as late as February 2010, Volume 19, Number 1.

Table 9.27 lists the most influential predictors of each of the 7 dependent variables from each cluster of health determinants, comparison standards and domain satisfaction scores. Examining rows across the 7 columns, some repeated entries stand out. From the first row one learns that for 5 of the 7 dependent variables (71%), biological determinants had no statistically significant impact. As one would have expected, age had a negative impact on Average Health. For 5 of 7 dependent variables, among the social/economic determinants (row 2), the Good

Table 9.27 Most influential predictors

	General health	Hap.	Life sat.	QOL sat.	SWLS	CLAS	SWB
Biological determinants	Age	0	Gender	0	0	0	0
Social/economic det.	Income	SS	GNI	GNI	GNI	GNI	GNI
Health behaviour det.	Pain pills	Sleep	Drink	Pain pills	Meals	Sleep	Drink
Health services det.	See dr.	Own HC	Own HC	Own HC	Own HC	Own HC	Own HC
All health det.	Pain pills	Sleep/SS	SS	GNI	GNI	GNI	GNI
Comparison standards	SB	SW	SW	SW	SW	SW	SW
Domain satisfaction	Rec. sat	Life meaning	Friend sat	Local treat.	Life achieve	Life achieve	Fin.sec./life mean.
All determinants	Rec. sat	SW	Friend sat	Life meaning	SW	SW	Life meaning

0 no significant impact, age, gender, income total household income, GNI good neighbourhood index, SS social support index, pain pills # pain killers taken per week, sleep # hrs sleep per night, drink frequency of drinking, meals # times skipping meals per week, see dr. # times seeing doctor past year, Own HC respondents' rating their own health care, SB comparison between self now and best ever experienced, SW comparison between self now and self wanted, Rec. Sat satisfaction with your recreation activities, life meaning satisfaction with your sense of meaning in life, Friend sat satisfaction with your friendships, local treat. satisfaction with how local people treat you, life achieve satisfaction with what you achieve in life, Fin.Sec. satisfaction with your financial security

Neighbourhood Index had the largest impact. Although we were aware of quite a bit of research indicating the importance of neighbourhoods to various aspects of the quality of people's lives (e.g., Dittmann and Goebel 2010; Sirgy and Cornwell 2002; Fernandez and Kulik 1981), because we invented the GNI and had not used it before, we were delighted to discover that it had substantial explanatory power for so many key measures of overall quality of life. Among all the health determinants (row 5), GNI was most influential for 4 of 7 (57%) of dependent variables. What is equally interesting about GNI is that it never appeared as the most influential predictor in the final regression equations for any of the dependent variables (row 8).

For 6 of 7 (86%) dependent variables, among comparison standards, the gap between what respondents have and want (self-wants gap) was most influential (row 6). This was largely expected from earlier studies (Michalos 1985, 1991a, b, 1993a, b). We did not know what to expect from this determinant in the context of all our explanatory variables (row 8), but were pleased to find that it was most influential for 3 of the 7 dependent variables.

For 6 of 7 health services determinants, respondents' rating of their own health care were most influential (row 4). However, these ratings never appeared in the equations for all health determinants (row 5) or the final equations involving all determinants (row 8).

Besides the interesting phenomena of a few determinants displaying relatively strong explanatory power for several dependent variables, it was interesting to see the variety of most influential predictors across the 7 dependent variables. Regarding health behaviour determinants, for example, the average number of pain pills taken per week was most influential for 2 dependent variables (Average Health and satisfaction with the overall quality of life), average hours of sleep per night was most influential for 2 others (happiness and CLAS), frequency of drinking alcoholic beverages for 2 more (life satisfaction and subjective wellbeing), and skipping meals for one (SWLS).

Variety was also apparent for domain satisfaction determinants (row 7) and for the final equations (row 8). Satisfaction with recreation activities appears as most important for domain satisfaction determinants and for all determinants for Average Health. As well, satisfaction with friendships appears as most important for domain satisfaction determinants and for all determinants for life satisfaction. Beyond these cases, inspection of the other entries in rows 7 and 8 reveals considerable variety. Row 7 has 6 different most influential determinants and row 8 has 4 (like row 3).

Conclusion

The aim of this investigation was to obtain some baseline self-reported data on the health status and overall quality of life of a sample of residents of the city of Brandon, Manitoba aged 18 years or older, and to measure the impact of a set of designated health determinants, comparison standards and satisfaction with diverse domains of life on their health and quality of life. In May and June 2010, 2,500 households from the city of Brandon, Manitoba were randomly selected to receive a mailed out questionnaire and 518 useable, completed questionnaires were returned. Baseline health status data were obtained using the 8 SF-36 dimensions of health and 13 items from the United States Centers for Disease Control and Prevention, Behavioral Risk Factor Surveillance System. Determinants of health and overall quality of life included measures of socializing activities, a Good Neighbourhood Index, Social Support Index, Community Health Index, a measure of freetime exercise levels, health-related behaviours, use of drugs, health care issues, a set of domain-specific quality of life items, a set of measures concerning criminal victimization, worries and behaviours concerning victimization and the basic postulates of Multiple Discrepancies Theory (Michalos 1985). Overall life assessment, dependent variables included Average Health, happiness, a single item measure of satisfaction with life as a whole, a single item measure of satisfaction with the overall quality of life, the Satisfaction With Life Scale, Contentment with Life Assessment Scale and a Subjective Wellbeing Index.

Using stepwise multiple regression, we were able to explain as much as 75% of the variance in SWB scores and as little as 45% in happiness scores. Four clusters of health determinants explained from 20% (Happiness) to 44% (Average Health) of the variance in the dependent variables. Adding comparison standards and domain satisfaction scores to the set of health determinants increased our total explanatory power by 2% points for Average Health (from 44 to 46%), but by 36% points for satisfaction with the overall quality of life (from 31 to 67%) and 35% points for Subjective Wellbeing (from 39 to 74%).

For 5 of 7 dependent variables, biological determinants had no statistically significant impact. Among all of the health determinants, the Good Neighbourhood Index was most influential for 4 of 7 dependent variables, although this index never appeared as the most influential predictor in the final regression equations for any of the dependent variables. For 6 of 7 dependent variables, among comparison standards, the gap between what respondents have and want (self-wants gap) was most influential, and managed to be most influential in the final regression equations for 3 of the 7 dependent variables. For 6 of 7 health services determinants, respondents' rating of their own health care were most influential, but these ratings never appeared in the equations for all health determinants or the final equations involving all determinants. While a few determinants displayed relatively strong explanatory power for several dependent variables, there was considerable variety in the most influential predictors across the 7 dependent variables.

The three most important take-home messages from this investigation are (1) in assessing the relative influence of any alleged determinants of health and the quality of life, different sets of alleged determinants will appear to be more or less influential for different dependent variables. Therefore, (2) researchers should use diverse sets of determinants and dependent variables and (3) it is a big mistake to use measures of health status like SF-36 as a measure of the perceived quality of life.

Acknowledgements We would like to thank the Rural Development Institute of Brandon University, Brandon Regional Health Authority, City of Brandon, Manitoba Agriculture, Food and Rural Initiatives and Brandon University for supporting this project, as well as Nancy McPherson, Sandy Trudel, Bev Lischka and Deandra Tousignant for their administrative work and the people of Brandon who generously gave us their time to complete our questionnaire.

References

Brandon Regional Health Authority. (2009). *Community health assessment*. Manitoba: Brandon.

CDC. (2000). *Measuring healthy days*. Atlanta, Georgia, U.S.: Centers for Disease Control and Prevention.

Diener, E., Emmons, R. A., Larsen, R. J., & Griffin, S. (1985). The satisfaction with life scale. *Journal of Personality Assessment, 49*(1), 71–75.

Dittmann, J., & Goebel, J. (2010). Your house, your car, your education: The socioeconomic situation of the neighborhood and the impact on life satisfaction in Germany. *Social Indicators Research, 96*(3), 497–513.

Fernandez, R. M., & Kulik, J. C. (1981). A multilevel model of life satisfaction: Effects of individual characteristics and neighborhood composition. *American Sociological Review, 46,* 840–850.

Garratt, A. M., Ruta, D. A., Abdalla, M. I., Buckingham, J. K., & Russell, I. T. (1993). The SF-36 health survey questionnaire: An outcome measure suitable for routine use within the NHS? *British Medical Journal, 306,* 1440–1444.

Lavallee, L. F., Hatch, P. M., Michalos, A. C., & McKinley, T. (2007). Development of the contentment with life assessment scale (CLAS): Using daily life experiences to verify levels of self-reported life satisfaction. *Social Indicators Research, 83*(2), 201–244.

McHorney, C. A., Ware, J. E., Lu, J. F. R., & Sherbourne, C. D. (1994). The MOS 36-item short-formhealth survey (SF-36): III tests of data quality, scaling assumptions, and reliability across diverse patient groups. *Medical Care, 32*(1), 40–66.

McHorney, C. A., Ware, J. A., & Raczek, A. E. (1993). The MOS 36-item short-form health survey (SF- 36): II. Psychometric and clinical tests of validity in measuring physical and mental health constructs. *Medical Care, 31*(3), 247–263.

Michalos, A. C. (1985). Multiple discrepancies theory (MDT). *Social Indicators Research, 16*(4), 347–413.

Michalos, A. C. (1991a). *Global report on student well-being. Volume 1: Life satisfaction and happiness*. New York: Springer.

Michalos, A. C. (1991b). *Global report on student well-being, Volume 2: Family, friends, living partner and self-esteem*. New York: Springer.

Michalos, A. C. (1993a). *Global report on student well-being, Volume 3: Employment, finances, housing and transportation*. New York: Springer.

Michalos, A. C. (1993b). *Global report on student well-being, Volume 4: Religion, education, recreation and health*. New York: Springer.

Michalos, A. C. (2002). Policing services and the quality of life. *Social Indicators Research, 61*(1), 1–18.

Michalos, A. C. (2003). *Essays on the quality of life*. Dordrecht: Kluwer Academic Publishers.

Michalos, A. C. (2004). Social indicators research and health-related quality of life research. *Social Indicators Research, 65*(1), 27–72.

Michalos, A. C., Hatch, P. M., Hemingway, D., Lavallee, L., Hogan, A., & Christensen, B. (2007). Health and the quality of life of older people: A replication after six years. *Social Indicators Research, 84*(2), 127–158.

Michalos, A. C., Hubley, A. M., Zumbo, B. D., & Hemingway, D. (2001). Health and other aspects of the quality of life of older people. *Social Indicators Research, 54*(3), 239–274.

Michalos, A. C., & Kahke, P. M. (2010). Stability and sensitivity in perceived quality of life measures: Some panel results. *Social Indicators Research, 98*(3), 403–434.

Michalos, A. C., Thommasen, H. V., Read, R., Anderson, N., & Zumbo, B. D. (2005). Determinants of health and the quality of life in the Bella Coola Valley. *Social Indicators Research, 72*(1), 1–50.

Michalos, A. C., & Zumbo, B. D. (2000). *Quality of life in Quesnel, British Columbia.* UNBC: Institute for Social Research and Evaluation.

Michalos, A. C., & Zumbo, B. D. (2003). Leisure activities, health and the quality of life. In A. C. Michalos (Ed.), *Essays on the quality of life* (pp. 217–238). Dordrecht: Kluwer Academic Publishing.

Michalos, A. C., Zumbo, B. D., & Hubley, A. (2000). Health and the quality of life. *Social Indicators Research, 51*(3), 245–286.

Michalos, A. C., et al. (2010). *An approach to the Canadian index of wellbeing*. Toronto: Atkinson Charitable Foundation.

Pedhazur, E. J. (1982). *Multiple regression in behavioral research*. New York: Holt, Rinehart and Winston.

Provincial Health Officer. (1994). *A report of the health of British Columbians: Provincial health officer's annual report 1994*. Victoria, B.C.: Ministry of Health and Ministry Responsible for Seniors.

Sirgy, M. J., & Cornwell, T. (2002). How neighborhood features affect quality of life. *Social Indicators Research, 59*(1), 79–114.
Ware, J. E., Kosinsky, M., & Keller, S. D. (1994). *SF-36 physical and mental health summary scales: A user's manual*. Boston, MA: The Health Institute, New England Medical Center.
Ware, J. E., & Sherbourne, C. D. (1992). The MOS 36-item short-form health survey (SF-36): I. Conceptual framework and item selection. *Medical Care, 30*(6), 473–483.
Ware, J. E., Snow, K. K., Kosinski, M., & Gandek, B. (1993). *SF-36 health survey: Manual and interpretation guide*. Boston, MA: The Health Institute, New England Medical Center.
Zumbo, B. D., & Michalos, A. C. (2000). Quality of life in Jasper, Alberta. *Social Indicators Research, 49*(2), 121–145.

Chapter 10
A Note on Student Quality of Life

Alex C. Michalos and Julie Anne Orlando

The *University of Northern British Columbia Act* was passed in June 1990, creating the university. In August 1994, Her Majesty the Queen Elizabeth II officially opened the Prince George campus. The Institute for Social Research and Evaluation was opened at the university in June 1998 and in the Fall of that year we began administering annual Student Quality of Life surveys. The university student body is still relatively small, numbering about 3500 students, and the annual survey samples average about 400. Because most of the information in the survey questionnaires is designed for in-house monitoring and assessment purposes, no results have ever been published from these surveys. However, because we have always had some fairly standard quality-of-life items in our questionnaires (e.g., Michalos 2003) and we recently decided to aggregate data from seven surveys (1998–2005, omitting 2004 for technical reasons), it was possible to produce this short note disclosing some results that may have some interest to people outside our university. The aggregated sample had a size of $n = 3407$.

Table 10.1 lists the means and standard deviations of the main variables of interest here. The variables covering satisfaction and happiness are all formatted in 7-point Likert scales running from "very dissatisfied/unhappy = 1 point" to "very satisfied/happy = 7 points". The Subjective Well-Being (SWB) Index is formed by summing the scores on four variables (satisfaction with life as a whole, with the

---

Michalos, A.C., & Orlando, J.A.: 2006. A note on student quality of life. Social Indicators Research, 79, pp. 51–59.

A.C. Michalos (✉)
University of Northern British Columbia, Prince George, BC, Canada
e-mail: michalos@brandonu.ca

J.A. Orlando
University of Northern British Columbia, 3333 University Way, Prince George, BC V2N 4Z9, Canada
e-mail: orlando@unbc.ca

A.C. Michalos, *Connecting the Quality of Life Theory to Health, Well-Being and Education*, DOI 10.1007/978-3-319-51161-0_10

Table 10.1 Descriptive statistics, N $\geq$ 2416*

Topic	Mean	St. dev.
Life satisfaction	5.4	1.4
Happiness	5.7	1.4
Sat. with quality of life	5.3	1.3
Sat. w standard of living	5.4	1.3
Subjective well-being	18.0	7.7
Sat. w housing	5.3	1.6
Sat. w family relations	5.6	1.5
Sat. w friendships	5.5	1.4
Sat. w recreation	4.5	1.6
Sat. w financial security	3.8	1.7
Sat. w self-esteem	5.4	1.4
Sat. w instructors	4.9	1.4
Sat. w course offerings	4.2	1.5
Sat. w student services	4.5	1.4
Sat. w library services	4.6	1.5
Sat. w food services	3.7	1.7
Sat. w fitness services	4.2	1.6
Sat. w bookstore services	4.5	1.5
Univ. useful preferred work	4.0	1.3
Univ. useful any work	4.1	1.2
Age	24.3	7.4
# Academic credits earned	51.1	40.0

*Satisfaction and happiness items run 1–7 points; SWB = 4–28; useful work = 1–5

overall quality of life and with one's standard of living, and overall happiness). It runs from 4 to 28, and has a Cronbach internal reliability (a) score of 0.89. There are two items asking "How useful do you think your university experience will be for gaining future work?", one focusing on "obtaining [any] work" and one focusing on "obtaining work I'd like to do". The scale of responses ran from "not at all useful = 1" to "extremely useful = 5". The ages of respondents ran from 16 to 69, with a mean of 24.3. Seventy-three percent of the students were 25 years old or younger. On average, respondents had earned 51.1 academic credits, with a range running from 0 to 186.

As usual for the set of six life domain items (housing, family, friends, recreation, financial security and self-esteem), the mean score for satisfaction with one's family relations (5.6) is higher than all others and that for satisfaction with one's financial security (3.8) is lower. There are seven university-related satisfaction items listed in the table, from satisfaction with UNBC instructors to satisfaction with bookstore services. On average, the university-related satisfaction scores are lower than the life domain scores, 4.4 compared to 5.0, respectively. The former run from a high of 4.9 for satisfaction with UNBC instructors to a low of 3.7 for satisfaction with food services. For the four global items in the Subjective Well-Being Index, the mean happiness score (5.7) is highest and mean score for satisfaction with the overall quality of life is lowest (5.3).

One idea of the relative size of the life domain and global scores may be obtained by comparing them with the last fall survey taken of adults 18 years and older in the city of Prince George in November 2004. The sample was relatively small ($n = 387$), but, for example, the mean satisfaction scores were for family relations (5.8), financial security (4.8), overall quality of life (5.6) and happiness (5.9). Each of these mean scores was higher than its student counterpart. Another interesting comparison may be made between the average of the mean life satisfaction (4.8) and happiness (4.7) scores for students ($n = 8849$) in my 39-country undergraduate student survey made in 1985–1987 (Michalos, 1991, pp. 91–92). The UNBC mean scores were clearly above the average.

Table 10.2 is a zero-order correlation matrix of all the variables used in our analyses, revealing several interesting associations. First, all of the seven university-related satisfaction items (last row, variables 11–17) are negatively associated with numbers of academic credits earned. The more credits students earned, the lower their levels of satisfaction became with each student service offered, in varying degrees. The variation in degrees is also interesting, running from a low of $r = -0.04$ for the correlation between credits earned and satisfaction with UNBC instructors to a high of $r = -0.28$ for the correlation between credits earned and satisfaction with food services. A glance across the second last row reveals that age alone did not account for these negative relationships. Only three of the seven university-related satisfaction items are negatively related to age. Second, the correlation of satisfaction with UNBC instructors and satisfaction with course offerings is relatively high, $r = 0.45$, but not as high as that between some components of SWB, e.g., satisfaction with life as a whole and happiness ($r = 0.73$) and satisfaction with the overall quality of life ($r = 0.71$). Third, satisfaction with student services is relatively highly correlated with satisfaction with library services ($r = 0.55$) and with food services ($r = 0.49$).

Each of the last four tables contains results of three stepwise regressions with a different dependent variable in each table. In each case, under the column headed Life Domains, scores on the dependent variable were regressed on (explained by) scores for satisfaction with one's housing, family relations, friendships, financial security, recreation activities, self-esteem and age. Under the column headed University Domains, scores on the dependent variable were regressed on scores for satisfaction with the seven university-related items, the total number of university credits earned, perceived usefulness of one's university education for obtaining any work (Any work use), and perceived usefulness of one's university education for obtaining work the respondent would like to do (Preferred work use). Under the column headed Life + Univ. Domains, scores on the dependent variable were regressed on scores for those independent (predictor) variables in the first two columns which were statistically significant in the first two regressions. Any of the variables listed above that had no statistically significant relation to any of the dependent variables are not listed in the tables.

Table 10.2 Correlation matrix for all variables, N $\geq$ 2414, $p \leq 0.05$*

Topics	1	2	3	4	5	6	7	8	9	10	11	12	13	14	15	16	17	18	19	20
Life sat	–																			
Happiness	73	–																		
Qual. Life	71	66	–																	
SWB	48	80	83	–																
Housing	32	30	36	36	–															
Family	51	41	46	50	36	–														
Friends	61	52	55	59	27	40	–													
Finances	34	35	44	43	23	27	29	–												
Recreation	40	40	56	49	26	28	42	37	–											
S-esteem	71	71	64	75	26	42	53	33	40	–										
Instructors	25	22	28	28	17	20	21	17	17	21	–									
Courses	23	17	22	24	17	17	17	19	17	17	45	–								
Stu. serv	24	20	29	27	20	20	21	22	21	19	41	55	–							
Lib. serv	19	15	21	21	16	18	15	16	12	16	30	46	55	–						
Food serv	17	14	20	21	18	15	13	21	17	15	21	38	49	44	–					
Fit. serv	15	15	20	20	11	12	16	17	17	17	21	29	37	36	38	–				
Book. serv	21	18	24	26	18	19	18	20	17	18	26	39	50	45	51	48	–			
Pref. work	19	15	15	04	10	13	14	09	09	16	14	18	15	12	09	10	11	–		
Any work	11	10	09	ns	06	07	11	06	08	09	11	11	12	08	08	04	08	63	–	
Age	03	03	06	15	08	ns	ns	08	09	ns	06	ns	06	ns	07	10	ns	03	ns	–
# Credits	ns	ns	04	ns	ns	ns	ns	13	ns	ns	04	14	21	16	28	17	24	ns	ns	16

1 = Satisfaction with life as a whole, 2 = Happiness with whole life, 3 = Sat. with overall quality of life, 4 = Subjective well-being, 5 = Sat. with one's housing, 6 = Sat. with family relations, 7 = Sat. with friendships, 8 = Sat. with financial security, 9 = Sat. with recreation activities, 10 = Sat. with self-esteem, 11 = Sat. with UNBC instructors, 12 = Sat. with course offerings, 13 = Sat. with student services, 14 = Sat. with library services, 15 = Sat. with food services here, 16 = Sat. with fitness services here, 17 = Sat. with bookstore services, 18 = University experience useful for getting work student would like to do, 19 = University experience useful for getting any work, 20 = age, 21 = # of university credits earned, ns = not statistically significant

*Decimals omitted, underlined numbers are negative

If our independent variables were sufficient to account for all the variation in scores in any dependent variable, there would be 100% of variance explained. The 4 tables show that we could explain from 8 to 72%, depending on which dependent and array of independent variables used. The tables also show that when the university domains are added to the life domains, practically no explanatory power is added, from 0 to 1% point. In the case of happiness, there is a 1% point reduction. Anyhow, practically speaking, the university-related domains have no impact when they are examined in combination with the life domains.

The β values are standardized regression coefficients with means of zero and standard deviations of one. Figuratively speaking, one can think of the dependent variable moving some percentage of a unit step for every full unit step change in the independent variable, when the values of all other variables are held constant. For example, in Table 10.3, under the Life Domains column next to Self-esteem, one finds that if there were an increase of one unit in the mean score for satisfaction with one's self-esteem ($\beta = 0.47$), there would be an increase of 47% of a unit in the mean life satisfaction score. So, for example, in that particular set of independent and dependent variables, satisfaction with one's self-esteem is much more influential than all the other significant predictors. If you glance at the other tables, you will see that it is always the most influential predictor when it is in the equation to begin with. That is not always the case for all groups, but it is very often the case for adult samples of Prince George residents.

Table 10.3 shows that for life satisfaction, students' satisfaction with their instructors is the most influential predictor ($\beta = 0.15$) among the university-related

Table 10.3 Explaining life satisfaction by satisfaction with domains of life, university domains and their combination

Topics	Life domains	University domains	Life + Univ. domains
n	2151	2226	2060
% Variance explained	61	11	62
	β value	β value	β value
Housing	0.04	a	0.04
Family relations	0.19	a	0.19
Friendships	0.24	a	0.23
Financial security	0.03	a	b
Recreation activities	0.05	a	0.05
Self-esteem	0.47		0.47
UNBC instructors	a	0.15	0.04
Student services	a	0.12	b
Bookstore services	a	0.10	b
Preferred work use	a	0.14	0.05
Age	0.05	b	0.05
Total # credits	a	0.06	b

a = Not in equation; b = not statistically significant

domains (in the middle column). However, examining the third column scores one finds that the relative influence of this variable is significantly reduced ($\beta = 0.04$) and slightly surpassed by students' belief that their university experience would be useful for obtaining a job that they would like to do ($\beta = 0.05$). The relative influence of satisfaction with one's selfesteem ($\beta = 0.47$) is undiminished.

Table 10.4 shows that for satisfaction with the overall quality of life, the most influential explanatory variable is satisfaction with one's self-esteem ($\beta = 0.35$), and this variable's influence is undiminished when combined with the significant university-related domain variables (third column). Among the university-related domains, satisfaction with UNBC instructors was most influential ($\beta = 0.17$), and it remained most influential among those variables in a diminished state ($\beta = 0.06$) when combined with the life domain scores.

Table 10.5 shows that for overall happiness, among the life domain variables the most influential one is satisfaction with one's self-esteem ($\beta = 0.57$), and this variable remains supreme when it is combined with the university-related variables, though at a slightly diminished state ($\beta = 0.55$). Among the university-related variables, satisfaction with UNBC instructors is most influential ($\beta = 0.14$), and it is the only such variable in the final regression, in a diminished state ($\beta = 0.03$).

Table 10.6 shows that for Subjective Well-Being, satisfaction with self-esteem is most influential across the board, from $\beta = 0.49$–0.48. Satisfaction with UNBC instructors runs from $\beta = 0.17$ among university-related variables to $\beta = 0.04$ among the combined set of predictors.

Table 10.4 Explaining satisfaction with one's overall quality of life by satisfaction with domains of life, university domains and their combination

Topics	Life domains	University domains	Life + Univ. domains
n	2150	2224	2059
% Variance explained	59	13	59
	β value	β value	β value
Housing	0.10	a	0.09
Family relations	0.11	a	0.10
Friendships	0.14	a	0.13
Financial security	0.14	a	0.13
Recreation activities	0.26	a	0.25
Self-esteem	0.35	a	0.35
UNBC instructors	a	0.17	0.06
Student services	a	0.15	0.04
Bookstore services	a	0.10	b
Preferred work use	a	0.09	0.05
Age	−0.03	−0.07	−0.04
Total # credits	a	0.04	b

a = Not in equation; b = not statistically significant

Table 10.5 Explaining happiness by domains of life, university domains and their combination

Topics	Life domains	University domains	Life + Univ. domains
n	2146	2220	2263
% Variance explained	56	8	55
	β value	β value	β value
Family relations	0.07	a	0.07
Friendships	0.15	a	0.14
Financial security	0.07	a	0.07
Recreation activities	0.07	a	0.07
Self-esteem	0.57	a	0.55
UNBC instructors	a	0.14	0.03
Student services	a	0.08	b
Bookstore services	a	0.08	b
Preferred work use	a	0.12	b

a = Not in equation; b = not statistically significant

Table 10.6 Explaining subjective well-being by university domains and their combination

Topics	Life domains	University domains	Life + Univ. domains
n	2157	2231	2036
% Variance explained	72	14	72
	β value	β value	β value
Housing	0.11	a	0.10
Family relations	0.14	a	0.14
Friendships	0.17	a	0.16
Financial security	0.12	a	0.11
Recreation activities	0.14	a	0.14
Self-esteem	0.49	a	0.48
UNBC instructors	a	0.17	0.04
Student services	a	0.11	0.04
Food services	a	0.06	b
Bookstore services	a	0.13	b
Preferred work use	a	0.11	b
Age	−0.03	−0.08	−0.03

a = Not in equation; b = not statistically significant

It would have been interesting to know what percentage of variation in scores for satisfaction with one's university education or one's university experience could be explained by our university—related variables. Unfortunately, and much to our regret, we never thought of including such important summary variables in our student surveys. From our point of view, one of the most important products of this aggregate analysis is the discovery of this huge omission. Beginning in the fall of 2005, at least one such summary variable will be included. In the 39-country survey, using a similar set of potentially explanatory life domains, satisfaction with one's university education ($\beta = 0.19$) was nearly as influential as satisfaction with one's self-esteem ($\beta = 0.20$) for life satisfaction (Michalos 1991. p. 100). Until such data have been gathered for the UNBC student community, we can only say that of all the particular aspects of university life, satisfaction with one's instructors is almost always the most influential predictor of students' overall perceived well-being.

Acknowledgements We would like to thank some of the people who reviewed our annual surveys over many of the 8 years covered by this study, and who routinely offered suggestions about items to add, polish or drop. Thanks very much Joan Ross, Susan McIntyre, Rob Van Adrichem, William Zhang and Bruno Zumbo.

References

Michalos, A. C. (1991). Global report on student well-being. Volume 1: Life satisfaction and happiness. New York: Springer.
Michalos, A. C. (2003). *Life*. Dordrecht: Kluwer Academic Publishers.

Chapter 11
Quality of Life of Some Under-Represented Survey Respondents: Youth, Aboriginals and Unemployed

Alex C. Michalos and Julie Anne Orlando

Introduction

Since the opening of the Institute for Social Research and Evaluation in 1998 at the University of Northern British Columbia in Prince George, a steady stream of publications has been produced based on mailout surveys of residents of this city. In most of these surveys people who are relatively young (18–24 years of age), unemployed or with Aboriginal ethnic backgrounds have been disproportionately under-represented. So, in the interest of being able to provide some analyses of these particular groups in comparison to the wider community, results were aggregated from 16 surveys. As the figures show, even the aggregated figures for these three groups are still relatively small. Still, they are large enough to help close some of our perceived information gaps, although there is no guarantee that the few respondents we have from each under-represented group are very much like those who failed to respond across the wide range of issues examined. A complete list of the surveys may be found in the Appendix.

Michalos, A.C., & Orlando, J.A.: 2006. Quality of life of some under-represented survey respondents: youth, aboriginals and unemployed. Social Indicators Research, 79, pp. 191–213.

A.C. Michalos (✉)
University of Northern British Columbia, Prince George, BC, Canada
e-mail: michalos@brandonu.ca

J.A. Orlando
University of Northern British Columbia, 3333 University Way, Prince George, BC V2N 4Z9, Canada

A.C. Michalos, *Connecting the Quality of Life Theory to Health, Well-Being and Education*, DOI 10.1007/978-3-319-51161-0_11

Data Sources and Descriptive Statistics

All of the surveys undertaken for the city by the Institute have a relatively small core of demographic and quality-of-life items attached to a relatively large wide variety of issues of particular interest to members of City Council and/or the City Administration. The particular issues have included such things as evaluations of city services, park facilities, budget allocations, value for tax dollars, criminal victimization, police services, ethnic relations, health and health care, gambling and public housing. Discussions of these kinds of issues may be found in published papers listed in the Appendix and References. The focus of this paper is on the quality-of-life variables. More precisely, it is on measures of people's satisfaction with specific domains of their lives, namely, their housing, neighborhoods, family relations, living partners, jobs, friendships, health, religion (spiritual fulfillment), financial security, recreation activities, self-esteem, federal government, provincial government and local government, and on more global measures of their whole lives. The latter include satisfaction with life as a whole, satisfaction with the overall quality of life and happiness. As we will see, when a person reflects upon his or her whole life from the perspective of its overall quality, its satisfaction or happiness, slightly different sets of features of life become more or less salient and influential on the judgments a person makes. All of the satisfaction and happiness items are formatted in 7-point Likert scales, with response categories running from "very dissatisfied/unhappy = 1 point" to "very satisfied/happy = 7 points". (Readers interested in the history and psychometric properties of such scales may consult Michalos (1991a, 2003)).

Table 11.1 summarizes the basic demographics of the aggregated dataset. In broad strokes, we have a total sample *N* of about 8800, about 53% of whom are females. The median age is 47 years, with a range running from 18 to 96. Ten percent have some university experience and 19% have some kind of degree. The median household income for the group is $55,000. Sixty-one percent are married, and 47% are employed full-time with another 10% employed part-time. Fifty-three percent described their ethnic background as Canadian and another 40% described it as European. One hundred and fifty-three (1.9%) described their ethnic background as First Nations and 133 (1.7%) described it as Metis. Regarding the two other groups selected for special attention, there are 416 (4.8%) respondents aged 18–24 and 304 (3.5%) unemployed. Among the unemployed, there are 8 (2.9%) people with First Nations and 13 (4.7%) with Metis backgrounds. Thus, although fewer than one in 10 members of our unemployed group have Aboriginal backgrounds, Aboriginal people are disproportionately over-represented among the unemployed. They constitute 7.6% of the latter group but only 3.6% of all respondents. Young people are also overrepresented in the unemployed group, since 10.3% of the latter are aged 18–24 while only 4.8% of the total sample are in that age group.

Table 11.2 lists the mean satisfaction and happiness scores and the minimum sample sizes for the nine groups of interest to us here, i.e., all respondents, females

Table 11.1 Sample description

	N	%
Gender		
Female	4589	52.7
Male	4117	47.3
Total	8706	100.0
Age		
18–24	416	4.8
25–34	1334	15.5
35–44	1933	22.4
45–54	2061	23.9
55–64	1486	17.2
65	1384	16.2
Total	8614	100.0
Education		
Elem. Incomplete	86	1.0
Elem. Complete	163	1.9
Sec. Incomplete	769	8.9
Sec. Complete	1343	15.5
Some trade	1399	16.1
Diploma/Certif.	2395	27.6
Some University	904	10.4
Univ. Degree	1621	18.7
Total	8680	100.0
Income		
0–$15,999	643	8.8
16,000–27,999	741	10.1
28,000–39,999	861	11.7
40,000–49,999	735	10.0
50,000–59,999	826	11.3
60,000–69,999	827	11.3
70,000–79,999	693	9.4
80,000–89,999	570	7.8
90,000–99,999	378	5.2
100,000–119.999	575	7.8
120,000 or more	486	6.6
Total	7335	100.0
Marital status		
Now married	5291	61.1
Common law	892	10.3
Single/never mar.	877	10.1
Divorced	682	7.9

(continued)

Table 11.1 (continued)

	N	%
Separated	339	3.9
Widowed	583	6.7
Total	8664	100.0
Employment status		
Unemployed	304	3.5
Retired	1726	19.9
Part-time empl.	905	10.4
Full-time empl.	4104	47.2
Homemaker	497	5.7
Student	305	3.5
Disabled	118	1.4
Self-employed	489	5.6
Other	245	2.8
Total	8693	100.0
Ethnic background		
African	12	0.2
American	46	0.6
Asian	77	1.0
Australian/oceanic	12	0.2
Canadian	4226	53.4
European	3191	40.3
First Nations	153	1.9
Metis	133	1.7
Middle Eastern	48	0.6
South American	16	0.2
Total	7914	100.0

versus males, youth (18–24) versus the complementary class (non-youth) of all others, unemployed versus all others (non-unemployed), and Aboriginals (First Nations and Metis) versus all others (non-Aboriginals). Because most of the sample sizes are fairly large, most mean comparisons are statistically significant at $p < 0.05$. For every group, highest levels of satisfaction are reported for living partners and lowest levels of satisfaction are reported for the provincial government. For females, males, youth and unemployed, second highest levels of satisfaction are reported for family relations and third highest for friendships. For respondents in the Aboriginal group, the second highest level of satisfaction was reported for friendships, followed by satisfaction with family relations. The relatively high levels of living partner, family and friendship satisfaction are typical for people all over the world (Michalos 1991a, 2003).

Of the three levels of government included in our surveys, for every group, highest levels of satisfaction were reported for local government, leaving the federal

Table 11.2 Mean satisfaction and happiness ratings

Topics	All	Females	Males	Youth[a]	All others	Unemployed	All others	Aboriginals[b]	All others
$N \geq$	7085[c]	3479	3474	345	6593	217	6793	223	6091
Home	5.64	5.61	5.68	5.17	5.67	5.03	5.67	5.03	5.68
N'b'hood	5.55	5.50	5.61	4.84	5.59	5.01	5.57	4.93	5.61
Family	5.82	5.83	5.82	5.60	5.84	5.31	5.84	5.43	5.83
Partner	6.13	6.02	6.25	5.92	6.15	5.53	6.15	5.69	6.14
Job	5.24	5.22	5.26	4.67	5.27	3.28	5.31	4.98	5.24
Life sat.	5.67	5.66	5.68	5.39	5.68	4.83	5.70	5.31	5.67
Friends	5.72	5.79	5.65	5.54	5.73	5.14	5.74	5.57	5.72
Health	5.32	5.29	5.35	5.35	5.32	4.71	5.34	4.90	5.33
Religion	5.23	5.24	5.22	4.92	5.25	4.70	5.25	5.01	5.23
Finance	4.49	4.37	4.63	3.60	4.54	3.18	4.54	3.55	4.52
Recreation	4.94	4.83	5.05	4.68	4.95	4.35	4.96	4.40	4.97
S-esteem	5.43	5.30	5.58	5.13	5.44	4.62	5.46	5.02	5.44
Fed. Gov't	2.89	2.87	2.90	3.06	2.88	2.56	2.90	2.65	2.91
Prov. Gov't	2.50	2.52	2.47	2.76	2.49	2.30	2.50	2.52	2.50
Local Gov't	3.52	3.41	3.64	3.51	3.53	3.10	3.54	3.23	3.53
Qual. Life	5.48	5.48	5.49	5.32	5.49	4.64	5.51	5.13	5.48
Happiness	5.65	5.64	5.67	5.61	5.66	4.81	5.68	5.28	5.68

All Satisfaction and Overall QOL and Happiness scales range from 1 to 7 points

[a]Youth = respondents 18–24 years of age

[b]Aboriginals = respondents self-identifying as First Nations or Metis

[c]For each group, the reported N is the minimum number of responses for any rating topic

government with mean scores between the other two. The first 11 surveys in our dataset were undertaken with the New Democratic Party forming the government and the other 5 were undertaken under a Liberal government. Since governments tend to be public punching bags for many people, it might be wise to think of their assessments as rather special cases. Setting aside all government assessments, the lowest levels of satisfaction were reported for financial security, for every group. This is also quite typical for these kinds of measures.

Examining the female and male scores, practically speaking, there do not appear to be any remarkable differences, although for satisfaction with living partners, finances, recreation, self-esteem and local government the differences are statistically significant at $p < 0.001$. In each of these domains, mean levels of satisfaction are lower for females than for males. Haring et al. (1984) examined male and female differences in well-being scores in 146 studies, and reported that gender accounted for about 1% of the variance in such scores.

Comparing the scores for our three under-studied groups (youth, unemployed and Aboriginals), one finds that youth had the highest levels of reported satisfaction for 8 specific domains of life plus the highest mean scores on the 3 global indicators, while the unemployed had the lowest levels of reported satisfaction for 12 domains plus the lowest mean scores on the 3 global indicators. The Aboriginal group had the highest scores for 3 domains (jobs, friendships and religion) and did not have the lowest score for any domain. So, generally speaking, these scores indicate that of the three groups, the quality of life of youth is best, that of the unemployed is worst, and that of Aboriginals is between these two. Lest anyone jump to the conclusion that young people are better off than everyone else, inspection of the comparative scores for youth versus those for people of all other ages (i.e., the complementary class of non-youth) reveals that, setting aside government assessments, mean satisfaction scores for respondents of all other ages are higher than those for youth for every domain except health. In the latter domain, the scores for the two groups are practically the same, although the score for youth is numerically higher by 0.03 points.

Setting aside government assessments, the mean of every domain satisfaction score and every global indicator for the unemployed is significantly lower ($p < 0.001$) than its counterpart for all other respondents (nonunemployed). The significance level for differences in the mean federal and provincial satisfaction scores for the unemployed and all others is $p < 0.05$. The level of satisfaction with every level of government is lower for the unemployed than for youth or respondents with Aboriginal backgrounds. Our guess is that the unemployed believe that governments are not doing enough for people in their circumstances. Government assessments aside, unemployed respondents' satisfaction with their financial security is not only lower than that for every other domain, as already remarked, but also lower than that of youth and Aboriginal respondents for the same domain. Many of the unemployed responded to our job satisfaction question with a relatively low score, presumably indicating their dissatisfaction with their employment status.

Setting aside only the measure of satisfaction with provincial government, the mean of every domain satisfaction score and every global indicator for respondents with Aboriginal backgrounds is significantly lower ($p < 0.001$) than its counterpart for all other respondents (non-Aboriginals). The levels of satisfaction with provincial government are practically the same for both groups.

While our main focus of attention was on the three mentioned groups in comparison with their complementary classes, and incidentally on female/male comparisons, we also made some comparative observations of people aged 65 years or more and people with self-reported disabilities. The mean scores for unemployed people on all but three of the 14 variables were found to be lower than those for the disabled group ($N = 118$). The latter had lower mean scores than the unemployed for satisfaction with their own health, recreation and the overall quality of life. Because we had evidence from our 1999 survey of older people in the Northern Interior Health Region (mostly from Prince George) indicating that older people's scores on most of our study variables were higher than those for other adults (Michalos et al. 2001), we expected to find these results replicated. When we compared the scores on all variables for people 65 years or more to those of all others, we found the expected results, as indicated below.

Bivariate Relations

Table 11.3 lists the Pearson Product Moment Correlations for our variables, revealing the usual mild to moderate relationships for most variables and more robust relationships for the three global variables. There are only three associations that are not statistically significant at $p < 0.05$, and only two negative relationships. The latter relate age to health satisfaction and income negatively, as expected.

There is a very large body of research on relations between people's reported income and a variety of quality of life measures, especially measures of life satisfaction, happiness and subjective well-being (Diener and Oishi 2000; Easterlin 2001; Diener and Biswas-Diener 2002). Generally speaking, the research shows that income is positively correlated to most global measures of quality of life, with fairly modest correlations within countries (particularly industrially developed countries) and larger correlations among countries (involving developed and developing countries). The mean correlation between our domain satisfaction scores and income in Table 11.3 is 0.12, and that for global scores and income is 0.18. Squaring these figures to get the coefficient of determination for each pair, one finds that (ignoring all the other relations among our quality of life variables) income might explain from 1 to 3% of the variation in our quality of life scores. However, when we examined the impact of income on our three global quality of

Table 11.3 Correlation matrix for all variables, all respondents, $N \geq 5961$, $p < 0.05$*

Topics	1	2	3	4	5	6	7	8	9	10	11	12	13	14	15	16	17	18	19
Home	–																		
N'b'hood	59	–																	
Family	39	33	–																
Partner	34	24	52	–															
Job	31	24	31	32	–														
Life sat.	39	31	47	48	53	–													
Friends	34	29	45	38	42	61	–												
Health	27	23	30	27	32	50	44	–											
Religion	24	21	33	29	30	43	41	36	–										
Finances	42	34	32	31	43	46	33	37	35	–									
Recreation	35	28	31	30	34	47	44	46	37	50	–								
S-esteem	35	27	40	39	42	64	52	49	44	45	53	–							
Fed. Gov't	10	11	08	05	12	14	09	13	11	24	14	13	–						
Prov. Gov't	05	06	05	ns	09	10	04	08	06	18	10	06	70	–					
Local Gov't	15	20	13	09	16	19	14	15	13	25	19	16	57	49	–				
Qual. Life	44	37	42	42	46	68	50	52	40	53	50	60	20	14	24	–			
Happiness	32	25	39	43	40	63	44	41	33	41	40	54	15	10	18	61	–		
Age	18	19	13	09	15	08	10	06	14	23	11	10	04	04	10	06	ns	–	
Income	20	18	10	12	17	14	04	13	ns	30	15	16	05	03	07	21	19	14	-

1 = Sat. with house, apartment, or mobile home, 2 = Sat. with neighbourhood, 3 = Sat. with family relations, 4 = Sat. with living partner, 5 = Sat. with job, 6 = Sat. with life as a whole, 7 = Sat. with friendships, 8 = Sat. with health, 9 = Sat. with religion/spiritual fulfilment, 10 = Sat. with financial security, 11 = Sat. with recreational activities, 12 = Sat. with self-esteem, 13 = Sat. with federal government, 14 = Sat. with provincial government, 15 = Sat. with local government, 16 = Overall quality of life, 17 = Overall happiness, 18 = Age, 19 = Income, ns = not statistically significant. *Decimals omitted, underlined numbers are negative

life variables in the presence of all the other domain satisfaction variables for our three special groups, we found that income had no statistically significant impact at all. For females and males analyzed separately, income had no significant impact on life satisfaction scores, and for happiness and satisfaction with the overall quality of life, income's influence was near the bottom of the list of predictors (from ninth to twelfth place).

In a fine longitudinal study based on personal interviews of 942 Australians at five points in time from 1981 to 1989, Heady and Wearing (1992) examined the so-called 'mid-life crisis' phenomenon and came to the conclusion that "the mid-life crisis is a myth, or at most is confined to professional men, and does not occur at a specific age" (p. 153). They divided their respondents into three groups aged 18–34, 35–54 and 55 or over, and found (among other things) life satisfaction scores of 72.5, 75.0 and 77.5, respectively. Since their scales ran from 0 to 100, with larger numbers indicating greater satisfaction, their conclusion was apparently warranted for their panel.

We looked for signs of a mid-life crisis in our dataset, and selected three age-groups for our investigation, namely, youth (18–24), mid-life (38–44) and retirement (65 or more). The graphs assembled in Fig. 11.1 clearly show that our results are consistent with those of Headey and Wearing. For the 3 global indicators and for the 9 domain satisfaction indicators, ratings of the mid-life group are as high as or higher than those of the youth group. Furthermore, ratings of the retirement group are highest of the lot, except for satisfaction with one's own health. If there is a mid-life crisis phenomenon, it seems to have missed our respondents in Prince George.

Using much larger databases, other researchers have found that age has very modest to practically negligible impact on quality of life measures. For example, Stock et al. (1983) undertook an extensive review of research on the relation between age and subjective well-being, and concluded on the basis of 221 estimates from 119 different American sources published before 1980 that "the amount of variance in SWB [subjective well-being] explained by age…never rises above 1%" (p. 297). Inglehart (1990) examined age and self-reported well-being scores for 169,776 people in 16 nations, and reached a similar conclusion. On the basis of their review of several studies, Myers and Diener (1995, p. 11) concluded that "knowing someone's age gives no clue to the person's average sense of well-being". All of these investigations reminded me of a passage written by Marcus Tullius Cicero in about 45 B.C.E.

> Life's race-course is fixed; Nature has only a single path and that path is run but once, and to each stage of existence has been allotted its own appropriate quality; so that the weakness of childhood, the impetuosity of youth, the seriousness of middle life, the maturity of old age – each bears some of Nature's fruit, which must be garnered in its own season (Cicero 2001, p. 43).

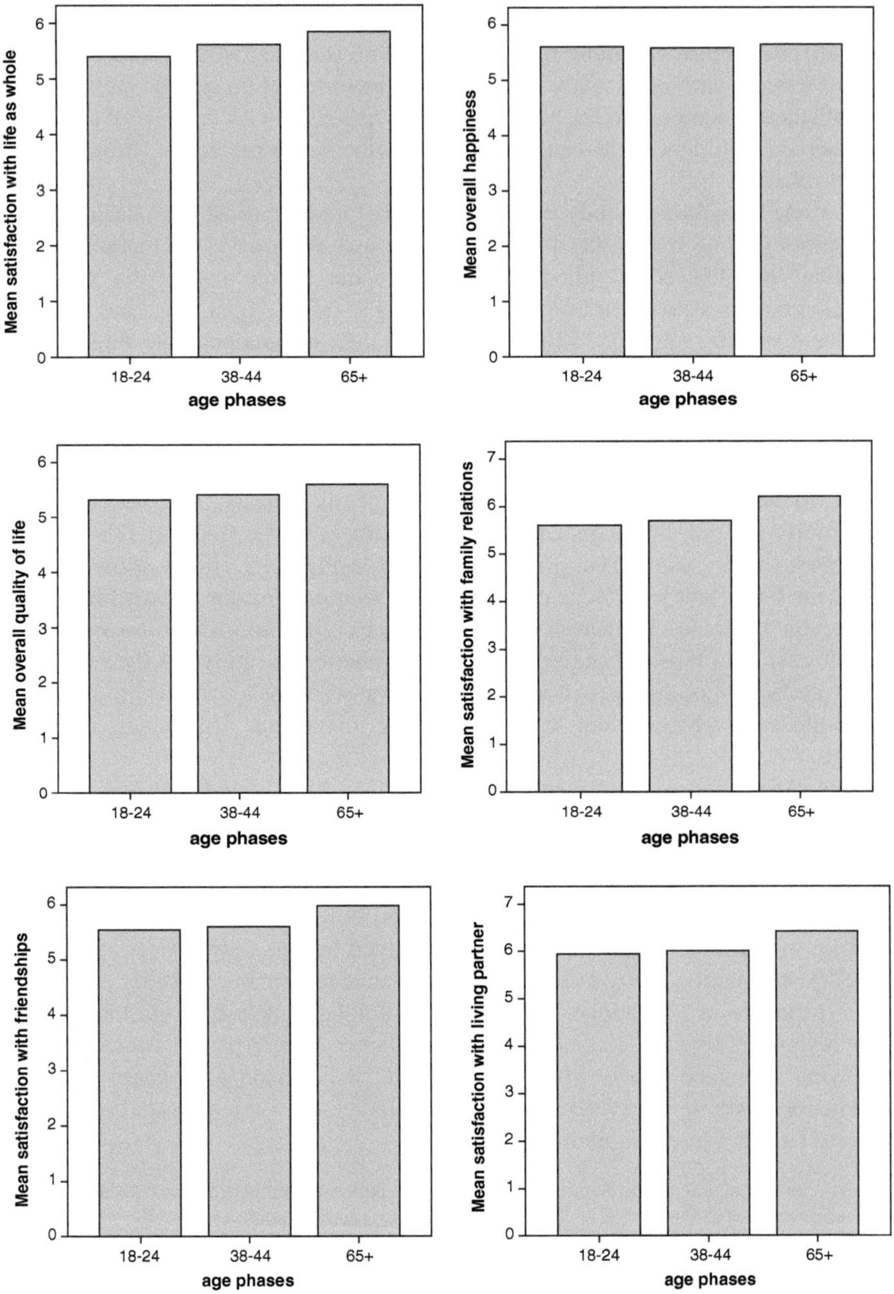

Fig. 11.1 Quality of life by age: youth (18–24), mid-life (38–44) and retirement (65 or more)

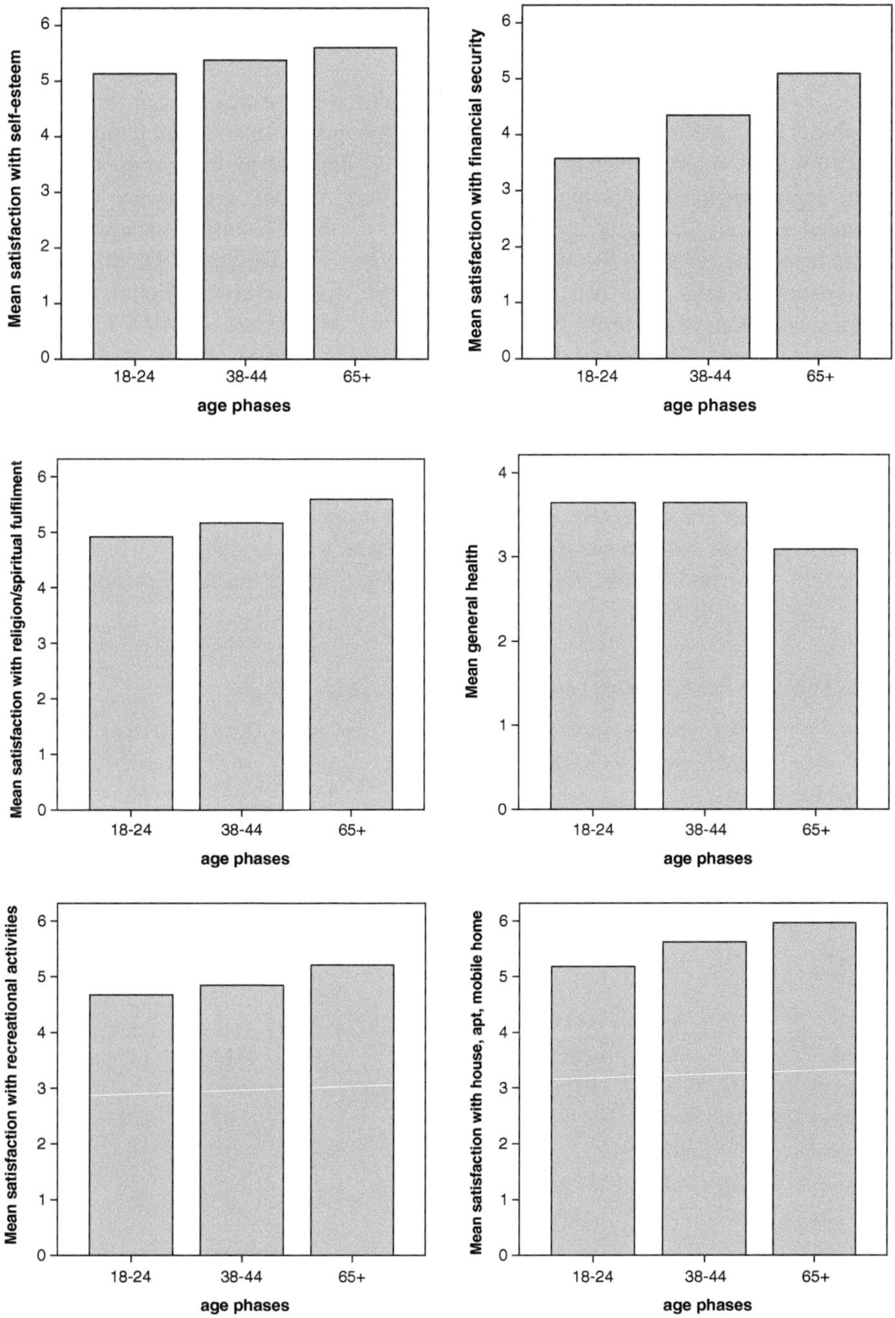

Fig. 11.1 (continued)

Multivariate Relations

Tables 11.4, 11.5 and 11.6 give the results of regressing scores for our three global variables (satisfaction with life as a whole and the quality of life, and happiness) on scores for 14 domain satisfaction variables, using stepwise multiple regression with mean replacement of missing values. This very simple explanatory model, a so-called Bottom-Up linear model, remains as a very live option despite considerable research, evidence for and discussions about Top-Down, Bi-Directional and discrepancy models. For literature reviews, see, for example, Michalos (1985), Headey and Wearing (1992), Veenhoven (1994), Mallard et al. (1997), Inglehart and Klingemann (2002) and Diener and Seligman (2004). While multiple discrepancies theory (Michalos 1985) provides a deeper understanding and a more promising explanatory model than Bottom-Up, Top-down or Bi-Directional models, the latter three are all useful. Using data gathered on 18,000 undergraduates from 39 countries by Michalos (1991a, b, 1993a, b). Mallard et al. (1997) showed that of the latter three models, a Bi-directional model provided the best fit for the Canadian data on domain satisfaction-life satisfaction relationships for the domains of health, finances, family relations, friendships, living partner, recreation and

Table 11.4 Life satisfaction explained by domain satisfaction variables

Topic	Total	Female	Male	Youth	Others	Aborig.	Others	Unempl.	Others
N	8832	4588	4116	423	8197	285	7627	303	8388
% var. Ex.	59	59	59	57	59	65	59	60	57
Sat. with:	Beta	Beta	Beta	Beta	Beta	Beta	Beta	Beta	Beta
Housing	0.04[c]	0.02[c]	0.04[c]	[b]	0.04[c]	[b]	0.04[c]	[b]	0.04[c]
Neighb.	[b]	[b]	0.02[c]	[b]	[b]	0.17	[b]	[b]	[b]
Family	0.08	0.08	0.06[c]	0.09	0.08	[b]	0.09	0.13	0.08
Partner	0.10	0.11	0.09	0.12	0.10	0.19	0.10	[b]	0.12
Job	0.15	0.14	0.15	0.12	0.15	0.14	0.14	[a]	[a]
Friends	0.23	0.23	0.23	0.27	0.23	0.39	0.22	0.26	0.26
Health	0.12	0.14	0.09	[b]	0.13	0.14	0.12	[b]	0.13
Religion	0.03[c]	0.03[c]	0.03[c]	[b]	0.03[c]	[b]	0.03[c]	[b]	0.04[c]
Finances	0.08	0.06	0.08	0.14	0.07	[b]	0.07	0.08	0.10
Recreation	[b]	0.03[c]	[b]	[b]	[b]	0.14	0.02[c]	[b]	[b]
Sf-esteem	0.28	0.26	0.30	0.33	0.28	0.25	0.28	0.48	0.29
Fed. Gov.	[b]	[b]	0.03[c]	[b]	[b]	[b]	[b]	[b]	[b]
Prov. Gov.	[b]	[b]	[b]	[b]	[b]		0.02[c]	0.11	[b]
Local Gov.	0.02[c]	0.02[c]	[b]	0.07	0.02[c]	[b]	[b]	[b]	0.03[c]

[a]Not in equation
[b]Not statistically significant
[c]Contribution to R^2 change < 0.01

Table 11.5 Happiness explained by domain satisfaction variables

Topic	Total	Female	Male	Youth	Others	Aborig.	Others	Unempl.	Others
N	8832	4588	4116	423	8197	285	7627	303	8388
% var. Ex.	38	37	40	34	39	42	39	42	37
Sat. with:	Beta	Beta	Beta	Beta	Beta	Beta	Beta	Beta	Beta
Housing	0.03[c]	[b]	0.04[c]	[b]	0.03[c]	[b]	0.03[c]	[b]	0.03[c]
Neighb.	[b]	[b]	[b]	[b]	[b]	[b]	[b]	0.11	[b]
Family	0.07[c]	0.08	0.06[c]	[b]	0.08	[b]	0.08	[b]	0.08
Partner	0.13	0.15	0.11	0.22	0.12	0.26	0.12	0.11	0.14
Job	0.08	0.07[c]	0.09	[b]	0.08	[b]	0.09	[a]	[a]
Friends	0.10	0.09	0.10	0.18	0.09	0.26	0.09	0.19	0.10
Health	0.10	0.09	0.11	[b]	0.11	[b]	0.10	[b]	0.11
Religion	[b]	[b]	[b]	[b]	[b]	[b]	[b]	[b]	[b]
Finances	0.10	0.10	0.10	0.15	0.10	0.18	0.09	0.17	0.10
Recreation	0.02[c]	0.04[c]	[b]	[b]	0.02[c]	[b]	[b]	[b]	0.02[c]
Sf-esteem	0.26	0.26	0.28	0.27	0.26	0.22	0.27	0.34	0.27
Fed. Gov.	0.03[c]	b	0.06[c]	[b]	0.03[c]	b	0.02[c]	[b]	0.03[c]
Prov. Gov.	[b]	0.04[c]	[b]	[b]	[b]	[b]	[b]	[b]	[b]
Local Gov.	0.02[c]	[b]	[b]	[b]	0.02[c]	[b]	0.03[c]	[b]	0.03[c]

[a]Not in equation
[b]Not statistically significant
[c]Contribution to R^2 change < 0.01

education. If such results turn out to be true of adults generally or of Canadian adults in particular, our Bottom-Up results may be only half the story about causal relations among these variables.

Because practically all studies involving regressions of our global variable scores on domain satisfaction plus demographic variable scores have shown that less than 10% of the variation in the former can be explained by the latter (Michalos 1991a), we did not include demographic data in our reported analyses below. Our results and those of others concerning age, and the relative impact of income in the presence of our domain satisfaction scores, were obtained in separate analyses, as reported above. We also found in separate analyses that of the six categories of marital status, married people have the highest scores on the three global indicators. This is also consistent with most other studies. According to Myers and Diener (1995, p. 15), "Throughout the Western world, married people of both sexes report more happiness than those never married, divorced, or separated". On the same page these authors noted that "The traffic between marriage and happiness…appears to be two-way: Happy people are more appealing as potential marriage partners and more likely to marry (Mastekaasa 1992; Scott 1992)". After reviewing 58 American studies, Haring-Hidore et al. (1985) concluded that marital status explains about 2% of the variance in overall subjective well-being.

Table 11.6 Satisfaction with the overall quality of life explained by domain satisfaction variables

Topic	Total	Female	Male	Youth	Others	Aborig.	Others	Unempl.	Others
N	8832	4588	4116	423	8197	285	7627	303	8388
% var. Ex.	54	53	55	51	54	53	54	51	53
Sat. with:	Beta	Beta	Beta	Beta	Beta	Beta	Beta	Beta	Beta
Housing	0.08	0.08	0.08	[b]	0.08	[b]	0.08	[b]	0.09
Neighb.	0.06[c]	0.06[c]	0.07[c]	0.11	0.06[c]	0.18	0.06[c]	0.20	0.06[c]
Family	0.04[c]	0.05[c]	0.03[c]	0.11	0.04[c]	[b]	0.06[c]	[b]	0.05[c]
Partner	0.07	0.07	0.07	[b]	0.07	0.11	0.06	0.09	0.07
Job	0.07	0.06[c]	0.08	[b]	0.07[c]	[b]	0.07[c]	[a]	[a]
Friends	0.10	0.10	0.08	0.25	0.09	0.18	0.10	0.16	0.11
Health	0.17	0.18	0.16	[b]	0.17	0.13	0.17	[b]	0.17
Religion	0.02[c]	[b]	0.02[c]	[b]	0.03[c]	[b]	[b]	[b]	0.03[c]
Finances	0.16	0.16	0.17	0.16	0.17	0.13	0.17	0.18	0.17
Recreation	0.06[c]	0.07[c]	0.06[c]	0.09	0.06[c]	[b]	0.07[c]	[b]	0.06
Sf-esteem	0.23	0.24	0.25	0.27	0.23	0.31	0.23	0.37	0.23
Fed. Gov.	[b]	[b]	[b]	[b]	[b]	[b]	[b]	[b]	[b]
Prov. Gov.	0.03[c]	[b]	0.04[c]	b	0.03[c]	0.12	0.02[c]	0.10	0.02[c]
Local Gov.	0.05[c]	0.06[c]	0.06[c]	0.12	0.05[c]	[b]	0.05[c]	[b]	0.06[c]

[a]Not in equation
[b]Not statistically significant
[c]Contribution to R^2 change < 0.01

Because the sample sizes for most of our groups are fairly large, some very small associations are statistically significant. Explanatory variables whose contribution to changes in the percent of variation explained in a dependent variable (R^2 changes) were less than 0.01 are flagged with a superscript ‘c’. Column entries are standardized regression coefficients (Beta values) with means of zero and standard deviations of one. Beta values are sample-specific insofar as they are sensitive to the particular array of variables and variables’ variances in any equation, but they have the virtue of providing easy comparisons of the relative impact of significant predictors in any particular set. Figuratively speaking, one can think of a dependent variable moving some percentage of a unit step for every full unit step change in the independent variable, when the values of all other variables are held constant. For example, in Table 11.4, in the column headed ‘Total’, one finds that if there were an increase of one unit in the mean score for satisfaction with one’s self-esteem ($\beta = 0.28$), there would be an increase of 28% of a unit in the mean life satisfaction score. Because the complementary groups of non-youth, non-Aboriginal and non-unemployed are quite similar, one would not expect to find great differences in results, although there are some differences.

Table 11.4 shows that scores on our 14 proposed explanatory variables in fact explained from 57 to 65% of the variation in scores for satisfaction with life as a whole. These percentages are typical for this particular array of predictors and dependent variable (Michalos 2003). This is the first time this relatively old explanatory model has been applied to a good-sized group of respondents with Aboriginal backgrounds, and it is interesting to find that the model works very well with such a group ($R^2 = 0.65$). Essentially the same model was applied to a sample of undergraduates ($N = 4886$) in 16 countries, producing an $R^2 = 0.50$ (Michalos 1991a, p. 100), which is a bit lower than the $R^2 = 0.57$ obtained for our youth group. However, the Canadian part of that international sample ($N = 451$) had an $R^2 = 0.55$, which is very close to the value obtained here (Michalos 1991a, p. 191).

With the exception of our Aboriginal respondents, satisfaction with one's own self-esteem is the strongest predictor of satisfaction with life as a whole for every group, i.e., the better one feels about oneself, the better one is likely to judge one's whole life to be. For those with an Aboriginal background, satisfaction with one's friendships is the strongest predictor of life satisfaction ($\beta = 0.39$), followed by satisfaction with self-esteem ($\beta = 0.25$). Unfortunately, although unemployed respondents have the lowest levels of satisfaction with their self-esteem compared to all other groups (Table 11.2), the influence of scores for this variable on life satisfaction scores is greater for unemployed respondents than for any other group ($\beta = 0.48$). As much as self-esteem satisfaction means to all respondents, from the point of view of its impact on life satisfaction, it means even more to those whose supply is most limited. For the international sample of undergraduates ($N = 4886$), self-esteem satisfaction was also the strongest predictor of life satisfaction ($\beta = 0.20$), followed closely by a variable that was not in our equations (satisfaction with one's university education) and then by satisfaction with one's finances ($\beta = 0.16$) (Michalos 1991a, p. 100). For the Canadian part of that sample ($N = 451$), the three most influential predictors of life satisfaction were satisfaction with one's own self-esteem ($\beta = 0.34$), family relations and friendships (each $\beta = 0.13$) (Michalos 1991a, p. 191).

For every group except Aboriginals, the second most influential explanatory variable is satisfaction with friendships. Curiously, although we saw that mean scores for living partner satisfaction are higher than all other domain satisfaction scores for all groups, only for Aboriginal respondents were living partner satisfaction scores ($\beta = 0.19$) among the three most influential predictors of life satisfaction scores. For the total group, males, and the two near-total groups of non-youths and non-Aboriginals, job satisfaction scores were the third most influential predictors of life satisfaction scores. (The job satisfaction variable was left out of the equation for the unemployed versus all others comparisons.) For females, job satisfaction tied with health satisfaction ($\beta = 0.14$) as a predictor of life satisfaction.

Table 11.5 shows that scores on our 14 proposed explanatory variables in fact explained from 34 to 42% of the variance in scores for happiness. These percentages are also typical for this particular array of predictors and dependent variable. Again, this is the first time this model has been applied to such a sizable group of respondents with Aboriginal backgrounds, with results at least as strong as those for other groups (R^2 = 0.42). When this model was applied to the international sample of undergraduates (N = 4819) in 16 countries, it produced an R^2 = 0.29 (Michalos 1991a, p. 100), which is again a bit lower than the R^2 = 0.34 obtained for our youth group. However, the Canadian part of that international sample (N = 455) had an R^2 = 0.40, higher than that for our youth group.

Looking across all the columns in Table 11.5, one finds that satisfaction with one's own self-esteem is the most influential predictor of happiness in every case except that of Aboriginal respondents. For the latter, there is a tie for first place between satisfaction with friends and living partner (β = 0.26). For the total group, females, youth, non-youth, non-Aboriginals and non-unemployed, the second most influential predictor is living partner satisfaction. For Aboriginal respondents, the second most influential predictor is satisfaction with one's own self-esteem (β = 0.22), for the unemployed group it is satisfaction with friendships (β = 0.19) and for males there is a tie between satisfaction with living partners and health (β = 0.11). For the international sample of undergraduates (N = 4819), the strongest predictor of happiness was satisfaction with one's living partner (β = 0.18), followed by a tie between satisfaction with one's self-esteem and family relationships (β = 0.14) (Michalos 1991a, p. 100). For the Canadian part of that sample (N = 455), self-esteem satisfaction came first (β = 0.31), followed by satisfaction with family relationships (β = 0.20) (Michalos 1991a, p. 191).

Table 11.6 shows that scores on our 14 proposed explanatory variables explained from 51 to 55% of the variance in scores for satisfaction with the overall quality of life. Because this particular dependent variable has only been used by ISRE researchers and mainly in Prince George, we don't know how it would compare in applications elsewhere. The result for Aboriginal respondents (R^2 = 0.53) indicates that the model is as applicable to this group as to any other. Inspecting all the columns, one finds that the question about one's satisfaction with the overall quality of life elicits a somewhat different array of responses from those elicited by the questions about life satisfaction and happiness. For every group, self-esteem satisfaction has the greatest impact on overall quality-of-life satisfaction, with Beta values running from β = 0.23 to β = 0.37. As in the cases of life satisfaction and happiness, the unemployed group's self-esteem satisfaction had a greater impact than the domain satisfaction for any other group on overall quality-of-life satisfaction. There is more variety among the second most influential predictors of this dependent variable than for either of the other two. For the total group (β = 0.17) and females (β = 0.18), the second most influential predictor is satisfaction with one's own health. For males, second place goes to satisfaction with finances (β = 0.17); for youth it is friendships (β = 0.25) and for the unemployed it is one's neighborhood (β = 0.20). Each of the remaining four groups has ties for second place. For non-youth, non-Aboriginals and non-Unemployed, satisfaction with health and financial security are tied (β = 0.17), and for Aboriginal respondents it is friendships and neighborhood (β = 0.18).

Concluding Comments

The primary reason for this note was to obtain a general overview of the quality of life of residents of Prince George in the period from November 1997 to February 2005, including especially the three groups in our community that are typically under-represented in our annual surveys. Although our aggregated samples for young, Aboriginal and unemployed residents are still relatively small, they were large enough to undertake some analyses that were previously impossible. Broadly speaking, we found that the quality of life of unemployed residents is lower than that of residents with Aboriginal backgrounds and that the quality of life of the latter is still lower than that of young people. Nevertheless, the quality of life of young people was significantly lower than that of the total sampled population, as well as that of the selected mid-life and retirement groups.

There is a considerable body of research devoted to the well-being, generally speaking, of unemployed people; e.g., see Clark and Oswald (1994), Van Bruggen (1997), Winkelmann and Winkelmann (1998) and Easterlin (2002a, b). Unemployment has significant negative effects beyond the loss of income, including increases in mortality and morbidity, risks of suicide, criminal activity, marital problems, depression and loss of social status and self-esteem. Diener and Biswas-Diener (2002, p. 151) claimed that "It appears that unemployed people on average would be dissatisfied even if they had a relatively high income—presumably because they are not doing a task that is respected in the culture." Using a very large dataset ($N = 264{,}710$) from survey research in 12 European countries covering the period from 1975 to 1991, Di Tella et al. (2001) examined the relative impact of the two components of the misery index (the sum of unemployment and inflation rates) on human well-being measured by life satisfaction and happiness scales roughly similar to those used here. Their conclusion is worth repeating in full.

> At the margin, unemployment depresses reported well-being more than does inflation. In a panel that controls for country fixed effects, year effects, and country-specific time trends, the estimates suggest that people would trade off a 1-percentage-point increase in the unemployment rate for a 1.7-percentage-point increase in the inflation rate. Hence, according to these findings, the famous 'misery index' $W(\pi + U)$ underweights the unhappiness caused by joblessness (p. 340).

Reflecting on these results, Easterlin (2002a, b, p. xiii) quite justifiably wrote,

> Recent decades have seen the increasing subordination of employment to price-level concerns as a goal of monetary and fiscal policy. This article implies that policy makers, if their ultimate interest is social welfare, have got it backward.

In many if not most studies of the well-being costs of unemployment, comparisons are made only between those in the labour force who are unemployed versus those who are employed (full-time, part-time or selfemployed). When we analyzed our data on this basis, we found that for 9 indicators the mean scores of the employed group were slightly lower (0.04% points on average) than those for the complementary class of non-unemployed, and for 3 indicators the mean scores of the employed group were slightly higher (0.01–0.02% points). The satisfaction with health mean score for the employed group was 0.12% points higher than that of the complementary class of non-unemployed. The relative status of the unemployed compared to the employed was essentially no different from its status compared to the non-unemployed.

Regarding predictors of our three global dependent variables for the three groups and the total population, we found that the Aboriginal group was most different from all others. Satisfaction with one's own self-esteem was the most influential predictor of each global indicator for every group except Aboriginal residents. For the latter, self-esteem satisfaction was only the strongest predictor of satisfaction with the overall quality of life. The strongest predictor of life satisfaction for the Aboriginal group was satisfaction with friendships, and there were two domain satisfaction scores tied (friendships and living partner) for most influential predictors of happiness. Self-esteem satisfaction ranked second in strength of influence on Aboriginal happiness and life satisfaction. Staats et al. (1995, pp. 108–109) claimed that "Self-esteem is a central component of personality and much of clinical psychological practice is aimed at increasing individual well-being through improving self-esteem…" Results from our Aboriginal sample suggest that there may be some cultural differences worth exploring on this score.

Inspecting the columns of predictors of global indicator scores, one finds that for satisfaction with the overall quality of life, living partner satisfaction is never among the top four predictors for any group, and it only reaches third place for one group (Aboriginal respondents) in the list of predictors of life satisfaction. Also for life satisfaction, living partner satisfaction appears in fourth place for females and the non-unemployed group, and it is tied for fourth place for males and youth. However, living partner satisfaction appears as the second (once tied) most influential predictor of happiness for seven of the nine groups (Table 11.5). Examining the list of predictors of life satisfaction more carefully, one finds that satisfaction with one's financial security is mentioned only once in the top four predictors for all groups. Although one might have thought that satisfaction with one's financial security would loom large for the unemployed, it is not among the top four predictors for that group. It is, however, the third most influential predictor of life satisfaction for our group of young residents. Clearly, then, although there is some overlap or similarity of meaning for our three global indicators for Prince George respondents, significant differences appear when one looks for explanations of global indicator scores among domain satisfaction scores.

Acknowledgements We would like to thank Nathan Cardinal, Greg Halseth, Seth Klein and Maurine Hatch for their suggestions and other help with this paper.

Appendix

Data Sources

1998 (June), "Quality of Life Survey Summary Statistics", Institute for Social Research and Evaluation, University of Northern British Columbia. 1998 (November), "Regional District of Fraser-Fort George Survey Summary Statistics", Institute for Social Research and Evaluation, University of Northern British Columbia.

2000 (April), "City Trails Survey Summary Statistics", Institute for Social Research and Evaluation, University of Northern British Columbia.

2000 (November), "Communication and Quality of Life Survey Summary Statistics", Institute for Social Research and Evaluation, University of Northern British Columbia.

2001 (June), "Foster Parents' Survey Summary Statistics", Institute for Social Research and Evaluation, University of Northern British Columbia. 2003 (October), "Solid Waste Collection Survey", Institute for Social Research and Evaluation, University of Northern British Columbia.

2004 (November), "Prince George Quality of Life Survey", Institute for Social Research and Evaluation, University of Northern British Columbia.

2005 (February), "Prince George Quality of Life Survey", Institute for Social Research and Evaluation, University of Northern British Columbia. Michalos, A.C.: 2002, "Policing services and the quality of life", *Social Indicators Research,* 60, pp. 1–18.

Michalos, A.C.: 2005, "Arts and the quality of life", *Social Indicators Research,* 71, pp. 11–59.

Michalos, A.C. and B.D. Zumbo: 2000, "Criminal victimization and the quality of life", *Social Indicators Research,* 50, pp. 245–295.

Michalos, A.C. and B.D. Zumbo: 2000, "Health and the quality of life", *Social Indicators Research,* 51, pp. 245–286.

Michalos, A.C. and B.D. Zumbo: 2000 (November), "British Columbians' expectations and attitudes going into the third millennium", Institute for Social Research and Evaluation, University of Northern British Columbia. Michalos, A.C. and B.D. Zumbo: 2001, "Ethnicity, modern prejudice and the quality of life, *Social Indicators Research,* 53, pp. 189–222.

Michalos, A.C., A.M. Hubley, B.D. Zumbo and D. Hemingway: 2001, "Health and other aspects of the quality of life of older people", *Social Indicators Research,* 54, pp. 239–274.

Michalos, A.C. and B.D. Zumbo: 2003, "Leisure activities, health and the quality of life", in Alex C. Michalos, *Essays on the Quality of Life* (Kluwer Academic Publishing, Dordrecht) pp. 217–239.

References

Cicero, M. T. (2001). *On old age, on friendship. On divination* (W.A. Falconer Trans.). Cambridge: Harvard University Press.
Clark, A. E., & Oswald, A. J. (1994). Unhappiness and unemployment. *The Economic Journal, 104,* 648–659.
Diener, E., & Biswas-Diener, R. (2002). Will money increase subjective well-being? A literature review and guide to needed research. *Social Indicators Research, 57,* 119–169.
Diener, E., & Oishi, S. (2000). Money and happiness: Income and subjective well-being across nations. In E. Diener & E. M. Suh (Eds.), *Culture and subjective well-being* (pp. 185–218). Cambridge: MIT Press.
Diener, E., & Seligman, M. E. P. (2004). Beyond money: Toward an economy of well-being. *Psychological Science in the Public Interest, 5*(1), 1–31.
Di Tella, R., MacCulloch, R. J., & Oswald, A. J. (2001). Preferences over inflation and unemployment: Evidence from surveys of happiness. *The American Economic Review, 91,* 335341.
Easterlin, R. A. (2001). Income and happiness: Towards a unified theory. *The Economic Journal, 111,* 465–484.
Easterlin, R. A. (Ed.). (2002a). *Happiness in economics.* Cheltenham: Edward Elgar.
Easterlin, R. A. (2002b). Introduction. In: R.A. Easterlin (Ed.), *Happiness in economics* (pp. iv–xv). Cheltenham: Edward Elgar.
Haring, M. J., Stock, W. A., & Okun, M. A. (1984). A research synthesis of gender and social class as correlates of subjective well-being. *Human Relations, 37,* 645–657.
Haring-Hidore, M. J., Stock, W. A., Okun, M. A., & Witter, R. A. (1985). Marital status and subjective well-being: A research synthesis. *Journal of Marriage and the Family, 47,* 947–953.
Heady, B., & Wearing, A. (1992). *Understanding happiness: A theory of subjective wellbeing.* Melbourne: Longman Cheshire.
Inglehart, R. (1990). *Culture shift in advanced industrial society.* Princeton: Princeton University Press.
Inglehart, R., & Klingemann, H.-D. (2002). Genes, culture, democracy and happiness. http://www.worldvaluessurvey.org/library/index.html).
Mallard, A. G. C., Lance, C. E., & Michalos, A. C. (1997). Culture as a moderator of overall life satisfaction. *Social Indicators Research, 40,* 259–284.
Mastekaasa, A. (1992). Marriage and psychological well-being: Some evidence on selection into marriage. *Journal of Marriage and the Family, 54,* 901–911.
Michalos, A. C. (1985). Multiple discrepancies theory (MDT). *Social Indicators Research, 16,* 347–413.
Michalos, A. C. (1991a). *Global report on student well-being. Volume One: Life satisfaction and happiness.* New York: Springer.
Michalos, A. C. (1991b). *Global report on student well-being. Volume Two: Family, friends, living partner and self-esteem.* New York: Springer.
Michalos, A. C. (1993a). *Global report on student well-being. Volume Three: Employment, finances, housing and transportation.* New York: Springer.
Michalos, A. C. (1993b). *Global report on student well-being. Volume Four: Religion, education, recreation and health.* New York: Springer.
Michalos, A. C. (2003). *Essays on the quality of life.* Dordrecht: Kluwer Academic Publishers.
Michalos, A. C., Hubley, A. M., Zumbo, B. D., & Hemingway, D. (2001). Health and other aspects of the quality of life of older people. *Social Indicators Research, 54,* 239–274.
Myers, D. G., & Diener, E. (1995). Who is happy? *Psychological Science, 6,* 10–19.
Scott, C. (1992). Personality versus the situational effect in the relation between marriage and subjective well-being. Unpublished doctoral dissertation. University of Illinois, Champaign.
Staats, S., Armstrong-Stassen, M., & Partilo, C. (1995). Student well-being: Are they better off now? *Social Indicators Research, 34*(1), 93–112.

Stock, W. A., Okun, M. A., Haring, J. J., & Witter, R. A. (1983). Age differences in subjective wellbeing: A meta-analysis. *Evaluations Studies Review Annual, 8,* 279–302.
Van Bruggen, A. C. (1997). Social participation and subjective well-being of long-term unemployed. In H. L. Meadow (Ed.), *Developments in quality-of-life studies* (Vol. 1, pp. 96–123). Blacksburg: International Society for Quality of Life Studies.
Veenhoven, R. (1994). Is happiness a trait? Tests of the theory that a better society does not make people any happier. *Social Indicators Research, 32*(2), 101–160.
Winkelmann, L., & Winkelmann, R. (1998). Why are the unemployed so unhappy? Evidence from panel data. *Economica, 65,* 1–15.

Chapter 12
Education, Happiness and Wellbeing

Alex C. Michalos

Introduction

Judging from the title of the conference, it appears that we were gathered to examine the science and philosophy involved in happiness studies, and to assess its significance for making public policy. Some of the invited speakers have devoted much of their life's work to addressing precisely these two broad topics and their views, sympathies and/or biases are well-known to people working in the trade. Diener and Seligman (2004) have a fine paper devoted precisely on the topic. As one would expect from any group of scholars, there are plenty of areas of agreement and disagreement among us. Anyone interested in more detailed overviews of work in this field and the progress made since the 1960s should have a look at Michalos (2005).

Judging from the proposed titles of contributions, it appears that we are proceeding from relatively broad overviews of happiness studies to more detailed discussions. In my case, the focus is supposed to be on the particular role of education in influencing happiness and what significance, if any, that might have for public policy. I will give a brief summary of my understanding of the basic questions and my answers now, and a more detailed investigation afterward.

Michalos, A.C.: 2008. Education, happiness and wellbeing. Social Indicators Research, 87(3), pp. 347–366.

The first version of this paper was written for the International Conference on 'Is happiness measurable and what do those measures mean for public policy?', at Rome, 2–3 April 2007, University of Rome 'Tor Vergata', organized by the Joint Research Centre of the European Commission, OECD, Centre for Economic and International Studies and the Bank of Italy. I would like to thank the organizers of the conference for the invitation and the participants for helping me clarify some things.

A.C. Michalos (✉)
University of Northern British Columbia, Prince George, BC, Canada
e-mail: michalos@brandonu.ca

A.C. Michalos, *Connecting the Quality of Life Theory to Health, Well-Being and Education*, DOI 10.1007/978-3-319-51161-0_12

The basic scientific and philosophical questions for this session seem to be: Does education influence happiness and if so, how and how much?

My answer is: It depends on how one defines and operationalizes 'education', 'influences' and 'happiness'. More precisely, if one defines and operationalizes (1) 'education' as highest level of formal education attained including primary, secondary and tertiary education leading to diplomas and degrees, (2) 'happiness' as whatever is measured by standardized single-item or multi-item indexes of happiness or life satisfaction, and (3) 'influences' as a direct and positive correlation between such measures of education and happiness, then the answers to the basic scientific and philosophic questions are well-known. Given these definitions, education has very little influence on happiness.

On the other hand, if one defines (1) 'education' more broadly to include formal education as specified above, non-formal education of the sort that might involve learning through course-work not connected to any diplomas or degrees, and informal education of the sort that might involve learning outside of any course-work, from news media, works of art and culture, work-related training and experiences, social interaction and routine as well as extra-ordinary life experiences, (2) 'happiness' as an Aristotelian *eudaimonia* or general wellbeing involving, in his phrase, "living well and doing well" by enjoying goods of the mind (e.g., wisdom, moral virtue and pleasure), goods of the body (e.g., physical beauty, health and pleasure again) and external goods (e.g., wealth and adequate material resources, good parents and families, good friends, peace and security within and between communities, and well-governed communities), and (3) 'influences' as indirect as well as direct associations among the diverse kinds of education and learning and the diverse features of a happy or good life, then the answers to the basic questions are more complicated and for that reason, less well-known. Given these more robust definitions of 'education', 'influences' and 'happiness', education has enormous influence on happiness.

Given the three essential variables related to our questions and the minimum number of alternative values of each variable, we could construct $2^N = 2^3 = 8$ research scenarios using the (1) narrow view of education, happiness and influence, (2) robust view of education, narrow view of happiness and influence; (3) narrow view of education, robust view of happiness, narrow view of influence, etc. to (8) robust view of education, happiness and influence. Of course this would be the tip of the iceberg of possible research scenarios because there are many more than two alternative values for each of our three variables, many more views about the nature of education, happiness and influence. Below I am only going to talk a bit about the first and last of the minimum eight scenarios.

Given the great variety of research scenarios that may be constructed from our three essential variables, one should expect plenty of different answers to the basic political question before us. What public policies one ought to adopt and implement regarding the influence of education on happiness depends minimally on which of the great variety of research scenarios one adopts and maximally on lots of other things as well, e.g., what is politically possible, financially possible, technically possible, morally possible, and so on (Michalos 1978). There are good reasons for people pursuing only either the first or last of the minimum eight scenarios. My personal preference is for the last, but I have done quite a bit of work with the first too. Compared to the last scenario, the first is far easier to manage. The last scenario costs a lot more in many ways than the first and, as usual, it costs more because it is worth more in the long run. It promises to deliver much more value in many more senses of this word (value) than the first, minimal research scenario. There is good evidence that most of the governments of most countries of the world perceive and have endorsed a political agenda that pretty clearly follows from those robust definitions.

Education as Learning

If the distinguishing feature of anything regarded as education is the fact that learning occurs, then it is a gross oversimplification to define 'education' as merely formal education leading to some kind of certification. Human beings must learn to eat and what to eat, to grasp and what to grasp, to stand, walk and talk, to talk this language and/or that, wisely or foolishly, rudely or politely, loudly or softly, a lot or a little, at the right time and in the right way to successfully communicate. Quite generally, individuals and communities must learn many different kinds of things in a wide variety of circumstances, and there are a wide variety of teachers (Michalos 2003). If the difference between knowledge and mere opinion or belief is that knowledge requires that one's opinions or beliefs must be true in the first place and well-warranted in the second place (Michalos 2006), then probably much of what one learns formally, non-formally and informally as characterized earlier is not knowledge. For example, Hayward et al. (2005, p. 118) reported that "A British study, cited in the *Journal of Internal Medicine,* found that 'much of the information patients receive about health and health care is misleading, outdated or biased'.

Every individual and community has a lifelong learning project involving perhaps at a minimum learning to know, to do, to live together and to be, as the Canadian Council on Learning says, following one of the social indicators research pioneers, Jacques Delors. I say "at a minimum" because a fourfold classification of reasons, motives, purposes or general goals for learning is only one of many classificatory schemes one might construct. Maybe, for example, the UN Millennium Development Goals and all the themes of the UN Decade of Education for Sustainable Development can be squeezed into one of the four pigeon holes, but I suspect it would be a tight squeeze.

I suppose it is not necessary to labour this point. Using the narrow definition of 'education', one would have to say that education appeared very late in human history and that a great deal of important learning that goes on across the whole lifespan of individuals and communities is not, after all, education. I suppose very few, if anyone at all, would be prepared to accept these consequences. So, I will assume most people will find a research scenario involving a more robust rather than a more narrow definition of 'education' most interesting.

Happiness, Quality of Life and Wellbeing

As some have heard me say too many times already, in very broad strokes one may think of the quality of life or wellbeing of an individual or community as a function of the actual conditions of that life and what an individual or community makes of those conditions. What a person or community makes of those conditions is in turn a function of how the conditions are perceived, what is thought and felt about those conditions, what is done and, finally, what consequences follow from all these inputs. People's perceptions, thoughts, feelings and actions, then, have an impact on their own and others' living conditions. This general model is illustrated in Fig. 12.1.

Taking the two main variables together (conditions of life and what people make of them), one can construct four scenarios which, with some exaggeration, may be described as different kinds of Paradise and Hell.

1. If people's living conditions are good, and people accurately perceive and think about them, feel good, act appropriately with good results, we may describe that as Real Paradise.
2. If people's living conditions are bad, and people accurately perceive and think about them, feel bad, act appropriately but still with bad results, we may describe that as Real Hell.
3. If people's living conditions are bad, and people inaccurately perceive and think about them, feel good, but act inappropriately with bad results, we may describe that as the classical Fool's Paradise.
4. If people's living conditions are good, and people inaccurately perceive and think about them, feel bad, act inappropriately but still get good results, we may describe that as a Fool's Hell.

Although some complicated epistemological and evaluative material was smuggled into the four scenarios, it may be neglected for present purposes. The most important point to be made here is that the classical notion of a Fool's Paradise requires at least the sort of two-variable model mentioned in the first paragraph. This notion is based on the common sense (epistemological realist's) view that

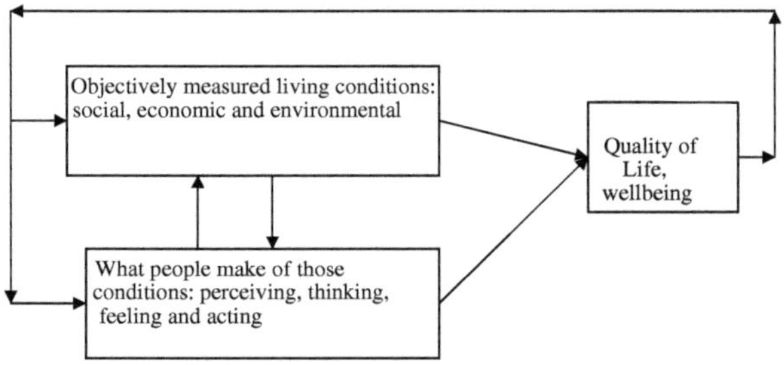

Fig. 12.1 General quality of life model

there is a real world, however roughly apprehended and partially constructed, and that there are good reasons for believing that some perceptions, etc. are more warranted, reliable, valid and reasonable than others. Unfortunately, the common sense, realist's view of the human condition is not universally appreciated and accepted. While anyone with any democratic sensitivity would grant that each person's assessment of his or her own life should be accorded some privileged status, it is far from obvious that such privilege should over-ride all other considerations. Nevertheless, for some of the ancients and their modern followers, it is apparently supposed that people's personal assessments of the quality of their lives are not only privileged, but ultimately definitive. So, for example, it seems to be supposed that if some people are satisfied living in unsanitary environments, breathing polluted air and drinking polluted water, abusing and being abused by family members and strangers, suffering imposed restrictions on opportunities for personal achievement and development, and generally facing an array of life chances promising a life that is relatively nasty, brutish and short rather than pleasant, elegant and long, then that is acceptable. It seems to be supposed, wittingly or not, that however constrained the perceptions, beliefs and so on of the people living in such conditions and assessing them as satisfactory, their assessments are paramount. For people holding such populist and somewhat post modernist views, there can be no Fool's Paradise, because there can be no fools foolish enough to misjudge their own satisfaction. For people holding such views, the quality of life, the good life or wellbeing, is completely internalized or psychologized as elaborated more fully below, and determined by each person's own experiences. Then, since each person has privileged access to his or her own experiences, personal reports of those experiences must be equally privileged.

For the purposes of this essay, it does not matter if one accepts the one or two-variable view of the basic elements required for a proper assessment of the quality of life. In keeping with an old sociological tradition of revealing one's most important assumptions rather than trying to eliminate them, it is worthwhile to present the options and the author's biases up front. I believe it is important to remember that the world contains many people living in poverty, lacking adequate food, shelter and medical care, and facing life chances offering little hope of relief. The good life that we must want and achieve for all people is not, I think, just a life in which people feel good, no matter how terrible their real life conditions are, but one in which they feel good with the best of all reasons, because the objectively measurable conditions of their lives merit a positive assessment.

Well, you might ask, who are those researchers who might neglect the objectively measurable conditions of people's lives and focus all their attention on personal reports of how people feel about their lives? They are not just members of the Economist's (2005) Intelligence Unit, the folks who produced the Quality of Life Index with life satisfaction as the dependent variable. There are many people working in the medicalized version of this entirely internalized or psychologized view of the quality of life, i.e., people working in the health-related quality of life research tradition, which I critiqued at length in Michalos (2004a).

Michalos (1991a, pp. 20–28) summarized the Profile of a Happy Person drawn from several studies cited in that book. A happy person is likely to have low levels of fear, hostility, tension, anxiety, guilt and anger; high degrees of energy, vitality and activity; a high level of self-esteem and an emotionally stable personality; a strong social orientation; healthy, satisfying, warm love and social relationships; an active lifestyle with meaningful work; and to be relatively optimistic, worry-free, present-oriented and well-directed. Although one would be hard-pressed to condemn the life of someone with this sort of psychological profile, it is just that, a psychological profile. One might reasonably ask about someone with such a profile, Is it well-warranted or not? Is the person living in a life-threatening and quite unsustainable situation, but unaware of it? Is the person a moral rogue, but quite free of guilt? Is his or her social orientation devoted to preserving something imagined to be a genetically superior white race? Does the person optimistically discount warnings of global warming and practically any science that disturbs his or her tranquility? Is the tranquility the product of special drugs or, closer to our topic, of some wonderfully effective but essentially perverse education? Exactly what are the real living conditions of this happy person, and does it matter to his or her happiness?

To take a more recent example, Kahneman (1999) resurrected the hedonism from Plato's fourth century BCE *Protagoras* (1924) and Bentham's more familiar treatise of 1789 to construct a concept called "objective happiness", which is rooted in subjective experience and involves only a narrow sense of happiness. The following passages capture its essential nature.

> Being pleased or distressed is an attribute of experience at a particular moment. I will label this attribute *instant utility,* borrowing the term 'utility' from Bentham (1789/1948)… Satisfaction questions refer to more inclusive domains of life, such as family life or work… At the highest level of integration we find dimensions such as happiness, or well-being, which encompass all domains of life… The perspective of the present chapter is bottom-up. It takes the instant utility of the moment as the basic unit of analysis and seeks an objective and normatively justified definition of 'true' well-being that is based mainly on information about instant utility… *Objective happiness* is derived from a record of instant utility over [a] relevant period… Objective happiness, of course, is ultimately based on subjective data: the Good/Bad experiences of moments of life. It is labeled objective because the aggregation of instant utility is governed by a logical rule and could in principle be done by an observer with access to the temporal profile of instant utility (Kahneman et al. 1997; Kahneman 1999, pp. 4–5).

Kahneman's definition of 'happiness' thoroughly psychologizes the concept. What is even worse from the point of view of our investigation of the relations between learning and happiness, his aggregation method is biased against learning. If every moment of instant utility measured by randomly selected experience sampling is equally valid, then each of them must be regarded as essentially incorrigible. The logical possibilities of a Fool's Paradise and a Fool's Hell have been eliminated. Pleasures and pains just are what they are and it does not matter how they are produced. If the pleasures of the uneducated can be at least as intense and plentiful as those of the educated, then it would be irrational for anyone without an education to pay any price for education. So, Mill was wrong. It is not the case that "It is better to be a human being dissatisfied than a pig satisfied; better to be Socrates dissatisfied than a fool satisfied" (Mill 1863).

In a fine critique of Kahneman's proposal, Alexandrova (2005, p. 315) wrote that

> In more general terms, the averaging method imposes equal weights on all aspects of person's experiences, while still hoping to claim the benefits of the subjective approach - yet these two goals are in obvious tension just when the subject does not endorse such an equal weighting.

Of course, it is precisely and especially when one thinks one has "learned one's lesson", has "seen the light", "finally got it right" that one repudiates one's earlier experiences. On reflection, we can all recognize the difference between a good time and a good life. To suggest that the results of such reflection should be replaced by an unreflective averaging of pleasures and pains is tantamount to suggesting that one cease to be a rational agent.

To take an even more recent example from one of my best friends, Diener and Seligman (2004, p. 2, 21) wrote that,

> Our proposed system of well-being indicators would not supplant economic or other current social indicators, but would supplement and enhance their value by placing them within an over-arching framework of well-being, underscoring the shortcomings of economic indicators… A national indicator [system] should include several global indicators, such as life satisfaction, but it should also target positive and negative emotions in specific areas, such as work life, health, social relationships, and mental health, and it should be fine-grained, breaking life satisfaction down into its constituent parts… The most important contribution of a national system of well-being indicators would be that they could focus the attention of policymakers and the public specifically on well-being, and not simply on the production of goods and services; one of the main benefits of well-being measures is that they add a valuable perspective beyond a cost-benefit market analysis in evaluating society structures and interventions.

In these passages and in that article "well-being" means something like 'well-being as experienced and/or reported', 'psychological wellbeing' or 'subjective wellbeing'. In an earlier article, Diener et al. (1998, pp. 35–36) claimed

> …that subjective well-being is a necessary ingredient of the healthy life, but not a sufficient one… subjective well-being is one value among many, but one that is widespread because it allows people to judge their own lives based on their own values and standards. Although people do not cherish subjective well-being to the exclusion of other values, most think it is important.

It seems to me that the 1998 article was nearer to the truth than the 2004 article, but the former was still inadequate from the point of view of correctly identifying a good life or a life with a good quality, all things considered. In the 1998 article, as the quoted passage suggests, a "healthy life" seems to be the ultimate dependent variable, i.e., the good life or a good quality of life is identical to a "healthy life". As explained in Michalos (2004a), this will not do because, among other things, it begs the question of the impact of good health on a good life. For many years researchers have tried to measure the relative impact of diverse domains of life (e.g., one's job, marriage, housing, neighborhood, income, friendships, personal security and health) on one's perceived quality of life. If one's perceived quality of life is identified with one's health or, more particularly, one's self-reported health, then this particular research question is answered a priori by one's construction of the dependent variable. No empirical research is necessary because the question at issue was answered by definition.

I was an active member of and completely agree with the unanimous view of the committee of the International Society for Quality of Life Studies (Hagerty et al. 2001) that a robust set of wellbeing indicators should include a vast array of important measures of subjective wellbeing, including happiness, life satisfaction, job satisfaction and so on. Nobody was more disappointed than I was to see the OECD (1982) list of social indicators with only one subjective indicator or the more recent Federation of Canadian Municipalities Quality of Life Reporting System (Flett 2002) without any subjective indicators. In my view, it makes no sense to measure people's wellbeing without asking the people themselves what they think or how they feel.

What I find dangerous and unacceptable is, first, the idea that 'wellbeing' might be interpreted merely as 'subjective wellbeing'. Second, I worry about the idea that measures of subjective wellbeing might be exhausted by measures of how people *feel* and neglect measures of people's *perceptions* about the world and its inhabitants (e.g., do they see people with different skin pigments as alien and/or threatening, and why), measures of what people *think* about what they perceive (e.g., do they think that skin pigments cause good or bad social and economic conditions), measures of what people actually *do* about what they perceive, think and feel (e.g., do they engage in political action and if so, of what sort) and, finally, measures of what real-world *consequences* follow from different combinations of perceptions, beliefs, feelings and actions.

With special reference to issues of health and health care, Vingilis and Sarkella (1997, pp. 163–164) illustrated the general sorts of concerns I have.

> A challenge for researchers and practitioners alike is the education of society on the determinants of health and well-being and the linkages among them. Without the knowledge and understanding of these broad determinants and their interrelatedness: without the appreciation that factors such as housing, unemployment, poverty and lone-parent family status predict rates of smoking, teen pregnancy, crime, disease, hospitalization and premature mortality communities will be limited in the programs and policies they have in their arsenal to sustain or improve on current levels of health and well-being... Indeed, knowledge is the crucial first step in planned approaches to enhancing community health... *As long as there are major discrepancies between a community's perceived health issues and the actual health issues, the sustainability and enhancement of well-being can be jeopardized* (emphasis added).

To these observations one might add,

> It is crucial for health and sustainability that the population knows where its food comes from, the implications of long-distant transportation of food products, the additives, toxins, and *actual* nutrition values of the food, implications for local farmers and local economies, and the environmental impacts created by the production system (Hayward et al. 2005, p. 123).

Such information, information about exactly what a particular population *knows* requires survey research with a rich array of questions probing much deeper than happiness and satisfaction. At a recent meeting of the Community Indicators Consortium in Jacksonville, Florida one speaker boldly proclaimed that "We need factual indicators, not indicators of people's perceptions and feelings". This is a big mistake for two reasons. First, what people perceive, think, feel and know are themselves important facts, and second, people's intentional or deliberate behaviour is largely a function of such facts. If we want to change people's behaviour, we must know what the world is like from their perspective. Otherwise, our interventions may be entirely counter-productive.

In the early days of the social indicators movement, most researchers were determined to resist economists' determination to economize the idea of human wellbeing, i.e., to imagine at least, what they could not actually demonstrate, that there is some kind of monetary or financial root for happiness. We were quite happy to share our research beds with psychologists, sociologists, health practitioners and an occasional geneticist even though we believed that human wellbeing is too multifaceted to be captured by a single discipline. I guess the presence of economizers, psychologizers, medicalizers, biologizers and so on in the research beds of our field proves again that politics produces strange bedfellows. From the beginning of the movement, we all knew that the field was essentially politicized in at least two ways. First, there was a discipline-based desire by non-economists to increase their influence in public policy making, which probably pleased everyone but the economists. More profoundly, the determination of the idea of human wellbeing, who is well off, better or worse off, who gets to make these determinations, according to what principles and rules, and who gets to decide what is to be done by, to and for whom, have always been particularly political as well as generally philosophical issues. In this section, the psychologizers have been criticized, but it is vitally important for the scientific integrity and the democratic usefulness of our research field that we try to balance all the legitimate interests of researchers, policy makers and everyone else affected by our decisions.

Happiness as Eudaimonia

There is an old view of the nature of happiness that is decidedly not merely psychological and quite consistent with the broad, two-variable account sketched above. It is based on the Greek word EUDAIMONIA, which literally means something like 'favoured by the DAIMONES (near-gods or gods)'. It is usually translated as 'happiness' but it connotes something closer to what people nowadays would call wellbeing rather than happiness. Today, in common parlance 'happiness' is frequently and perhaps more often than not psychologized. It is often taken to mean something very close to an extended feeling of pleasure or an extended good mood or pleasant affect. Because the English 'happiness' is linguistically more versatile than 'wellbeing', translators of ancient Greek texts typically prefer the former, e.g., we can talk about happy people, happy lives and happy gardening, but not wellbeing people, lives and gardening. Nevertheless, readers should remember that our modern notion of 'wellbeing' is closer to the ancient Greeks' notion of 'happiness' than to our modern notion of 'pleasure', and our modern notion of 'happiness' is closer to our modern notion of 'pleasure' than to the ancient Greeks' notion of 'happiness'. Moral philosophers working in the *eudaimonist* tradition (e.g., Socrates, Plato and Aristotle) agreed that people should reflect on their lives as a whole, discover what is most important or valuable (i.e., life's final end or TELOS), and plan and live their lives to achieve that end.

Some of the most frequently quoted passages in the history of philosophy come from a fourth century BCE treatise, namely, Aristotle's *Nicomachean Ethics* (1999) and concern our topic directly. For example,

> Every craft and every line of inquiry, and likewise every action and decision, seems to seek some good; that is why some people were right to describe the good as what everything seeks…
>
> Suppose, then, that the things achievable by action have some end that we wish for because of itself, and because of which we wish for the other things, and that we do not choose everything because of something else—for if we do, it will go on without limit, so that desire will prove to be empty and futile. Clearly, this end will be the good, that is to say, the best good…
>
> What is the highest of all the goods achievable in action? As far as the name goes, most people virtually agree; for both the many and the cultivated call it happiness [EUDAIMONIA], and they suppose that living well and doing well are the same as being happy. But they disagree about what happiness is, and the many do not give the same answer as the wise (Aristotle 1999, p. 3).

The situation was even more complicated than Aristotle's remarks suggest, for "the wise" had (and probably still have) significantly different views among themselves. However, it is clear from Aristotle's phrase "that living well and doing well are the same as being happy" that he is not talking about a mere extended feeling of pleasure. In fact, shortly after the passages quoted above, he wrote,

> The many, the most vulgar, would seem to conceive the good and happiness as pleasure, and hence they also like the life of gratification. In this they appear completely slavish, since the life they decide on is a life for grazing animals (Aristotle 1999, p. 4).

A couple thousand years later, Einstein picked up the same theme when he wrote that "I have never looked upon ease and happiness as ends in themselves—such an ethical basis I call more proper for a herd of swine" (quoted from Michalos 2004b, pp. 344–345).

Regarding views of "the many", Aristotle's best account is given in the *Rhetoric* (1926) and runs as follows.

> …for the sake of illustration, let us ascertain what happiness, generally speaking, is, and what *its parts consist* in;… Let us then define happiness [EUDAIMONIA] as well-being combined with virtue, or independence of life, or the life that is most agreeable combined with security, or abundance of possessions and slaves, combined with power to protect and make use of them; for nearly all men admit that one or more of these things *constitutes*

> happiness. If, then, such is the nature of happiness, *its component parts* must necessarily be: noble birth, numerous friends, good friends, wealth, good children, numerous children, a good old age; further bodily excellences, such as health, beauty, strength, stature, fitness for athletic contests, a good reputation, honour, good luck, virtue. For a man would be entirely independent, provided he possessed all internal and external goods; for there are no others. Internal goods are those of mind and body; external goods are noble birth, friends, wealth, honour.
>
> To these we think should be added certain capacities and good luck; for *on these conditions* life will be perfectly secure. Let us now in the same way define each of these in detail. Noble birth… (Aristotle 1926, pp. 47–49, emphasis added).

These passages are merely the beginning of several pages of more detailed definitions of *components and/or conditions* of a happy life or of a life of someone "living well and doing well". Logically speaking, Aristotle was not as tidy as one would have preferred in constructing his definitions, and he was no more adept than we are at sorting out *components or constituents* from *conditions or determinants* of happiness. The trouble is that he knew as well as we do that some things, like health, are good in themselves (intrinsically good) as constituents of individual wellbeing and also instrumentally good in producing other good things. Nevertheless, he certainly provided an excellent list of candidates for components and conditions of happiness. What's more, as a report of the common views of his contemporaries' (i.e., "the many"), he gave us a gem of sociological and psychological observation. For present purposes, one should notice especially that there are relatively few items in his list that most people today would exclude from our list, e.g., slaves certainly, and possibly noble birth, numerous children and "fitness for athletic contests".

Aristotle was by all accounts one of the most conventional of all ancient philosophers, always respectful of previous and current thinkers and mindful of the need to appropriately contextualize his own contributions. For example, in Book 1 of the *Nicomachean Ethics* he tells his readers that "the facts harmonize with a true account" of any particular subject and that "all the features that people look for in happiness appear to be true of the end described in our account" (Aristotle 1999, p. 10). Nevertheless, his own views were not entirely consistent with conventional wisdom. Following conventional wisdom, he seems to have accepted the notion that some sort of independence is necessary for a good life. He apparently believed that, in the first place, one chooses to live a particular way of life because one regards that way as not requiring anything beyond itself. Today we might say that it is both sustainable and worthy of being sustained, e.g., we choose understanding because it is good in itself but also because it contributes to our general wellbeing, to "living well and doing well". If someone asked, "But why do you choose to live well and do well?" we might wonder if the questioner understood English, because the question seems to presuppose that the alternative of preferring to live poorly and do poorly is reasonable. It is, after all, a logical truism that living well and doing well is better than living poorly and doing poorly, just as breathing well is better than breathing poorly.

Unfortunately, Aristotle's two major treatises on ethics, the *Nicomachean Ethics* and the *Eudemian Ethics*, do not provide unambiguous guides to filling in his "sketch" of a good life. Contrary to the somewhat academic, contemplative good lives sketched in the final chapters of the *Nicomachean Ethics* and *Eudemian Ethics*, the preceding chapters of both treatises sketch good lives requiring considerably more variety. In Book 1 of the former, readers are told that "a human being is a naturally political animal" (Aristotle 1999, p. 8). In Book 6, one finds that "Political science and prudence are the same state, but their being is not the same" (p. 92). A few pages earlier, "It seems proper to a prudent person to be able to deliberate finely about things that are good and beneficial for himself, not about some restricted area… but about what sorts of things promote living well in general" (p. 89).

In Book 1 of the *Politics*, Aristotle provided a naturalistic account of the origin of city-states that runs from the natural unions of men and women "for the sake of procreation" and natural rulers and natural slaves "for the sake of survival", to households "to satisfy everyday needs", and to villages promising still greater security and finally, to city-states "for the sake of living well". City-states are characterized as "complete communities" displaying "total self-sufficiency" (Aristotle 1998, pp. 2–3). An ordinary human being cannot flourish outside of a city-state. "Anyone who cannot form a community with others," he says, "or who does not need to because he is self-sufficient, is no part of a city-state—he is either a beast or a god" (p. 5). Clearly, then, Aristotle's requirement for self-sufficiency in a good or happy life is not absolute, but relative to a community which would be absolutely self-sufficient. Being able to live in such a community constitutes an important external good. The similarities between his and Plato's views on community and individual interdependence are striking (Michalos 2008).

Several times in the *Nicomachean Ethics* Aristotle insisted on the necessity of external goods for a completely happy life. For example, after noting that "happiness is… activity in accord with virtue", he wrote,

> Nonetheless, happiness evidently also needs external goods to be added, as we said, since we cannot, or cannot easily, do fine actions if we lack the resources. For, first of all, in many actions we use friends, wealth, and political power just as we use instruments. Further, deprivation of certain [externals] - for instance, good birth, good children, beauty - mars our blessedness… And so, as we have said, happiness would seem to need this sort of prosperity added also (Aristotle 1999, p. 11).

A few pages later, he asked "Why not say that the happy person is one whose activities accord with complete virtue, with an adequate supply of external goods, not for just any time but for a complete life?" (Aristotle 1999, p. 14).

All things considered, Aristotle's characterization of a good or happy life is the clearest example we have from the ancients of the view that the quality of a person's or of a community's life is a function of the actual conditions of that life and what a person or community makes of those conditions. Conceptually, he could clearly distinguish Real Paradise and Hell from a Fool's Paradise and Hell. Most importantly, he regarded all four cases as essentially and objectively involving human action that would be praiseworthy or blameworthy. A good or happy life is not simply given by nature, God or gods. It requires internal and external gifts and good luck beyond our control, but it also requires individual and communal initiative. For example, individuals naturally have the capacity to reason and to act bravely and justly more or less. With the right education, training and hard work, one may come to exercise these capacities excellently. A good or happy life, according to Aristotle, is achieved exactly insofar as one deliberately engages in the unimpeded excellent exercise of one's capacities for the sake of doing what is fine, excellent or noble (KALON), provided that the deliberation and activities are undertaken from a developed disposition (i.e., a virtuous character) and accompanied by an appropriate amount of external goods and pleasure. In short, a good or happy life consists of a harmonious mixture of internal and external goods in the first place, and regarding the former, an equally harmonious mixture of reason, appetite and emotion. From his perspective, a discordant or inactive life would not be worth living and the idea of a happy scoundrel would be an oxymoron.

The Influence of Education on Happiness

One does not have to look far to find plenty of evidence of the influence of education on many important aspects of people's lives. So, if 'happiness' is understood in the robust *eudaimonist* sense of overall human wellbeing, then education evidently has an enormous impact. Without providing any particular order or categorization, here is a brief sample of impact statements drawn from Hayward et al. (2005) and others as indicated.

- the well-being of modern society is dependent not only on traditional capital and labour but also on the knowledge and ideas possessed and generated by individual workers. Education is the primary source of this human capital (Crocker 2002, p. 1).
- Educational attainment is positively associated both with health status and with healthy lifestyles. For example, in the 1996–1997 [Canadian] National Population Health Survey, only 19% of respondents with less than high school education rated their health as 'excellent', compared with almost 30% of university graduates. Self-rated health, in turn, has been shown to be a reliable predictor of health problems, health-care utilization, and longevity. From a health determinant perspective, education is clearly a good investment that can reduce long-term health care costs (pp. 37–38).
- According to Statistics Canada, workers with higher education were more likely to have secure, high-wage, high-benefit jobs. Employees with less than high school education were more likely to have insecure work, low wages and no benefits… poverty and inequality are acknowledged to be the most reliable predictors of poor health outcomes, and they are also closely linked to low educational attainment and unhealthy lifestyles (p. 39).

- GPI *Atlantic's* Cost of Obesity report found that Canadians with less education are much more likely to be overweight than those with higher education… 0.36% of Canadians with less than a high school education are overweight compared to 22% of those with a university education (p. 40).
- In 2001, 75.4% of female university graduates had a job, compared with 79.3% of male graduates. By contrast, women with less than a Grade 9 education are less than half as likely to be employed as their male counterparts—13.6% of women compared to 29.4% of men (p. 41).
- According to the GPI *Atlantic* Cost of Crime report, only 19% of the Canadian population as a whole have less than a grade 10 education. However, 36% of all inmates, 34% of provincial inmates, and 46% of federal prisoners, who are the most serious offenders, have less than a grade 10 education (p. 42).
- After controlling for variables such as cognitive abilities and personality-scale measures, the tacit knowledge measures are the best predictors of actual performance in jobs and at school (Sternberg 2001, p. 61).
- One study (Coulombe et al. 2004) looking at economic growth (based on the GDP) found that the *average* literacy score in a population is a better indicator of economic growth than a score based only on high-level skills (p. 64).
- According to the OECD (2006, p. 27), The estimated long-term effect on economic output of one additional year of education in the OECD area is generally between 3 and 6%.
- …(Bauer et al. 2000) have shown that the level of political knowledge one has a major impact on 'political preferences, likelihood of voting and a whole host of other important behaviours, attitudes and beliefs' (p. 106).
- Using panel data analysis for 35 developing countries for the years 1990, 1995 and 2000… [it was shown] that the set of functionings enabled by educational attainment—being able to read, count, communicate, make informed choices, have a sense of self-worth, have greater degree of control over one's life and so on—have a substantial impact on life expectancy. Significantly, the direct effect of those educational functionings on longevity is almost equivalent to their effect by way of resource accumulation (Wigley and Akkoyunlu-Wigley 2006, pp. 287–301).

On top of all the studies and data, one should also recognize the continuing commitment of the international community of nations represented in the United Nations Educational, Scientific and Cultural Organization (UNESCO). The Preamble of the Constitution of UNESCO, ratified in 1946, says that "since wars begin in the minds of men, it is in the minds of men that the defences of peace must be constructed". Since its inception, UNESCO has been faithful to its mandate and produced a huge stockpile of "weapons of mass instruction". Among its programmes relevant to this conference, one should mention UNESCO's programmes of Education For All and the most recent work implementing the UN Decade of Education for Sustainable Development, 2005–2014 (UNESCO 2005). I have the privilege of serving on the Monitoring and Evaluation Expert Group which is responsible for creating some of the overall assessment procedures and survey instruments. Although our work is only in its initial stages and considerable work has been done by the UN Economic and Social Council (2006), the Asia-Pacific Region (2006) and the Sub-Saharan Africa Region (2006), it is fair to say that the initiatives undertaken in the interest of achieving real changes in all forms of education across the decade are unprecedented.

> The overall goal of the DESD is to integrate the principles, values, and practices of sustainable development into all aspects of education and learning. This educational effort will encourage changes in behaviour that will create a more sustainable future in terms of environmental integrity, economic viability, and a just society for present and future generations (UNESCO 2005, p. 6).

While the nearly universal commitment of governments to the achievement of the DESD overall goals is not evidence of the influence of education on wellbeing, it is evidence of nearly universal belief in such influence. If this belief were misguided, it would be difficult to imagine a more colossal human error. Given the robust sense of 'education', I do not believe it is misguided.

Notwithstanding all the well-supported and publicized information just reviewed, the most frequently told story about the influence of education on happiness is that there is little, if any, influence. "On the basis of a review of 90 American studies," I wrote in Michalos (1991a, p. 61), "Witter et al. (1984) concluded that educational attainment accounts for between 1% and 3% of the variance in adult subjective well-being." In their broad overviews of things that contribute to happiness or wellbeing, Myers and Diener (1995) and Diener and Seligman (2004) did not even mention education. Layard (2005, p. 62) wrote that "education has only a small direct effect on happiness, though of course it raises happiness by raising a person's income." His cited source was Helliwell (2003). In the final section of the 2002 version of Helliwell's paper, he claimed that

> This paper has attempted to illustrate rather than exhaust the possibilities for using international well-being data to measure and explain differences in well-being within and among nations... The well-being data themselves have fairly good claims as measures of individual welfare. Insofar as these claims are justified, the coefficients can be used to combine what might otherwise be incommensurable results into an overall welfare assessment of changes in policies and institutions... Analysis of wellbeing data provides means for combining income, employment, governmental effectiveness, family structure and social relations together in ways that permit the external effects of institutions and public policies to be assessed... The well-being data show that the effects flowing directly from the quality of the institutions may dwarf those that flow through productivity and economic growth (Helliwell 2002, pp. 29–31).

Although Helliwell is generally cautious and modest in his claims for subjective wellbeing research, he clearly believes that subjective wellbeing measures might not only do the work of what I call overall wellbeing or quality of life measures, but particularly do the very hard work of providing an alternative to troublesome composite indexes of wellbeing. I have argued against the first assumption in this paper and in favour of composite indexes in Michalos et al. (2006). Without entering into the debate about composite indicators, I would like to say that moving Pandora's Box of aggregation problems from the visible world to the invisible Black Box inside people's heads does not strike me as a progressive research programme.

It is important to notice that most of the studies of the influence of education on happiness or some form of subjective wellbeing only measure direct effects, although the possibility of indirect effects is often mentioned. It seems to me that to construct an allegedly causal model that posits some measure of happiness or subjective wellbeing as simply the direct effect of highest level of formal education attained is to create a seriously misspecified model. At a minimum, one ought to consider and search for indirect and total effects. As a matter of fact, Michalos (1985) did propose a general theory of satisfaction involving direct and indirect effects of education as predictors, and tested this theory on over 18,000 undergraduates, with results reported in Michalos (1991a, b, 1993a, b). A brief summary of some of those results will illustrate what the most frequently told story about the influence of education on happiness typically fails to notice.

A few months ago, while Diener and I were exchanging email messages on something else, I confessed that so much good information (i.e., knowledge) was being accumulated about subjective wellbeing by him and others that I pretty well despaired of being able to produce a single theory capable of doing justice to everything known about subjective wellbeing today. He was, as one would expect, sympathetic. Setting my despair aside, here are the postulates of Multiple Discrepancies Theory (MDT) as stated in Michalos (1985, pp. 347–413) with a minimal number of additions in italics that subsequent research has shown ought to be included. I do not know if the suggested ways of including the new variables are the best ways and I do not know the best ways to accommodate longitudinal data. Currently I have three waves of data for three independent panels, but the analyses are incomplete.

H1 Reported net satisfaction is a function of perceived discrepancies between what one has and wants, relevant others have, the best one has had in the past, expected to have 3 years ago, expects to have after 5 years, deserves and needs.

H2 All perceived discrepancies, except that between what one has and wants, are functions of objectively measurable discrepancies, which also have direct effects on satisfaction and actions.

H3 The perceived discrepancy between what one has and wants is a mediating variable between all other perceived discrepancies and reported net satisfaction.

H4 The pursuit and maintenance of net satisfaction motivates human action in direct proportion to the perceived expected levels of net satisfaction.

H5 All discrepancies, satisfaction and actions are directly and indirectly affected by age, sex, education, ethnicity, income, self-esteem, social support,

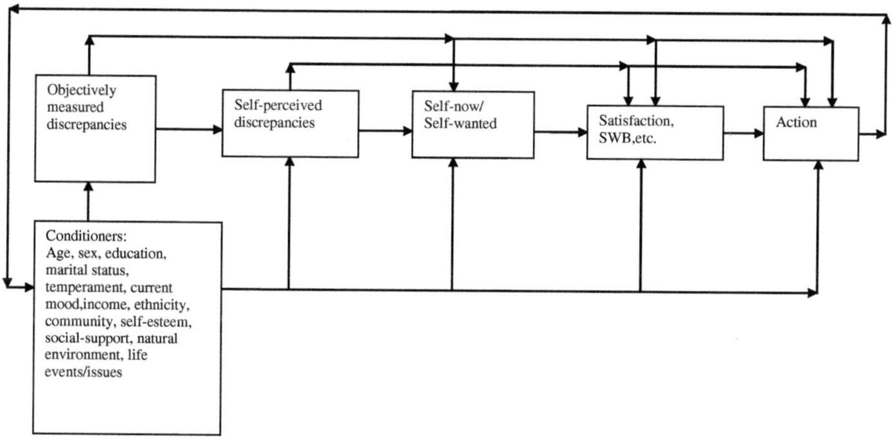

Fig. 12.2 Multiple discrepancies theory (MDT)

temperament, current mood, community, natural environment, life events/issues.

H6 Objectively measurable discrepancies are functions of human action and conditioners.

The relationships postulated in MDT are illustrated in Figs. 12.2 and 12.3. In Michalos (1991a, pp. 47–48) I inserted 'positive linear' or 'linear' in front of 'function', in response to Frank Andrews's suggestion that I set the bar too low if I did not specify some kind of function. Since some of the functions are not linear, as I reported in Michalos (1985, pp. 352–353), I should have resisted Frank's suggestion. Also in the 1991 version, I inserted '(happiness or subjective well-being)' after 'satisfaction' in H1 to emphasize the point that MDT was intended to be a

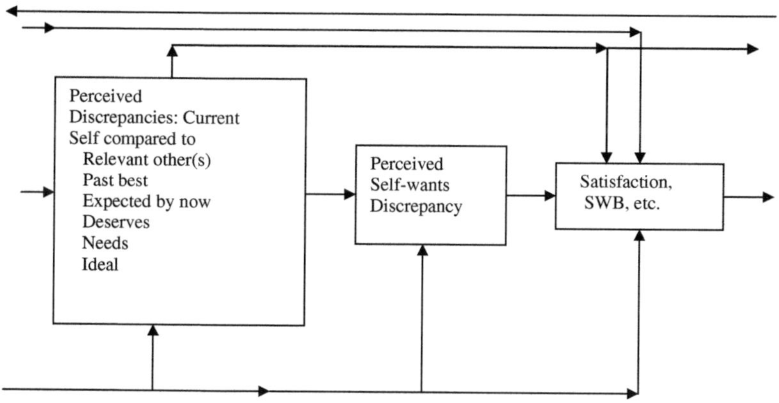

Fig. 12.3 Perceptual core of MDT

theory sufficient to explain all three notions. Based on the different relationships among these three concepts and a diverse array of other variables that have been revealed in many empirical studies, I have always thought these three concepts have somewhat distinct cores with overlapping connotations. Also, as indicated in Michalos (1991a, pp. 3–4), I believe that

> ...a fully developed scientific theory of subjective well-being would... be applicable to satisfaction or happiness with life as a whole (i.e., global satisfaction or happiness) as well as to satisfaction or happiness with specific domains of life (i.e., domain satisfaction) such as marital satisfaction and job satisfaction.

Thus, a general theory like MDT could be used on its own to explain global and domain satisfaction (happiness or subjective wellbeing) or it could be used in combination with the familiar simple linear, bottom-up model in which, say, life satisfaction is explained by aggregated domain satisfaction, and satisfaction in each of the domains is explained by MDT.

When MDT was used to explain happiness, life satisfaction and satisfaction with family, friends, living partner, self-esteem, employment, finances, housing, transportation, religion, education, recreation and health for the 18,000 undergraduates enrolled in 75 universities in 39 countries, the results concerning the direct versus total effects of education on levels of happiness or satisfaction were under-whelming. The educational attainment variable was not the usual one but one with predictably less variation. It was years-of-university-education and had seven response categories; one year of university, two, three, four, five, degree obtained and other. The results of applying MDT to measure happiness and life satisfaction, and satisfaction in 12 domains of life for the group as a whole are given in Table 12.1. MDT performed well, explaining an average of 54% of the variance in each dependent variable, with a high of 67% for satisfaction with one's living partner and a low of 42% for happiness. However, the average direct effect of years-of-university-education for the 14 variables was −0.006 and the average total effect was −0.0007. Even if we neglect considerations of the reliabilities of our measures, such values are hardly worth mentioning though they are curiously negative.

Out of a total of 2,162 applications of the theory, covering all the universities and countries, with separate applications for whole groups, males and females, there were some striking differences between direct and total effects. Since the general results were so unremarkable, I would not make much of the few remarkable results. Still, it should be noted that I sometimes got direct effects of zero and total effects as large as 0.20 or −0.29, and sometimes equal direct and total effects as large as 0.20 and −0.19. The main point of this story, then, is just that while the chances are very good that for any particular group of people and for any domain of life, educational attainment will not have a great impact on reported happiness or satisfaction, for some groups and some domains there may be relatively great effects and significantly different direct and total effects. Expecting small effect sizes, researchers should specify models and use sample sizes most likely to capture all relevant effects.

Table 12.1 Summary of direct and total effects of years of university education resulting from applying MDT to undergraduate sample for two global indicators and 12 domains of life

Variables	*N*	Direct effects	Total effects	% Variance explained
Happiness	7,502	−0.06	−0.06	42
Life satisfaction	7,703	−0.03	−0.03	45
Family satisfaction	7,934	0	0.02	55
Friendship sat.	8,091	0	0.01	50
Living partner sat.	4,728	0	0.04	67
Self-esteem sat.	7,813	0	0.02	52
Paid job sat.	3,710	0	−0.05	65
Finances sat.	7,912	0	0.03	54
Housing sat.	7,956	0	0.05	55
Transportation sat.	7,838	0	−0.01	60
Religion sat.	5,598	0	−0.01	63
Univ. education sat	7,950	−0.02	−0.04	50
Recreation sat.	7,939	0	0	52
Health sat.	8,076	0.02	0.02	51
Average	7,196	−0.006	−0.0007	54

Sources Michalos (1991a, b, 1993a, b)

Regarding the negative signs on the effect measures, there is what I call a *connoisseur effect* which has been recognized by others and reported in Michalos (1993b) and Michalos and Orlando (2006, p. 53). In the latter paper, we noted that for our sample of 3,407 students at the University of Northern British Columbia, "the more credits students earned, the lower their levels of satisfaction became with each student service offered". Applegate and Clark (1987, p. 133) reported that a survey of 92 visitors to a National Wildlife Refuge near Atlantic City, New Jersey showed that birders who were more knowledgeable had lower levels of satisfaction from bird watching than less knowledgeable birders. These authors concluded their article by remarking that their

> …study raises some concern over the utility of satisfaction data in resource management planning. It would seem intuitive that social benefits are increased by programs that increase the cumulative satisfaction of a recreation clientele. Here, however, we have provided evidence that the most committed segment of a user group is less satisfied than their more casual counterparts with on-site experiences. It is unreasonable to conclude that individuals have spent many preparatory hours in achieving competence, and commit many more hours to on-site experiences, in order to receive fewer benefits. In another context, it would make no sense for a refuge manager, interested in maximizing social benefits from the use of a resource, to initiate programs that would decrease the average competence of visitors. The obvious conclusion is that measures of satisfaction may be poor indicators of social benefits.

From the point of view of the general position defended here, especially the necessity of measures of the actual conditions that people live in as well as measures of what they make out of them, one need not be misled by the connoisseur

Table 12.2 Summary of direct and total effects of 12 predictors resulting from applying MDT to undergraduate sample for life satisfaction and happiness

Predictors	Life satisfaction (N = 7,703)		Happiness (*N* = 7,502)	
	Direct effects	Total effects	Direct effects	Total effects
Sex	−0.02	0.03	0	0.05
Age	−0.02	−0.04	0	−0.02
Work status	0.04	0.04	0.02	0.02
Years of university	−0.03	−0.03	−0.06	−0.06
Country of birth	−0.03	0	0.02	0.02
Self-other comparison	0.19	0.30	0.20	0.27
Self-deserved comp.	0.06	0.11	0.07	0.07
Self-needs comp.	0.05	0.11	0.05	0.09
Self-progress comp.	0.09	0.15	0.09	0.13
Self-future comp.	0	−0.02	0	−0.01
Self-best previous comp.	0.10	0.14	0.27	0.30
Self-wants comp.	0.38	0.38	0.23	0.23
% of variance explained	45		42	

Source Michalos (1991a, b, p. 116)

effect. One just has to aim for a maximally inclusive, comprehensive and balanced account of wellbeing, and then hope for the best. There are no guarantees of hitting the target.

Table 12.2 summarizes some results of using MDT to explain life satisfaction and happiness for the international undergraduate sample. In particular, the exhibit lists the variety of direct and total effects of education (years of university education) for the 12 key predictors of the theory. Five points are worth noting. First, the 12 predictors of MDT explained 45% of the variance in life satisfaction, while the 39 predictors in Helliwell's (2002, p. 41) most robust equation explained only 26%. Second, inspection of the figures in the exhibit reveals that there are often striking differences between direct and total effects, and third, that the rank order of predictors of life satisfaction and happiness are not the same. Considering only total effects, for life satisfaction, the most influential predictors are the gap between what respondents have now and want, then between what respondents have now and others of the same age and sex have, and then between what respondents have now and what, 3 years earlier, they hoped to have at this point in time. For happiness, the most influential predictors are the gap between what respondents have now and the best they ever had in the past, then between what respondents have now and others of the same age and sex have, and then between what respondents have now and want. Fourth, predictors can't do any work or reveal any effects at all if they are not in our survey instruments and equations. Granting that the equations of MDT have several important missing explanatory variables and that, therefore, these equations are also misspecified, it seems to me that judging from their relative explanatory power, they are less defective than the usual run of predictors. Fifth, it is, therefore, demonstrably worthwhile to consider a wide range of subjective indicators in any assessment of human wellbeing or the quality of life, and to actually include the most likely heavy hitters (most likely most influential) in one's explanations and analyses.

Conclusion

In this paper I have argued that answers to the questions 'Does education influence happiness and if so, how and how much?' depend on how one defines and operationalizes the ideas of 'education', 'influences' and 'happiness'. A great variety of research scenarios may be constructed from our three essential variables, and one should expect plenty of different answers to the basic questions. What public policies one ought to adopt and implement regarding the influence of education on happiness depends minimally on which of the great variety of research scenarios one adopts and maximally on lots of other things as well. While my personal preference is for a robust definition of 'education', 'influences' and 'happiness', other approaches are also legitimate and easier to manage. My preferred approach costs more in many ways because it is worth more in the long run. Nevertheless, it seems to me that most of the governments of most countries of the world have endorsed a political agenda that pretty clearly follows from those robust definitions.

References

Alexandrova, A. (2005). Subjective well-being and Kahneman's 'objective happiness'. *Journal of Happiness Studies, 6*(3), 301–324.

Applegate, J. E., & Clark, K. E. (1987). Satisfaction levels of bird-watchers: An observation on the con-sumptive-nonconsumptive continuum. *Leisure Sciences, 9,* 129–134.

Aristotle. (1926). *The 'art' of rhetoric* (J. H. Freese, Trans.). Cambridge: Loeb Classical Library, Harvard University Press.

Aristotle. (1998). *Politics* (C. D. C. Reeve, Trans.). Indianapolis: Hackett Publishing Company.

Aristotle. (1999). *Nicomachean ethics* (2nd ed., T. Irwin, Trans.). Indianapolis: Hackett Publishing Company.

Asia-Pacific Region. (2006). *Monitoring and assessing progress during the DESD in the Asia Pacific region: A quick guide to developing ESD indicators.* Sydney, Australia: The World Conservation Union, Commission for Education and Communication, and Macquarie University.

Bauer, M. W., Petkova, K., & Boyadjieva, P. (2000). Public knowledge of and attitudes to science: Alternative measures that may end the 'science war'. *Science, Technology and Human Values, 25*(1), 30–51.

Bentham, J. (1789). *An introduction to the principles of morals and legislation.* Oxford: Oxford University Press.

Coulombe, S., Tremblay, J.-F., & Marchand, S. (2004). *Literacy scores, human capital and growth across fourteen OECD countries.* Ottawa: Statistics Canada, Catalogue number 89–552-MIE200411.

Crocker, R. K. (2002). *Learning outcomes: A critical review of the state of the field in Canada*. Ottawa: Canadian Education Statistics Council.
Diener, E., Sapyta, J. J., & Suh, E. (1998). Subjective well-being is essential to well-being. *Psychological Inquiry, 9*(1), 33–37.
Diener, E., & Seligman, M. E. P. (2004). Beyond money: Toward an economy of well-being. *Psychological science in the public interest, 5*(1), 1–31. Washington: American Psychological Society.
Economist. (2005). The world in 2005. Retrieved from http://www.economist.com/media/pdf/QUALITY_OF_LIFE.pdf.
Flett. (2002). *Quality of life reporting system evaluation, final report*. Toronto: Prepared by the Flett Consulting Group Inc. and Fotenn Consultants Inc., (fcginc@rogers.com).
Hagerty, M. R., Cummins, R. A., Ferris, A. L., Land, K., Michalos, A. C., Peterson, M., et al. (2001). Quality of life indexes for national policy: Review and agenda for research. *Social Indicators Research, 55*, 1–96.
Hayward, K., Pannozzo, L., & Colman, R. (2005). *Draft: Developing indicators for the educated populace domain of the Canadian index of wellbeing, interim report*. Halifax: GPI Atlantic.
Helliwell, J. F. (2002). *How's life? Combining individual and national variables to explain subjective well-being*, working paper 9065. Cambridge: National Bureau of Economic Research.
Helliwell, J. F. (2003). How's life? Combining individual and national variables to explain subjective wellbeing. *Economic Modeling, 20*, 331–360.
Kahneman, D. (1999). Objective happiness. In D. Kahneman, E. Diener, & N. Schwarz (Eds.), *Well-being: The foundations of hedonic psychology* (pp. 1–25). New York: Russell Sage Foundation.
Kahneman, D., Wakker, P. P., & Sarin, R. (1997). Back to Bentham? Explorations of experienced utility. *Quarterly Journal of Economics, 112*, 375–405.
Layard, R. (2005). *Happiness: Lessons from a new science*. London: Penguin Books.
Michalos, A. C. (1978). *Foundations of decision-making*. Ottawa: Canadian Library of Philosophy.
Michalos, A. C. (1985). Multiple discrepancies theory (MDT). *Social Indicators Research, 16*(4), 347–413.
Michalos, A. C. (1991a). *Global report on student well-being, Vol. 1, Life satisfaction and happiness*. New York: Springer.
Michalos, A. C. (1991b). *Global report on student well-being, Vol. 2, Family, friends, living partner and self-esteem*. New York: Springer.
Michalos, A. C. (1993a). *Global report on student well-being, Vol. 3, Employment, finances, housing and transportation*. New York: Springer.
Michalos, A. C. (1993b). *Global report on student well-being, Vol. 4, Religion, education, recreation and health*. New York: Springer.
Michalos, A. C. (Ed.). (2003). *The best teacher I ever had: Personal reports from highly productive scholars*. London, Ontario: The Althouse Press.
Michalos, A. C. (2004a). Social indicators research and health-related quality of life research. *Social Indicators Research, 65*(1), 27–72.
Michalos, A. C. (2004b). Einstein, ethics and science. *Journal of Academic Ethics, 2*, 339–354.
Michalos, A. C. (Ed.). (2005). *Citation classics from social indicators research: The most cited articles, edited and introduced by A. C. Michalos*. Dordrecht: Springer.
Michalos, A. C. (2006). Logic, philosophy of science and the quality of life. *Encyclopedia of Life Support Systems*, UNESCO, online encyclopedia.
Michalos, A. C. (2008). The good life: Eighth century to fourth century BCE. In K. C. Land (Ed.), *Handbook of social indicators and quality-of-life studies*. New York: Springer.
Michalos, A. C., & Orlando, J. A. (2006). A note on student quality of life. *Social Indicators Research, 79*(1), 51–59.
Michalos, A. C., Sharpe, A., & Muhajarine, N. (2006). *An approach to a Canadian index of wellbeing*. Atkinson Charitable Foundation, Toronto: Draft paper for discussion.

Mill, J. S. (1863). *Utilitarianism*. London.
Myers, D. G., & Diener, E. (1995). Who is happy? *Psychological Science, 6*(1), 10–19.
OECD. (1982). *The OECD list of social indicators*. Paris: The OECD Social Indicator Development Programme.
OECD. (2006). *Education at a glance 2006*. Paris: OECD.
Plato. (1924). *Laches, Protagoras, Meno, Euthydemus* (W. R. M. Lamb, Trans.). Cambridge: Loeb Classical Library, Harvard University Press.
Sternberg, R. J. (2001). Why schools should teach for wisdom: The balance theory of wisdom in educational settings. *Educational Psychologist, 36*(4), 227–245.
Sub-Saharan Africa Region. (2006). *Towards the implementation of the decade of education for sustainable development (DESD) in sub-Saharan Africa (SSA), workshop report, November 27-30*. Namibia: Windhoek.
UN Economic and Social Council. (2006). *Indicators for education for sustainable development*, ECE/CEP/ AC.13/2006/5/Add.1, July 31.
UNESCO. (2005). *International implementation scheme, United Nations decade of education for sustainable development (2005–2014)*. Paris: UNESCO Education Sector.
Vingilis, E., & Sarkella, J. (1997). Determinants and indicators of health and well-being: Tools for educating society. *Social Indicators Research, 40*(1–2), 159–178.
Wigley, S., & Akkoyunlu-Wigley, A. (2006). Human capabilities versus human capital: Gauging the value of education in developing countries. *Social Indicators Research, 78*(2), 287–304.
Witter, D., Okun, M. A., Stock, W. A., & Haring, M. J. (1984). Education and subjective well-being: A meta-analysis. *Educational Evaluation and Policy Analysis, 6*, 165–173.

Chapter 13
A Developmental View of Liberal Education

Alex C. Michalos

Introduction

In the following pages I present four views of liberal education, which might be called pragmatic (following John Dewey), aristocratic (following Aristotle), residualist, and developmental. Casual observation and discussions with colleagues in several universities over the past twenty-one years has led me to believe that most academics think of liberal education as either some sort of a residual category (what one gets if one is not educated for anything in particular) or as some sort of entertainment (what one does if one is not preparing to do anything else). These views have some fairly long and prestigious historical roots and, I hope, practically no future at all. In contrast to these views, I propose a developmental characterization of liberal education. Its roots are in the pragmatic tradition of William James, Ralph B. Perry, C.I. Lewis and Dewey. Briefly, I propose that liberal education is any education designed with the dual aims of self and social development. Some paragraphs are devoted to explaining this view.

Michalos, A.C.: 1983. A developmental view of liberal education. Revised paper presented at a Conference on Logic and Learning at Carnegie-Mellon University, Pittsburgh, 1979.

A.C. Michalos (✉)
University of Northern British Columbia, Prince George, BC, Canada
e-mail: michalos@brandonu.ca

A.C. Michalos, *Connecting the Quality of Life Theory to Health, Well-Being and Education*, DOI 10.1007/978-3-319-51161-0_13

Historical Roots

People have long been divided on the question of the appropriate output of education. Just how long they have been divided and along what lines is indicated by the following quotation from Aristotle.

> For mankind are by no means agreed about the things to be taught, whether we look to virtue or to the best life. Neither is it clear whether education is more concerned with intellectual or with moral virtue. The existing practice is perplexing; no one knows on what principle we should proceed – should the useful in life, or should virtue, or should the higher knowledge, be the aim of our training; all three opinions have been entertained. Again, about the means there is no agreement; for different persons, starting with different ideas about the nature of virtue, naturally disagree about the practice of it. There can be no doubt that children should be taught those useful things which are really necessary, but not all useful things...[1]

In short, at least since Aristotle people have viewed education as a means to the development of character (moral virtue), useful (practical) skills and knowledge. If we may trust John Dewey's history, the idea of a liberal education for Aristotle's countrymen was that of an education for a free aristocrat. It was contrasted with that of vocational training in useful arts for mechanics. High social status was as much a part of the former as low social status was a part of the latter.[2]

Dewey laboured long and hard (correctly, I think) against any separation of liberal versus useful, practical, scientific-technological, vocational education. He advocated scientific-technological training directed by liberating humane studies, and the latter informed by the former.[3]

---

[1]Aristotle, Politics (c. 330 BC), Book VII, $1337^{a}35$–$1337^{b}5$.

[2]J. Dewey, Philosophy of Education (Ames, Iowa: Littlefield, Adams and Co., 1958), pp. 121–122, 144–145.

[3]Ibid., pp. 86–87. The following quotation from the "Report of the Committee on Evaluation of Engineering Education", chaired by L.E. Grinter, is very reminiscent of Dewey and very instructive. According to Grinter, a "well- educated engineer"

> ...must be not only a competent professional engineer, but also an informed and participating citizen, and a person whose living expresses high cultural values and moral standards. Thus, the competent engineer needs understanding and appreciation in the humanities and in the social sciences as much as in his own field of engineering. He needs to be able to deal with the economics, human, and social factors of his professional problems. His facility with, and understanding of, ideas in the fields of humanities and social sciences not only provide an essential contribution to his professional engineering work, but also contribute to his success as a citizen and to the enrichment and meaning of his life as an individual.

The quotation was taken from W.R. Lynn, "Engineering and Society Programs in Engineering Education," Science (1977), p. 152.

In his view, pragmatism or instrumentalism was little more than the application of all contemporary learning (science, technology and the arts) to social problems in the interests of what he called "social betterment" and what we might call a good quality of life.[4] His philosophy of education flowed naturally from his philosophy of life, not in detail but in principle. Although with prolific writers generally and Dewey in particular, one often finds apparently contradictory positions defended in different treatises, I think that much of what I think is consistent with the general sort of pragmatism usually associated with Dewey.

It is important to notice that there is an influential and older tradition of liberal education that is practically the opposite of the pragmatic tradition represented by Dewey. The origins of this alternative view may be found in Aristotle, while its most notable advocate was John Henry Newman. Newman summarized his discussion of liberal education and knowledge in his classic work[5] thus:

> All that I have been now saying is summed up in a few characteristic words of the great Philosopher. 'Of possessions,' he says, 'those rather are useful, which bear fruit; those liberal, which tend to enjoyment. By fruitful, I mean, which yield revenue; by enjoyable, where nothing accrues of consequence beyond the using.'

For Newman and followers of this tradition,

> ...cultivation of mind is surely worth seeking for its own sake, [and]... there is a knowledge, which is desirable, though nothing come of it, as being of itself a treasure, and a sufficient remuneration of years of labour.[6]

Given these two distinct traditions about liberal education, it is often confusing to use the very same phrase for both traditions. Besides, advocates of each tradition frequently grant most if not everything that the other recommends. Still, I think there is an important difference between recommending education in the interests of making individuals and communities better and recommending education in the interests of enjoyment. After all, having a good character is not the same as having a good time.[7]

---

[4]Ibid., p. 55.

[5]J.H. Newman, The Idea of a University (Oxford: Clarendon Press, 1976), p. 102.

[6]Ibid., p. 105.

[7]Good character has been recommended as a central aim of education by many educators. For example, Dewey wrote that "It is a commonplace to say that the development of character is the end of all school work." (J. Dewey, Moral Principles in Education (New York: Philosophical Library, 1959), p. 2). Robert Maynard Hutchins wrote that "Education is the deliberate attempt to form human character in terms of an ideal." (R.M. Hutchins, Education for Freedom (Baton Rouge: Louisiana State University Press, 1943), p. 104). Nathan M. Pusey claimed that "What Harvard wants more than anything now to give to our country and the world is educated men-and-women-of character." (N.M. Pusey, The Age of the Scholar (Cambridge: Harvard University Press, 1964), p. 204).

A Residualist View

In spite of Dewey's efforts and more recent movements toward the humanization of technical-professional programs in engineering, medicine and business, there remains a powerful inclination for some folks to think of liberal education as a residual category. That is, it's what a student gets when he or she doesn't quite know exactly what he or she wants or ought to get. Those who are not being educated specifically as sociologists, engineers, mathematicians and so on are being educated liberally, which some folks might identify with just barely.

Ignoring the pejorative identification of "liberally" and "just barely," the historical roots of this residualist view of a liberal education are traceable to the Aristotelian era mentioned above. In those days it was a residual sort of education insofar as it was the logical complement (the nonpractical, nonuseful, etc.) of the only other sort of formal education. Moreover, it may still be the case that insofar as one is prepared to dichotomize education into two mutually exclusive and exhaustive complementary classes characterized as practical and nonpractical, there is no other way to think of liberal education except residually. If so, I think that is a good reason not to dichotomize education at all.

There are, in fact, at least two reasons for rejecting the practical-nonpractical division of education. The first reason is, as I have just suggested, that it leads to thinking of liberal education as nothing but a residual category. This is objectionable because it is possible and worth-while to give liberal education a positive characterization. It doesn't have to be, indeed, should not be an old bucket good for nothing but the overflow of something called "practical" education. I will return to this characterization shortly.

The second, and itself sufficient, reason to reject the practical-nonpractical (or useful-nonuseful) division of education is that nothing is practical or useful in the abstract. Nothing is practical or useful simpliciter. Things are only practical or useful for certain purposes in certain circumstances. The study of the sentential calculus may be useless and impractical from the point of view of making automobiles, but it is precisely to the point (not the only point, of course) from the point of view of inspecting the structure of some arguments and patterns of inference. The study of automotive engineering may be useless and impractical from the point of view of making a living in the arctic, but it may be precisely to the point in Detroit—for a while. To set up any educational curriculum and say that it is practical or useful, or to say that it is not is to say both too little and too much. It is to say too much insofar as circumstances and the aims of some people may falsify one's claims immediately, and it is to say too little insofar as it is an incomplete essentially relative remark.

Self and Social Development

Suppose we abandon all talk of practical-nonpractical, useful-useless education with its misleading propensity to allow us to think of liberal education as a residual dumping ground. How should we characterize a liberal education? I would like to propose that we identify this sort of education by the two interdependent aims of self and social development. In other words, that I hope mean approximately the same thing, liberal education is education designed to increase the chances for the development of individuals and communities. To turn the view upside down, an educational system that is self-destructive or socially destructive is not liberal. Thus, for example, systems of indoctrination designed to produce uncritical parrots of a party line are not systems of liberal education, because the elimination of the possibility of rational criticism implies the elimination of rational planning and growth.[8]

Obviously such a proposal (or set of proposals) is not intended or expected to close discussion. Several features of the proposal require further comment.

First, it should be noticed that although it might be said that all education is somehow aimed at self and social development,[9] it is not the case that all education is designed with these general aims as its primary aims. People do say, for example, that the primary aim of education (i.e. that for the sake of which programs are designed and people enrol in them) is to prepare folks to enter the labour force; to make money; to expose students to different sorts of people with different backgrounds, values and aspirations; to socialize people; to develop specific expertise (computer programming, salesmanship, medical skills, etc.) and so on.

Attractive by-products of a productive system are just that, things one gets without necessarily trying to get. Moreover, they may well be the first things to be abandoned when production slows down. The following two quotations may be instructive for those who are inclined to think that the aims of self and social development are as acceptable as motherhood and apple pie, i.e., as <u>primary</u> aims.

At a 1972 conference on co-operative education, U.S. Senator Joseph M. Montoya said

> Students today are not content to put in an expensive apprentice-ship at a four-year liberal-arts institution, only to emerge with a worthless degree in terms of real earning capacity. ...Educational institutions must become more relevant in terms of skills and

---

[8]The following quotation from the University Grants Committee of England is worth repeating. "Here arises the responsibilities of the universities. They are the inheritors of the Greek tradition of candid and intrepid thinking about the fundamental issues involved in the life of the individual and of the community, and of the Greek principle that the unexamined life is no life for man." Quoted in Hutchins, <u>op. cit</u>., p. 101.

[9]For example, R.S. Peters claimed "It would be a logical contradiction to say that a man had been educated but that he had in no way changed for the better, or that in educating his son a man was attempting nothing worth-while," in <u>Ethics and Education</u> (Chicago: Scott, Foresman, Co.', 1967), p. 3. I have more to say about improving and developing shortly.

> earning payoffs, or they are doomed to become museum pieces in our future scheme of things.[10]

Frank Hallgren, Director of Placement at the University of Nebraska was quoted as saying

> People who support us - parents, alumni, legislators - have the basic feeling that college is supposed to get young people ready for the working world.[11]

Second, I have used the word ‘development’ instead of ‘fulfillment’ in order to avoid the essentialism that seems to be suggested by ‘fulfillment’.[12] I do not believe that people or communities have something like a package of potentialities just waiting to be actualized in appropriate circumstances. It is possible (in many senses of the word[13]) for people and communities to develop in many different ways; but it is not necessary, useful or even legitimate to jump from this simple fact to an Aristotelian metaphysics of potentialities and actualities.

Third, unlike Dewey,[14] I have characterized a liberal education in terms of the peculiar aims assigned to it, rather than its results. This allows me to evaluate such an education in terms of results. That is, we may say that a liberal education is good (excellent or distinguished) exactly insofar as it is self and socially constructive (or developing), and it is bad insofar as it is self or socially destructive (or debilitating). The evaluation of the goodness or badness of the quality of a liberal education is, therefore, an empirical matter. It is a question of the goodness of fit between aims and results. (More of this in section “Evaluation”.)

Fourth, it is extraordinarily difficult to decide exactly what is self and socially constructive or destructive. For example, consider the fundamental disagreement that people have toward work.[15] Some folks believe that work is in some ways inherently self-destructive or necessarily unpleasant, and that the proper attitude toward it is one of avoidance. Self-development for these folks implies decreasing one’s working time and increasing one’s leisure time. On the other hand, some folks believe that work is inherently self-constructive and that the proper attitude toward it is one of enthusiastic adoption. This is the attitude of the skilled craftsperson or professional who expresses himself or herself through work. Self-development for these folks practically implies increasing one’s working time and decreasing one’s

---

[10]“Catching on at Colleges: Earning While Learning,” U.S. News and World Report, February 19, 1973, p. 72.

[11]“After Graduation - Then What?” U.S. News and World Report, August 28, 1972, p. 35.

[12]A recent report of the Organization for Economic Co-operation and Development referred to liberal education as “essentially leisure time courses for self-fulfillment.” (O.E.C.D., Learning Opportunities for Adults (Paris: O.E.C.D., 1977) , p. 25).

[13]Problems with this word are examined in A.C. Michalos, Foundations of Decision-Making (Ottawa: Canadian Library of Philosophy, 1978), pp. 93–98.

[14]Dewey, op. cit., p. 83.

[15]A good review of this issue may be found in N. Chomsky, “Toward a Humanistic Conception of Education,” Work, Technology, and Education, ed. W. Feinberg and H. Rosemont, Jr. (Urbana, Illinois: University of Illinois Press, 1975), pp. 204–220.

leisure time. Or, perhaps a better description would be that it implies a radical blurring of most distinctions between work and leisure activity.[16]

If one adopts a positive attitude toward work as an element of self and social development, as is my own inclination, then a plethora of additional problems arise. One wants to know what kind of work, if any, is especially relevant for a liberally educated person. How much should such a person be exposed to his or her life's work during formal education? At what point should the training begin? By what means? And so on. Hard evaluatively-loaded decisions will have to be made in order to answer such questions.[17]

It should be noticed that in the preceding two paragraphs I did not say that the determination of the constructive or destructive nature of anything was not an empirical matter. As I have explained in other places,[18] I operate with a naturalistic view of the ontological status of value in the tradition of Perry, Lewis and Dewey. It has well-known limitations, as do all of the alternatives, but it also has the notable advantage of turning all evaluations into empirical claims. So evaluatively-loaded decisions may be very complicated, but they remain in principle subject to empirical investigation—which does not, of course, make them manageable, solvable, logically tidy or especially splendid. But it does leave them uncluttered by supernatural forces.

Just as we will have problems specifying what is to count as development at the level of individuals, we will have problems reaching agreement on what is to count as social development. For example, there will be a continuum of options between pure socialism and pure capitalism, between distribution of resources according to need and according to merit or contribution. Although it may be logically possible to consider such options in a more or less unbiased way, I doubt that one can design a program of liberal education as proposed here that does not involve some commitments in these matters. If, for example, anyone presented political assassination and terrorism as a routine process of settling conflicts of interest in a community, that person would be appropriately regarded by most people as a dangerous nut. On the other hand, those who present democratic processes as routine and rational are correctly regarded as sensible people. I see no reason to be squeamish about such commitments.

---

[16]An excellent variation on this theme may be found in C. Frankel, "The Nature and Sources of Irrationalism" (Science (1973) pp. 927–931). Frankel discusses what he calls "an ancient division in the Western soul." It is basically the division between those who see the good life as that of a passive Lotus-Eater and those who see it in the active image of Prometheus.

[17]It has recently been claimed that "Liberal education without a study of business will create a one-dimensional person. In a true liberal education process both the humanities and business are essential." The same author thought that "Without a knowledge of management, accounting, finance, law, and economics, one simply cannot make educated and valid decisions." (I.I. Varner, "A Liberal Education Should Include the Study of Business," The Chronicle of Higher Education, May 14, 1979, p. 23). I find this view farfetched, but thought-provoking.

[18]For example, see A.C. Michalos, "Measuring the Quality of Life," Values and the Quality of Life, ed. J. King-Farlow and W.R. Shea (New York: Science History Publications, 1976), pp. 24–37; Foundations of Decision-Making, Chapter 12.

Indeed, the full force of self and community preservation is behind them. "The first step in education is to give the mind good habits," Hutchins said. "The next step in the education of free minds is the understanding of what is good."[19]

Fifth, with the definition of a liberal education proposed here, any sort of vocational or technical education may also be liberal. If, for example, programs in electrical engineering are designed with the aims of developing humane engineers who are sensitive to the social consequences and responsibilities of their technical expertise, then such programs are liberal. They are liberal insofar as engineers trained with these aims in view will be trained in the interests of self and social development as understood here. Similar remarks may be made about liberal education and medicine or commerce. The selves and social groups we are interested in developing are human in the full sense of that word, i.e., thinking, feeling, creative persons capable of choosing and pursuing their own ends. To imagine developing such persons in less than humane ways or in the interests of less than humane aims would be to imagine self and social destruction.

Sixth, it is a consequence of my proposal that a program of studies in the humanities and arts may fail to be liberal. When, for example, tragedies are studied as art forms instead of as human tragedies, then education is in danger of becoming illiberal, I don't have a well thought out theory of esthetics or art criticism, but I think it is possible to miss the point of many works of art if one only attends to their mechanics. I was reminded of this fact when my daughter talked to me about the study of sonnets in her eleventh grade English course. Technique was virtually everything. What the author tried to do or say with that particular technique was somehow omitted from the discussion.

Seventh, my proposal is consistent with the ancient view that a liberal education is education for a free person in a free society.[20] The root ideas in development are growth, progress or enhancement of some sort. Liberal education should be, as Dewey insisted, liberating education.[21] It should "elicit and fortify creative impulses," as Chomsky might have said.[22]

Eighth, a liberal education as specified here should satisfy all three of the traditional demands put on education as outlined by Aristotle.[23] Insofar as such an

---

[19]Hutchins, op. cit., p. 91. Coming at the same view from a different side, he wrote that "…if we succeeded in teaching everybody to read, and everybody read nothing but pulp magazines, obscene literature, and Mein Kampf, the last state of the nation would be worse than the first. Literacy is not enough." (Ibid., p. 15).

[20]"Education for free men is what used to be called liberal education." (Pusey, op. cit., p. 41).

[21]Dewey, op. cit., p. 83.

[22]Chomsky, op. cit. , p. 204.

[23]A.N. Whitehead gave us a slightly different triad. "There are three main methods which are required in a national system of education, namely, the literary curriculum, the scientific curriculum, the technical curriculum. But each of these curricula should include the other two. What I mean is, that every form of education should give the pupil a technique, a science, an assortment of general ideas, and aesthetic appreciation, and that each of these sides of his training should be illuminated by the others." The Aims of Education (New York: Macmillan Co., 1929), p. 58. I don't know how he saw moral virtue getting into his triad.

education is concerned with social development, it will contribute toward the development of character and moral virtue, for the latter are in large measure the result of concern for the interests of other persons.

Insofar as knowledge is a prerequisite for anyone interested in increasing the self and socially constructive forces in the world, and decreasing their opposites, knowledge will be a necessary ingredient in a liberal education. Insofar as knowledge and good intentions are helpless to initiate social and individual change in the absence of sound techniques, some attention to the latter, to doing things, will also be required in a liberal education. Again, there will be enormous difficulties in specifying exactly what knowledge, techniques and character traits to be exposed, when, for how long, in what way, and so on.

Ninth, it is perhaps worthwhile to mention that development is not something that happens later, tomorrow or at the end. It is a process that goes on now, for any now, if it goes on at all. In the fairy tale, a beautiful maiden kisses a frog who immediately becomes a prince. In the real world, a similarly disposed maiden would end up with a face full of frog froth. The moral of this story is that there are no instant princes or princesses. Good character, wisdom and technique in individuals and societies have to be nursed along, day by day, event by event. Accordingly, one ought to develop a tendency to appreciate the present moment, in principle at least, as not merely a means toward something else, but as an end in itself, a moment in a lifetime that will never come again.[24]

Tenth, and finally, it may be helpful to think of self-development, and without too much stretching of the sense of the terms, even social development as a process of getting one's heart and head together. In more prosaic prose, development involves a process of co-ordinating the cognitive and affective elements in human beings and communities. From a biological point of view, human beings are developing creatures their entire lives. As they pass through the stages of infancy, childhood, adolescence, young adulthood, middle and old age, fundamental changes occur in their bodies whether they know it or not, want it or not, and like it or not. What we call intellectual maturation is largely a matter of getting a belief and attitude system that is appropriate to one's sociophysical circumstances. Such maturation is typically the result of pursuing the truth and avoiding falsehood, in trial and error fashion, as one continually tries to build a belief and attitude system that can accommodate his or her changing circumstances. For example, children reach puberty as a matter of biological development, but must learn through useful experiences and instruction about the new personal and social possibilities and responsibilities that accompany the biological changes. Formal education, from

[24]"Next, perhaps, to the evils of passive adsorption and of competition for external standing come, perhaps, those which result from the eternal emphasis upon preparation for a remote future. …I have in mind…the habitual procrastination that develops when the motive for work is future, not present; and the false standards of judgment that are created when work is estimated, not on the basis of present need and present responsibility, but by reference to an external result, like passing an examination, getting promoted, entering high school, getting into college, etc." (Dewey, Moral Principles in Education, p. 25.).

nursery school through university, has a significant role to play in the process of co-ordinating hearts and heads within and among human beings. Moreover, as I see it, a liberal education has precisely this sort of co-ordinating function as its primary aim.[25]

Evaluation

By now we should probably have an idea of liberal education that is clear enough to allow us to press on with the basic question before us. However, I want to clarify a point that I made earlier before addressing the main question.

You recall that I said we could evaluate a liberal education by the goodness of fit between its aims and results. This is really only half of the story, and the second half at that. In the first place we must undertake the sort of philosophical analysis I am initiating here (following many others to be sure). One has to consider alternative conceptions of a good life for individuals and groups, and how formal education might contribute toward such a life.[26] In another place[27] I tried to show that aims as well as means could be rationally chosen on the basis of a broad-based cost-benefit analysis.

Without reviewing that discussion here, let me just say that empirical science will have as much to do with the selection of aims as it does with means. No one, philosophers included, has the dubious luxury of ignoring scientific knowledge while trying to get a plausible notion of what a good life might look like.

When I mentioned the goodness of fit between the aims and results of a liberal education, I had in mind a standard model of experimental science. We select and/or design a battery of standardized tests that have some face validity or relevance to the sort of output of interest to us as liberal educationists. There are, for example, measures of tolerance, authoritarianism, liberalism, various aspects of cognitive ability, and so on.[28] We select control and experimental groups of first year students in some liberal and non-liberal education programs. Controlling as well as we can for contaminating variables, we try to measure the impact of the

---

[25]I suppose the roots of this co-ordinating view of development should be traced back to Book IV of Plato's Republic.

[26]"We want to lead the good life," Hutchins said. "We want the good state as a means to that life. Once more, to find the good life and the good state we must inquire into the nature of man and the ends of life." (Hutchins; op. cit., p. 24).

[27]Michalos, Foundations of Decision-Making, pp. 141–142.

[28]A good idea of the wealth of more or less standardized tests that are available may be found in K.T. Chun, Measures for Psychological Assessment: A Guide to 3,000 Original Sources and Their Applications (Ann Arbor, Michigan: Institute for Social Research, 1975) and U.K. Buros, Tests in Print (New York: Cryphon Press, 1961). See also Robert H. Ennis, "A Concept of Critical Thinking," Harvard Educational Review (1962), pp. 81–111 and "A Conception of Rational Thinking," the Presidential Address to the Philosophy of Education Society, Toronto, April 20, 1979.

programs by analyzing the test scores of our students at the beginning and end of their academic careers.

Variants of this sort of evaluative exercise have been undertaken with a variety of results.[29] Sophisticated attempts to discover the extra value-added that education in prestigious schools should contribute to graduates as a result of objective advantages just haven't been successful. That is, we have been unable to show that people who go to prestigious universities with relatively illustrious faculty, excellent laboratories and libraries, actually learn more than people who go to run-of-the-mill universities.[30] Whatever extra value-added that graduates of first rate institutions seem to show is apparently the result of the extra brains and background those people bring with them.

The character studies of university graduates have a similar pattern. University graduates are notoriously tolerant folks compared to non-graduates, but this seems to be more a result of a weeding out process than a development process.[31]

Obviously I would not be here addressing these problems if I thought that the studies that have been done are final and decisive. I'm only trying to suggest that the idea of systematically evaluating a proposed program of liberal education is by no means novel. There are useful precedents and models, and even some relevant results.

---

[29]Good reviews of the literature may be found in C.K. Kaapper et al. (ed.), If Teaching is Important: The Evaluation of Instruction in Higher Education (Toronto: Clark, Irwin and Co., Ltd., 1974). A.W. Astin concluded his study as follows.

> The principal purpose of this study was to determine the effects of certain traditional indices of institutional excellence on the intellectual achievement of the undergraduate student. Our analysis failed to confirm the hypothesis that the student's achievement in social science, humanities, or natural science is facilitated either by the intellectual level of his classmates or by the level of academic competitiveness or financial resources of his institution. Similarly, the evidence did not support the contention that the bright student benefits more than does the average student from exposure to these assumed indices of institutional "quality." Additional analyses indicated that differences in student achievement during the senior year were much more highly dependent upon variations in student characteristics that existed before entrance into college than upon the characteristics of the undergraduate college attended. The results of these analyses suggest that it may be wise to reexamine some of our traditional notions about institutional excellence, particularly as it relates to the intellectual development of the student.

"Undergraduate Achievement and Institutional Excellence," Science (1968), p. 667.

[30]Ibid., p. 667.

[31]For example, see M.D. Blumenthal, et al., Justifying Violence: Attitudes of American Men (Ann Arbor: Institute for Social Research, 1972), and M.R. Porter, J. Porter and B.R. Blishen, Does Money Matter? (Toronto: Institute for Behavioural Research, York University, 1973), p. 7.

Conclusion

In the previous sections I have tried to sketch four views of a liberal education, which might be called pragmatic (following Dewey), aristocratic (following Aristotle), residualist, and developmental. My own view is that a liberal education may be identified by its dual and distinctive aims of self and social development. It is not education for the hell of it or for the fun of it, but education in the interests of personal and communal growth. It is education designed to help individuals and species achieve the highest quality of life of which they are capable.

Acknowledgements I would like to thank Jay Newman, Douglas Odegard and Stewart Thau for helpful suggestions regarding an earlier version of this paper. Parts of another version were presented at a Conference on Logic and Liberal Learning at Carnegie-Mellon University, Pittsburgh, Pennsylvania, June 1979.

Chapter 14
Einstein, Ethics and Science

Alex C. Michalos

Introduction

One hundred years after Albert Einstein's famous string of relativity papers were published, it might have been expected that there would be and indeed it has already turned out to be the case that there have been many conferences, symposia and individual presentations and articles produced in celebration of those papers. The original version of this essay began as an invited contribution to just such a celebratory symposium, and it has been altered a bit to fit the specific scope of this journal. Because Einstein was both a brilliant scientist and a political activist, there should be some benefit for ordinary scholars in an examination of some of his basic assumptions and motives. I believe this presumption is warranted, as I will show below.

Einstein's Intellectuals

For any of the extraordinary, if not great, philosophers of the first half of the 20th century, the place to begin looking for an overview of their work is Paul Schilpp's famous *Library of Living Philosophers.* One can find excellent, comprehensive analyses of the likes of Bertrand Russell, Sri Radhakrishnan, Rudoph Carnap, G.E. Moore, Karl Popper and Einstein, to mention a few. Each volume has about 25

Michalos, A.C.: 2004. Einstein, Ethics and Science. Journal of Academic Ethics, 2, pp. 339–354. © Springer 2005.

A.C. Michalos (✉)
University of Northern British Columbia, Prince George, BC, Canada
e-mail: michalos@brandonu.ca

A.C. Michalos, *Connecting the Quality of Life Theory to Health, Well-Being and Education*, DOI 10.1007/978-3-319-51161-0_14

essays by experts on various aspects of the philosopher's work and life, and each has some sort of autobiography and replies to his critics.

The first thing that strikes one examining the Schilpp (1951) volume on Einstein is that of the 25 critical essays in the volume, only one deals with a subject not properly within the discipline of physics, namely, Hinshaw's essay on "Einstein's Social Philosophy." The second thing that strikes one is that in Einstein's replies to his critics in that volume, he did not reply to Hinshaw.

Hinshaw said it was "hard to discover, in Einstein's speeches and writings, any systematic position in social ethics" (p. 649). So, he preferred to talk about Einstein's "convictions" rather than Einstein's "position, in social philosophy." Among his convictions, Einstein thought that "intellectuals" should engage in social action. He never went as far as Gloria Steinem in favouring "anything that gets people off their asses" (a remark she made in a television interview), but typically he preferred action to inaction. He often used the term "intellectual" to refer to educated professionals of one sort or another. In contemporary terms, Einstein was a thorough-going elitist, who apparently accepted the special obligations of those having special talents, i.e., noblesse oblige. In 1931 or 1932 he wrote to Sigmund Freud, deprecating politicians and proposing an organization of intellectuals.

> Political leaders or governments" he said, "owe their position partly to force and partly to popular election. They cannot be regarded as representative of the best elements, morally or intellectually, in their respective nations. The intellectual elite have no direct influence on the history of nations in these days; their lack of cohesion prevents them from taking a direct part in the solution of contemporary problems. Don't you think that a change might be brought about in this respect by a free association of people whose previous achievements and actions constitute a guarantee of their ability and purity of aim? This association of an international nature,... might, by defining its attitude in the Press... acquire a considerable and salutary moral influence over the settlement of political questions. Such an association would, of course, be a prey to all the ills which so often lead to degeneration in learned societies, dangers which are inseparably bound up with the imperfections of human nature. But should not an effort in this direction be risked in spite of this? I look upon such an attempt as nothing less than an imperative duty (Einstein 1954, pp. 104–105).

I am not a populist. Forty years of driving the sharpest ideas from history's sharpest minds into the thick skulls of North America's most intellectually advantaged youth strongly militates against any populist inclinations I may have had. Apart from the lessons of my own experience, there is the plain logical fact that the moral requirement to tell the truth implies due diligence in the pursuit of truth and the avoidance of falsehood. After all, without the latter, one's ability to tell the truth is little more than a crap shoot, which would be considerably less than the moral maxim demands. Among other things, like moral courage and personal integrity, I suppose it is this willingness to pursue the truth with due diligence that distinguishes John Gardner's (1990) "responsibles" from run-of-the-mill populists.

Notwithstanding the fact that I am not a populist, I find Einstein's easy dismissal of the moral authority of democratically elected governments and easy acceptance of the moral authority of intellectuals troublesome. After all, there is no good reason to believe that the virtue of excellence displayed by a great physicist, philosopher, painter or musician is equivalent to, exchangeable or substitutable for moral virtue (notwithstanding the predilections of classical utilitarians and robust consequentialists). To imagine that the production of fine works of science, humanistic studies or art makes one morally virtuous or politically astute is to imagine a world that does not exist. To imagine that a group of highly productive scholars and artists would automatically be willing and able to craft a common political agenda for action is to believe in politics without tears. The Royal Society of Canada is a fine example of just such a group of scholars and in over a century of its existence, it is not a great exaggeration to say that its most obvious goals seem to have been to find someone in government to take "our" advice (whatever that might be and whoever might be able to discern it) and to pay the rent on our offices. Regarding the former point, writing to one of his friends, about five hundred years ago, Machiavelli complained that no matter how comprehensively and carefully he offered advice to his Florentine governors, they only used the parts that were consistent with policies that they seem to have adopted prior to receiving his advice. Writing to his friend Henrich Zangger in December 1917, Einstein said, "Our whole, highly praised technological progress … and civilization in general, can be likened to an ax in the hand of a pathological criminal." To this remark Levenson added, "If so, it was his friends who forged that ax while he watched, fully aware of what was happening around him" (Levenson 2003, p. 84).

After World War I Einstein accumulated additional evidence of the irresponsibility of some politicians and governments, as well as evidence that the social action of intellectuals is as likely as not to be not only narrowly self-serving but socially pernicious. When Hitler "took the oath as Chancellor of a republic about to become a reich" in January 1933, Einstein was in Pasadena about to travel to a conference in Belgium and from there back to his home in Berlin. He issued a public statement indicating that he would not return to Germany because it was no longer a country "where civil liberty, tolerance and equality of all citizens before the law prevail", and he sent a letter of resignation to the Prussian Academy of Sciences and later to the Bavarian Academy of Sciences, including "renunciation of German citizenship." According to Levenson (2003, pp. 3, 418–419), it was the second time in his life that he had renounced his German citizenship. Hitler's propaganda machine and several newspapers responded with bitter denunciations, which Einstein would have expected. What were perhaps less expected were the attacks from "his fellow members" of the Academies, and what was certainly unexpected was the way his dear old friend, idol and great physicist Max Planck joined the critics.

In Levenson's view, "Max Planck disgraced himself." In Planck's

> … public statement on Einstein's resignation from the Academy… He praised Einstein as a physicist without equal since the days of Kepler and Newton, but, he concluded, his exile was his own fault: 'It is … greatly to be regretted,' he said at the Academy meeting that day, 'that Mr Einstein through his political behavior himself rendered his continued membership in the Academy impossible'. Einstein's politics were to blame, not those of a German government that had chosen to destroy him. Planck's declaration was as clear a signal as Einstein needed of the state of affairs in Berlin. Planck had always ranked with the best of Germany's intellectuals, an honest, generous friend and an uncompromising

> scientist. But just as he had thrilled to the call of war in 1914, in 1933 he could not resist the siren lure of loyalty to the state, even one run by Hitler ... He became a kind of moral imbecile: not evil in himself, not at all, but still incapable of acknowledging evil's presence at the heart of his beloved state (Levenson 2003, p. 420).

Personally, I suspect that Levenson's characterization of Planck as a "moral imbecile" probably does not do justice to Hanna Arendt's (1976) persuasive analysis of the banality of evil and the role of such evil throughout history. This is not an issue that has to be pursued at length here, but it does merit some thought. Lucky enough for all of us, we seldom see evil in its most ugly and heartbreaking forms, e.g., as reported by Dallaire (2003) or as most of us saw on our television screens on September 11, 2001. Monstrous as these things are, and monumental as they are as highly visible signs that the world is not as it should be, they are not as dangerous to the body politic as the apparently banal, microbialsized evils that gnaw away at the fibre of our democracy.

In 1948, fifteen years after his mistreatment by the Prussian intellectuals, Einstein wrote a speech for the Intellectuals' Conference for Peace in which he said,

> By painful experience we have learnt that rational thinking does not suffice to solve the problems of our social life. Penetrating research and keen scientific work have often had tragic implications for mankind, producing, on the one hand, inventions which liberated man from exhausting physical labor ... but on the other hand, ... creating the means for his own mass destruction ... We scientists, whose tragic destination has been to help in making the methods of annihilation more gruesome and more effective, must consider it our solemn and transcendent duty to do all in our power in preventing these weapons from being used for the brutal purpose for which they were invented (Einstein 1950, pp. 24–25).

The Organizing Committee of the Conference rejected his contribution, which he published later anyhow. Still, Einstein never seems to have given up his faith in intellectuals. While he could always count on intellectuals like Bertrand Russell and George Bernard Shaw (which is more than any of their wives could say) as a collaborative class, the intellectuals of his day seem to have left a lot to be desired. Lest the parenthetical remark is missed, along with many privileged males before and since, Einstein, Russell and Shaw shared the unattractive moral flaw of being very good to people in the abstract, but very inconsiderate and thoughtless to their own wives. Levenson (2003, pp. 149–150) described this characteristic of Einstein as follows.

> He had no gift for empathy, no ability to imagine himself into the emotional life of anyone else. His behavior was of a piece, a symptom of that same deep gap in his understanding of people. He could reason himself to a powerful moral position and then rely on his strength of mind and will to hold it. He did oppose the war [both world wars]; he did defend his fellow Jews; he longed for justice and was willing to put himself to great pains and occasional real risk to uphold his beliefs. But to grasp what someone else felt, to understand the impact of his personal desires and deeds on the minds and hearts of the individual human beings around him - that was vastly more difficult. . . There is no question that he sought a real connection to his son [Hans Albert]. But he had scant resources to offer. The lasting message was that physics did outrank family for Einstein.

I digressed a bit into Einstein's personal life. The main point of reviewing the little bit of his history was to show that he had evidence of the fickleness of intellectuals in general and of the best and brightest of intellectuals in particular that extended over two-thirds of his life. Although he never gave up on them, he never forgave the non-German intellectuals for their "lack of courage" or the German intellectuals for behaviour he regarded as "no better than the common mob" (Levenson 2003, pp. 422, 427).

In the 120 years or so of the Royal Society's existence, I do not know of any case where Fellows had to face the sorts of conflicts of conscience and self-interest faced by those in the Prussian Academy in Hitler's Germany. Shortly after 9/11, the Royal Society of Canada was asked to organize a small conference on Research and Security, which took place in Ottawa in May 2002. A number of us were invited to suggest topics and speakers. I told the President that it was important to prevent the meeting from focusing on developing and spreading more lethal weapons, and to make sure that speakers were invited who would represent Canada's most profound proponents of building human security through the development of a culture of peace across the globe. I also suggested several names of the usual suspects from Project Ploughshares, Science for Peace and UNESCO. Anyone who attended that conference knows that nothing of the sort happened. At a time when our friends in the USA especially needed the wise counsel of their closest friends to remind them that the best road to lasting security begins with trust built on understanding, the Royal Society conference provided little more than assurance that our best and brightest Canadians "stood at the ready" as required. Officially, within the Society, that conference has been celebrated as a great success because, after all, the Society not only pulled it off in a relatively short time, but made a bundle of money on top of it. To me, it was a great failure, not a failure of imagination as described by Arendt in her account of the banality of evil, but a failure of moral courage and professional integrity. If Canada's best and brightest could be so easily co-opted in circumstances far less treacherous and dangerous than those faced by Einstein and his German colleagues, what would we do in those circumstances?

Plato saw the danger lurking in a form of government (democracy) that would allow people to elect scoundrels or weaklings merely because they were excellent representatives of the people themselves. Churchill was not joking when he said that democracy was a bad form of government, but preferable to all others. My own view is that democracy just barely works, and works very slowly at that, but it works exactly insofar as some people (Gardner's "responsibles" again), with whatever skills they happen to have, make the necessary personal investments in time, energy, research and so on. The rich mixture of ordinary and extraordinary resources and investments over time makes it work. As long as people from all walks of life are willing to step up to the plate and donate a fair share of their resources and their lives to making democracy work, it will work. The solution to the problems of an inadequate democracy lies not in some sort of an aristocracy of intellectuals, but in a greater, more fully developed and functional democracy of "responsibles." I am not sure that Einstein would have approved of this view.

Einstein's Ethics

I spent some time looking for the roots of Einstein's moral philosophy. In 1931, he wrote that

> To inquire after the meaning or object of one's own existence or of creation generally has always seemed to me absurd from an objective point of view. And yet everybody has certain ideals which determine the direction of his endeavours and his judgments. In this sense *I have never looked upon ease and happiness as ends in themselves—such an ethical basis I call more proper for a herd of swine.* The ideals which have lighted me on my way and time after time given me new courage to face life cheerfully, have been Truth, Goodness, and Beauty. Without the sense of fellowship with men of like mind, of preoccupation with the objective, the eternally unattainable in the field of art and scientific research, life would have seemed to me empty. The ordinary objects of human endeavour—property, outward success, luxury—have always seemed to me contemptible (Einstein 1979, p. 2, emphasis added).

When I saw the italicized part of this quotation, I figured he was pretty clearly not a utilitarian, and certainly not a hedonist. The italicized part reminded me of a comment of Aristotle's in the *Nicomachean Ethics* (c.350 B.C.E., p. 4).

> "The many," he wrote, "the most vulgar, would seem to conceive the good and happiness as pleasure, and hence they also like the life of gratification. In this they appear completely slavish, since the life they decide on is a life for grazing animals."

Like most of his contemporary Greeks and anyone who has ever had a morning hangover after a joyous party the night before, Aristotle knew the difference between having a good time and having a good life. In Aristotle's view, a good life, which he identified with a happy life, required a bundle of good things, which he collected under the general rubrics of "goods of the body" (e.g., health), "goods of the soul" (e.g., wisdom) and "external goods" (e.g., friends). This is not a topic to be pursued here, but it is worth mentioning because many people still seem inclined to confuse pleasure and happiness.

Einstein often mentioned happiness as a worthwhile and desirable end for human beings. In 1938 he wrote,

> To be a Jew, after all, means first of all, to acknowledge and follow in practice those fundamentals in humaneness laid down in the Bible – fundamentals without which no sound and happy community of men can exist (Einstein 1950, pp. 109–110).

In 1943 he wrote,

> Our Jewish forbears, the prophets and the old Chinese sages understood and proclaimed that the most important factor in giving shape to our human existence is the setting up and establishment of a goal: the goal being a community of free and happy human beings who by constant inward endeavor strive to liberate themselves from the inheritance of anti-social and destructive instincts (Einstein 1950, pp. 108–109).

In his 1947 memorial address for his friend Paul Langevin he said that Langevin's "desire to promote the happier life for all men was perhaps even stronger than his craving for pure intellectual enlightenment" (Einstein 1950, p. 87), and in 1949 about Steven Wise he said that "everybody knows that behind the enormous labors of this man there has always been the passionate desire to make mankind better and happier" (Einstein 1950, p. 116). Presumably he was not praising his departed friends for their interests in promoting a life suitable to "a herd of swine." Most likely, he had in mind a relatively robust notion of happiness along the lines of Aristotle.

In his 1949 paper on socialism, Einstein raised a fairly standard utilitarian type of question, namely, How should "the structure of society and the cultural attitude of man… be changed in order to make human life as satisfying as possible?" After a brief, straightforward Marxian analysis of the problem, he concluded that

> The economic anarchy of capitalist society as it exists today is, in my opinion, the real source of the evil … Unlimited competition leads to a huge waste of labor, and to that crippling of the social consciousness of individuals which I mentioned above. This crippling of individuals I consider the worst evil of capitalism. Our whole educational system suffers from this evil. An exaggerated competitive attitude is inculcated into the student, who is trained to worship acquisitive success as a preparation for his future career. I am convinced there is only one way to eliminate these grave evils, namely through the establishment of a socialist economy, accompanied by an educational system which would be oriented toward social goals. In such an economy, the means of production are owned by society itself and are utilized in a planned fashion … Nevertheless, it is necessary to remember that a planned economy is not yet socialism. A planned economy as such may be accompanied by the complete enslavement of the individual. The achievement of socialism requires the solution of some extremely difficult socio-political problems… (Einstein 1950, pp. 5–8).

Needless to say, he did not know how to solve the problems of a planned economy as far as he could see them. I am not going to get into his democratic socialism, though I am sympathetic to it. (Interested readers may read Michalos 1995, 1997). In fact, for most of the years he lived in Berlin (1914–1932), most Berliners were sympathetic to it. In those years, Berlin was something like the Regina of social democracy in Germany. (I'm sure they would have been impressed by the comparison).

Although one can find utilitarian language in Einstein, the roots of his moral philosophy came from the prophetic tradition in Judaism. He was very clear about this on more than one occasion. For example, in 1934 he wrote,

> The pursuit of knowledge for its own sake, an almost fanatical love of justice, and the desire for personal independence – these are the features of the Jewish tradition which make me thank my stars that I belong to it … Judaism seems to me to be concerned almost exclusively with the moral attitude in life and to life … The essence of that conception [of life] seems to me to lie in an affirmative attitude to the life of all creation.
>
> The life of the individual has meaning only in so far as it aids in making the life of every living thing nobler and more beautiful … 'serving God' was equated with 'serving the living.' The best of the Jewish people, especially the Prophets and Jesus, contended

> tirelessly for this. Judaism is thus no transcendental religion; it is concerned with life as we live it and can up to a point grasp it, and nothing else (Einstein 1979, pp. 90–91).

These remarks might have been as comfortably rooted in the prophetic tradition as they would have been in Spinoza's pantheism (as Einstein explicitly recognized) or Schweitzer's reverence-for-life philosophy. In any event, such remarks make it easier to think of his moral philosophy as having humanistic rather than theistic foundations, although the prophets themselves might have been appalled at the idea of divorcing the moral law from its creator.

Einstein often referred to the Jewish prophets and the ancient Greek philosophers in the context of remarks on the origins of ethics. unlike the prophets, many of the Greeks would not have found it extraordinary to insist upon moral virtue in the absence of a supernatural moral law maker. For example, among the fragments attributed to the philosopher-politician Solon (c.594 B.C.E.), one finds such maxims as "Never tell a lie. Pursue worthy aims. Do not be rash to make friends and, when once they are made, do not drop them. Learn to obey before you command. In giving advice seek to help, not to please, your friend. Be led by reason. Shun evil company. Honour the gods, reverence parents" (Diogenes Laertius c. 225 A.C.E., p. 61). So far as I know, there is no fragment in which Solon claims the gods as the authors of his moral maxims or the source of his own moral authority.

Einstein's Philosophy of Science

Granting his humanism, I was very surprised to find Einstein using some very unhumanistic, religious language to talk about science. In 1930, after describing a "state of religious experience" that he called "cosmic religious feeling," he said,

> The individual feels the futility of human desires and aims and the sublimity and marvelous order which reveal themselves both in nature and in the world of thought. Individual existence impresses him as a sort of prison and he wants to experience the universe as a single significant whole...The religious geniuses of all ages have been distinguished by this kind of religious feeling,... In my view, it is the most important function of art and science to awaken this feeling and keep it alive in those who are receptive to it ... I maintain that cosmic religious feeling is the strongest and noblest motive for scientific research (Einstein 1954, pp. 38–39).

I am not sure how we are to understand this paragraph, and especially the very last sentence. It seems quite out of character for a relatively hard-headed humanist, but it apparently captured some very important aspect of Einstein's own feelings and motives about his scientific work. I have never seen any research in the psychology or sociology of science that would confirm his claim. If I had to bet, my guess would be that among physicists, such feelings and motives might be found mostly among cosmologists, but I have never seen any systematically gathered evidence of that. Among psychologists and sociologists, and even more so among political scientists and economists, I think such feelings and motives would be relatively rare. Personally, I would never use such language to characterize my own motives and feelings about my social scientific research, or even my philosophical speculations for that matter. I began my graduate work studying comparative religion and abandoned work in that field because it seemed to me that the religious language that was so essential to most of the writers in the field was cluttering up my thinking. For me, the path to what I regarded as clear thinking about those aspects of the world of interest to me was a path free of religious language. Apparently, that was not the case for Einstein.

On the occasion of celebrating Max Planck's sixtieth birthday in 1918, Einstein suggested a remarkably escapist motive for scientific research, following Schopenhauer. At that time he wrote,

> I believe with Schopenhauer that one of the strongest motives that leads men to art and science is escape from everyday life with its painful crudity and hopeless dreariness, from the fetters of one's own ever shifting desires. A finely tempered nature longs to escape from personal life into the world of objective perception and thought;... With this negative motive there goes a positive one. Man tries to make for himself in the fashion that suits him best a simplified and intelligible picture of the world; he then tries to some extent to substitute this cosmos of his for the world of experience, and thus to overcome it. This is what the painter, the poet, the speculative philosopher, and the natural scientist do, each in his own fashion. Each makes this cosmos and its construction the pivot of his emotional life, in order to find in this way the peace and security which he cannot find in the narrow whirlpool of personal experience (Einstein 1954, p. 225).

Personally, I always found Schopenhauer a bit depressing, and it doesn't surprise me that he would have thought about science along the lines in this paragraph. Notice that even the so-called "positive" motive in this paragraph is escapist, and in that sense it is still negative. Unattractive as it is, I would bet that the escapist motive is much stronger than the "cosmic religious feeling" motive among most academics, although the two motives are not mutually exclusive. Again, my view is only based on 40 years of casual observation of colleagues in a handful of universities, not on systematic research. But I have the clear impression that one of the main reasons people become scholars and work in universities is that they much prefer the world of ideas to the real world. In principle, the world of ideas is much tidier, although in fact any individual's personally crafted cosmos may be a garbage bin of half–baked baloney. Still, I suspect people find such baloney easier to digest than the meat and potatoes of real life.

I suppose I am not the only person who has found his or her own office, if not the smaller space of his or her own head, to be the safest place in the world on some days. So, I suppose few of us would have trouble relating to the Schopenhauer-Einstein hypothesis. Nevertheless, I think it would be inaccurate and unfair to a lot of academics, as well as poets, painters and other creative people if we fail to mention altruistic motives. That is, some of the creative work that people do is designed to make the world a better place, or more precisely, to make life better for some people than it might otherwise be. While Oscar Wilde and Bernard Shaw may have written delightful plays largely in the interest of creating excellent art, Shaw was also motivated to write plays in the interest of getting people to see the evils of social injustice that were all around them and to motivate them to remedial action. And, of course, they both wrote to make a living. Regarding my own work, I know that some of it was motivated primarily by a desire to understand some things better (e.g., my *North American Social Report* 1980–82, and *Global Report on Student Well-Being* 1991–93), some was written to instruct students (e.g., *Principles of Logic* 1969, *Improving Your Reasoning* 1970), some was designed to motivate others to action (e.g., *Militarism and the Quality of Life* 1989, *Good Taxes* 1997), some was written for the fun of it (e.g., *Bernard Shaw and the Webbs,* Michalos and Poff 2002), and at least one was published to prove that Imre Lakatos was wrong and I was right about *The Popper-Carnap Controversy* (1971). Thus, even the briefest of reflections on some of my own work indicates a variety of motives for scientific research beyond those suggested by Einstein.

While Einstein's views about motives for scientific research seemed to be a bit extra-ordinary, his views about the nature of science itself were fairly prosaic. Along with many others, he thought of technology as applied science (Einstein 1950, p. 11, from a 1935 paper), although he must have known that very often technological advances precede and provoke scientific research. Without reviewing a longer treatment of this subject in Michalos (1981), it is probably enough to quote a remark made in 1971 by Caryl Haskins; "modern archaeological research leaves little room for doubt that the basic technological revolutions of mankind antedated the scientific revolution by many thousands of years" (quoted in Michalos 1981, p. 4). Regarding the frequently mentioned distinction between basic and applied science, I think the view expressed in the 1971–72 *Annual Report* of the Science Council of Canada was right on the button. Contrary to the view expressed by the Senate Special Committee on Science Policy, the Science Council questioned "the desirability of separating basic and applied research—in their performance, funding, administration, and communication. This is [the Council felt], a retrograde step, and runs counter to the whole weight of evidence on the advantages of interaction" (quoted in Michalos 1981, p. 3).

In 1949, Einstein expressed the view that "Science… cannot create ends and, even less, instill them in human beings; science, at most, can supply the means by which to attain certain ends" (Einstein 1950, p. 2). For a man whose whole adult life was spent working at the known frontiers of physical research and crafting solutions to problems that were only intelligible to other scientists working at the same frontiers, this is a remarkably limited view of the power of science, of scientific theories in particular, to create ends. Without reviewing discussions in Michalos (1971, 1981), Popper was certainly right when he insisted that scientists should try to construct bold theories, whose empirical content reaches beyond known data to predictions and observations of data hitherto unknown. Insofar as this conceptualization of good science or good scientific research is logically prior to actually producing such science or engaging in such research, the latter is driven by the former. That is, in the sense that good scientific research specifies and demands certain kinds of theorizing or hypothesizing, it creates appropriate ends. While it is possible and often happens that people engage in scientific research in the interest of obtaining marketable products or solving practical problems (e.g., octane enhancing fuel additives), it happens as well that the internal logic of science or of scientific theories creates both general and specific ends. For example, in my own field of research on personal satisfaction or happiness, it is no mere coincidence that scientists around the world focused their attention on exploring the psychometric properties of frequently used measures, examining the impact of such things as question phrasing, the order of questions, the length of questionnaires, the length of questions, introductory remarks preceding questions, the effects of personal interviews versus mailout questionnaires, effects of male versus female interviewers, numbers of response categories, off scale options, seasonal effects, gender effects, age effects and so on. The fact that scientific research in all disciplines has its own internal logic probably makes it more difficult for scientists and philosophers of science to appreciate the work of sociologists of science and others who take the external conditions or context of people's work more seriously. Since good cases can be and have been made for the so-called internalist and externalist histories of the growth of science (Durbin 1980), we need not press the internalist case any further.

Einstein's limited view of science as a creator of ends was matched by his view of the intellect itself.

> We should take care not to make the intellect our god;" he wrote in 1943, "it has, of course, powerful muscles, but no personality. It cannot lead, it can only serve; and it is not fastidious in its choice of a leader. This characteristic is reflected in the qualities of its priests, the intellectuals. The intellect has a sharp eye for methods and tools, but is blind to ends and values. So it is no wonder that this fatal blindness is handed on from old to young and today involves a whole generation (Einstein 1950, p. 108).

This he could not have learned from the Greeks, at least none of the most prolific and profound Greeks. It is an old problem, of course, the relations between our passions and our reason, and simply put it has an air of artificiality about it. That is, the very idea that human motives, inclinations, emotions, desires, thoughts and needs can be sorted out like fish and chips at a picnic smacks of academic artificiality. Still, the tradition out of Socrates and Plato, not to mention Solon who preceded them, was that reason could and ought to (prudentially and morally) govern one's actions. The contemporary cognitivist view of psychologists is that reason often, if not always, does govern one's actions and that it ought to (Michalos 1985). Einstein apparently followed Schopenhauer, who followed David Hume, who may have followed others unknown to me, in believing that one's passions govern one's actions, whether or not they ought to prudentially and morally. The contemporary anti-cognitivist view in psychology is represented very well by Zajonc (1980). Apart from the fact that I do not know how I would do it briefly, there is no need to try to resolve this problem here. It is enough to note that Einstein's view of the problem was consistent with his view of the nature of science. Given his position on this problem, it was remarkable that to his political opponents

> he represented intellect – mind, not heart. More broadly, he was the embodiment of reason as opposed to authority, reason that could compel changes in fundamental beliefs. That was

subversive enough, especially when there were German orators who argued in the 1920s that 'we suffer today from an excess of culture. Only knowledge is valued. …What we need is instinct and will' (Levenson 2003, p. 246; the quoted orator was Hitler in 1923).

If Einstein's position is true, then our "fundamental beliefs" are finally selected by our passions, merely aided and abetted by reason, and there may well be no good reason, logically speaking, to prefer anyone's "fundamental beliefs" to those of anyone else. Artificial though the problem may be, it does have some philosophical bite when you think about it.

Einstein was probably wrong when he said that science cannot instill ends in human beings. After all, one of the reasons that all of our research institutions must have Research Ethics Boards review proposed research on human subjects prior to the execution of research is that scientists have the means to instill ends in human beings, e.g., through the use of drugs, behavioural conditioning or outright deception. What's more, given the mixed motives with which most people tend to engage in most activities, including scientific research, he was probably wrong in thinking that "science, if it is to flourish, must have no practical end in view" (Einstein 1979, p. 30). At least since the time of Archimedes (c.250 B.C.E.), scientists, like artists, have always engaged in marketing their activities as practically useful (Gillings 1972). While it may be regarded as a nuisance to the artists and scientists, both art and science have managed to flourish in spite of such distractions. The resources invested by the Royal Society over at least the past twenty years trying to convince the federal government of the practical value of the Society's activities and the great potential for still greater value through federally funded, targeted research through the proposed Canadian Academies are not extraordinary in the history of science. What is perhaps extraordinary is how slow successive liberal and conservative governments have been to warm up to ideas that were accepted some time ago by governments of most industrialized countries. The proposed Academies can make a significant contribution to research in Canada, provided that they are operated in very transparent and even-handed ways, and do not become the vehicle for governments to reward their friends and punish their enemies or, what may be practically the same thing, for governments to fund industry-friendly research at the expense of research driven by the internal logic of the research theories and paradigms of diverse disciplines.

Conclusion

In a wonderfully provocative presentation at the 2004 Royal Society symposium on 'Life, Learning and the Arts', Alistair Macleod talked about the importance of *place* in literature. For example, it was not accidental or incidental to William Faulkner's work that none of his characters was ever threatened by frostbite in a frozen tundra, or by grizzly or polar bears. Reading Einstein's social and political papers, and his biography, it became obvious that Macleod's point could be made regarding the importance of *time*. All of Einstein's efforts to save what was best in Germany, including the cultural gem that was the Berlin he entered in 1914, only made sense because of the particular time in which he lived and the events that occurred in that period of time. "Einstein had next to nothing to do with the invention of nuclear weapons" (Levenson 2003, p. 426). Still, all of his work after 1945, addressing the "major moral problem of our age" (Hinshaw 1951, p. 651), trying to prevent the catastrophic further unleashing of nuclear weapons made sense for someone with his expertise and values in the years after the end of World War II. Even his transition from a conscientious objector to militarism and war in his Berlin years to an advocate for compulsory arbitration of international disputes backed up by the force of like-minded countries of his post-Berlin years is best understood against the historical events he witnessed. Similar remarks might be made about a variety of contextual features of Einstein's life, or any life, for that matter, as externalist historians of science and others have reminded us.

According to Levenson (2003, p. 429), "From the anti-Hitler efforts of the 1930s to his Zionism and his antinuclear campaigns of his last years, Einstein proved willing throughout his time in America to campaign to the point of exhaustion." He became an American citizen in 1940 but never abandoned his Swiss citizenship. Levenson thought that he was somewhat less active in his 22 years in America than he had been in his Berlin years. I suppose that is to be expected. He was 76 years old when he died in April 1955. He was a great physicist, perhaps the greatest since Newton. Expressing a view shared by many of the ancients, Diogenes Laertius (p. 519) regarded physics as "a branch of philosophy more ancient and important than the others." From that point of view, Einstein might have been the greatest philosopher since Newton. When Bertrand Russell was asked to compare the importance of his work in logic and mathematics with his social and political philosophy, he said that the latter was more important because if we got the latter wrong, all other human activities would become impossible. I am inclined to agree with Russell, but Einstein was an extraordinary man in either case. We can learn from his failures as well as from his successes. By any reasonable measure for a human being, I think it is fair to say that his was a life well-used and worth remembering.

Acknowledgements An earlier version of this paper was presented at a regional meeting of the Royal Society of Canada, held at the University of Guelph, Ontario, May 2, 2005. I would like to thank O.P. Dwivedi for inviting me to write the paper and Deborah C. Poff for helping me clarify some ideas in it.

References

Arendt, H. (1976). *Eichmann in Jerusalem: A report on the banality of evil*. New York: Penguin Books.

Aristotle. (c.350 B.C.E., 1999). *Nicomachean ethics* (2nd ed.) (T. Irwin, Trans.). Indianapolis: Hackett Publishing Co.

Dallaire, R. A. (2003). *Shake hands with the devil: The failure of humanity in Rwanda*. Toronto: Random House Canada.
Diogenes Laertius. (c. 225 A.C.E., 1925). *Lives of eminent philosophers* (Vol. 1) (R. D. Hicks, Trans.). Cambridge: Harvard University Press.
Durbin, P. T. (Ed.). (1980). *A guide to the culture of science, technology and medicine*. New York: The Free Press.
Einstein, A. (1950). *Essays in humanism*. New York: Philosophical Library.
Einstein, A. (1954). *Ideas and opinions*. New York: Wings Books.
Einstein, A. (1979). *The world as i see it*. New York: Wisdom Library.
Gardner, J. W. (1990). *On leadership*. New York: The Free Press.
Gillings, R. J. (1972). *Mathematics in the time of the pharaohs*. Cambridge: MIT Press.
Hinshaw, V. G. (1951). Einstein's social philosophy. In P. A. Schilpp (Ed.), *Albert Einstein: Philosopher-scientist*. New York: Tudor Publishing Co.
Levenson, T. (2003). *Einstein in Berlin*. New York: Bantam Books.
Michalos, A. C. (1969). *Principles of logic*. Englewood Cliffs: Prentice-Hall Inc.
Michalos, A. C. (1970). *Improving your reasoning*. Englewood Cliffs: Prentice-Hall Inc.
Michalos, A. C. (1971). *The Popper-Carnap controversy*. Hague: Martinus Nijhoff.
Michalos, A. C. (1980–82). *North American social report* (Vols. 1–5). Dordrecht: D. Reidel Publishing.
Michalos, A. C. (1981). *North American social report, vol. 3: Science, education and recreation*. Dordrecht: D. Reidel Publishing.
Michalos, A. C. (1985). Multiple discrepancies theory (MDT). *Social Indicators Research, 16*, 347–413.
Michalos, A. C. (1989). *Militarism and the quality of life*. Toronto: Science for Peace.
Michalos, A. C. (1991–93). *Global report on student well-being* (Vols. 1–4). Berlin, Heidelberg, New York: Springer.
Michalos, A. C. (1995). *A pragmatic approach to business ethics*. Thousand Oaks: Sage.
Michalos, A. C. (1997). *Good taxes: The case for taxing foreign currency exchange and other financial transactions*. Toronto: Science for Peace.
Michalos, A. C., & Poff, D. C. (Eds.). (2002). *Bernard Shaw and the Webbs*. Toronto: University of Toronto Press.
Schilpp, P. A. (Ed.). (1951). *Albert Einstein: Philosopher- scientist*. New York: Tudor Publishing Co.
Zajonc, R. B. (1980). Feeling and thinking: Preferences need no inferences. *American Psychologist, 35*, 151–175.

Chapter 15
Observations on Unacknowledged Authorship from Homer to Now

Alex C. Michalos

Introduction

The aim of this essay is to share some observations about the history and contemporary status of unacknowledged authorship or what is generally known as plagiarism. Some years ago I was advised as a scholarly journal editor to avoid using the "p word" and I have generally adhered to that practice. Brief sketches of three historical cases are offered partly to remind readers that unacknowledged authorship has been and still may be viewed in different ways given different contexts and purposes. The cases are also offered to prime the reader's thinking. Once I began thinking about such cases, I rapidly developed a fairly long list covering many famous writers in many different disciplines and it occurred to me that most scholars would probably have a similar experience. In the light of such experience, it is difficult to believe that the contemporary scene concerning unacknowledged authorship indicates a huge deterioration of research or publishing integrity. In any event, following the brief historical journey, overviews of two contemporary cases are presented that came across my desk. These illustrate some difficulties that editors and publishers have today that those in earlier historic periods could not have had, as well as some suggested procedures for managing such difficulties.

Michalos, A.C.: 2010. Observations on unacknowledged authorship from Homer to now. Journal of Academic Ethics, 8, pp. 253–258. © Springer Science+Business Media B.V. 2010.

A.C. Michalos (✉)
University of Northern British Columbia, Prince George, BC, Canada
e-mail: michalos@brandonu.ca

A.C. Michalos, *Connecting the Quality of Life Theory to Health, Well-Being and Education*, DOI 10.1007/978-3-319-51161-0_15

Three Familiar Historic Cases

Homer: Iliad and Odyssey

The short entry for 'Homer' in *Chambers Biographical Dictionary* (McGovern 1997, p. 745) informs us that "Homer was regarded in Greek and Roman antiquity as the author of the *Iliad*…and the *Odyssey*…[Although] It is now believed that the poems were developed from orally transmitted poems, which were much modified and extended by several hands. They are usually dated to the 8th century BC, …". According to McInerney (1998, pp. 14–16), in the period from 1200 to 900 B.C. epic poetry was developed and flourished in Greece with "Wandering poets [performing] these songs all over Greece, incorporating the accomplishments of local heroes. The greatest of the poems, the *Iliad* and the *Odyssey,* were written down around 725 B.C. The previously flexible oral tradition thus became solidified in a single, monumental version". In other words, someone named 'Homer' became famous for assembling under his name some versions of some poems by some poets without acknowledging the other poets. People sometimes say that in our electronic age, we must rethink the idea of plagiarism because so many of us have such free access to so much of the work of others. I suppose Homer would have been sympathetic to such suggestions.

Aesop: Fables

In one of the first conferences I went to over 40 years ago on the topic of social indicators, a man named Eli Goldston, who was the president of a big gas company in the New England States of the USA, told us a story that he said he got from his Rabbi who told him he got from the 6th century B.C. Greek poet Aesop. It's a great story about an old man, a boy and a donkey, and from it Aesop drew the wise moral that if you try to please everyone you will end up losing your ass. I have told that story dozens of times over the last 40 years and my wife has been telling it for many of the 30 years we have been together.

One day while I was browsing in a bookstore not long ago looking for some light reading, I stumbled upon a Penquin Classic called *The Complete Fables*, by Aesop (1998). Since I had never read the story I had been telling for so many years, I thought here was my chance to find out exactly what the old Greek had said, in translation at least. Among other things, what I found in a section called "A note on the text" was that this collection of 358 fables was based on a 1927 collection published in French, about which the editors and translators of this text wrote,

> We have taken Chambry's text to represent the 'complete' fables of Aesop for the purposes of this volume, although every scholar would probably alter the text by taking away some and adding others according to his or her own personal choices. There are many fables, some ancient, some not so ancient, which are not included in Chambry's edition, but since

> we have no knowledge whether any fables are by Aesop or not (or, if he did write them, whether any survive), the 'complete fables of Aesop' is whatever the editor of its Greek text chooses to say it is.... As for the various Victorian and Edwardian translations of Aesop, they were not only limited in their scope, inaccurate in their terminology and sentimental in their morals, but the famous 'translation' of Croxall was more than half written by the translator himself (Aesop 1998, pp. xxiv–xxv).

As disturbing as this information was, what followed was even more so. The great story of the old man, the boy and the donkey was not in the collection. There are lots of stories featuring an ass, e.g., The Ass, the Fox and the Lion, The Ass and the Frogs, The Ass Pronouncing the Horse Happy, The Ass Carrying Salt. But nothing about our favourite story. Since the main point of this case was to provide another historical example of a person (Aesop) becoming famous for telling, if not assembling, fables crafted by unacknowledged others, it does not matter that our favourite story was not in the collection, but it does remain something of a puzzle.

Bible: Synoptic Gospels

As part of a Bachelor of Divinity Program at the University of Chicago, all students had to pass exams covering the Bible and in particular so-called 'higher criticism' of Biblical texts. Among other things, we were introduced to the synoptic problem, which is the problem of explaining why the gospels according to Matthew, Mark and Luke are so similar to each other and so dissimilar to John. For present purposes, it only has to be noted first, that most scholars agree that both Matthew and Luke copied quite a bit from Marc and some additional source (called 'Q') without acknowledgement and second, that this is regarded as a "problem" rather than a scandal. The three synoptic gospels were written sometime between 60 and 115 A.D. (Cline 2010) and the tradition of citing one's sources was by then familiar to most scholars, but neither Matthew nor Luke nor their followers seems to have paid any attention to that tradition.

Fast Forward to Today

If we had the time and patience, the preceding three familiar cases could easily have been multiplied. I suppose most academics probably have their own favourites and the general message of such cases is simply that the problem of unacknowledged authorship is not new and has not always been regarded as a problem.

It is difficult for us today to see the world as Homer, Aesop, Matthew and Luke saw it. The closest things we have to their experience in this field are probably something like what I heard Pete Seeger say about some of his songs or like what sometimes happens now with massive letter-writing campaigns to government officials. Pete Seeger told an audience (recorded and later televised) that he wrote a song, then someone else changed the lyrics a bit, and someone else changed those, and so on, and in the end they all made sense conveying his original message. Somewhat similarly, I have received templates of letters to government officials (e.g., protesting NAFTA or the GST) urging me to make use of them in any way helpful to the campaign, without ever suggesting the need to let me know who authored the template or the need for me to put any of my own version of the template in quotes to recognize parts written by others. I think that for Seeger and the people urging me to write my MP, the "problem" of unacknowledged authorship would not have occurred to them. The important thing was the message, and getting the message out to people.

Of course as an academic, throughout my lifetime unacknowledged authorship has been regarded as a very serious problem. To me and to every teacher I have had, unacknowledged authorship or plagiarism is a kind of theft and must not be tolerated. Besides being a species of theft, it is evidence of a lack of academic integrity in general. In this section I will provide a couple examples that have come across my desk as a journal editor.

To put the examples in context, I should tell you that I have been the Editor and/or Co-editor and Founder of 6 journals. Their names, year of first publication, number of volumes published, average number of articles per volume and total number of articles published to date are all given in Table 15.1. Because *Social Indicators Research* and the *Journal of Business Ethics* have routinely published special issues and supplementary volumes, the total number of articles generated by these 6 journals is certainly larger than the 7210 listed in the lower right-hand corner of the table. Out of 7210+ articles published, there have been 3 cases of investigation for unacknowledged authorship, one case reported but not yet investigated and one case reported but lost. Since 100% of the investigated cases turned out to be not only reported but actual cases of unacknowledged authorship, it is more likely than not that those yet to be investigated will have the same fate. Still, all things considered, I think it is fair to say that the vast majority of authors of our 7210+ articles have displayed academic integrity so far as the acknowledgement of authorship is concerned. One might say that on my watch and that of some close

Table 15.1 Summary of journals initiated

Journal name	First year	# vols. Pub.	Ave. # a.p.v.	Total # articles
Social Indicators Research	1974	94	30	2820
Journal of Business Ethics	1982	90	40	3600
Teaching Business Ethics	1997	7	40	280
Journal of Happiness Studies	1999	10	40	400
Journal of Academic Ethics	2002	7	40	280
Applied Research on Quality of Life	2005	3	30	90
Total	NA	211	220	7210

collaborators, we have had a very modest reported crime rate of less than one offence for every 1000 articles published. It is important to keep this in mind as we review the following two cases, both of which occurred in 2009.

A & B Case

The following summary was taken from the website of the Committee on Publication Ethics (COPE). COPE was asked for its opinion about a decision reached about the dispute between A and B.

> *Date*: 2010
>
> *Case Number*: 10–23
>
> Keywords: authorship sanctions for misconduct
>
> "*Anonymised Text of the Case*
>
> Our case relates to a paper (by author's A and B) that was retracted because of lack of acknowledgement of the contribution of another author (C). The retraction statement noted: "While the A/B paper is largely the work of A and B, it includes some sentences and ideas that previously appeared in an unpublished paper and/or Power Point presentation only with A and C listed as authors. We regret that the paper was published without any acknowledgement of the earlier collaborative work." Author A has contacted the journal expressing concern that this retraction is damaging his reputation.
>
> The basis for the retraction was evidence from C that parts of the A/B paper were the same as parts of a paper started by A and C but never finalized or published. C provided six specific cases involving about 23 lines of duplication. While this represents a small percentage (about 4%) of the total number of lines in the paper, because they duplicated lines from some version of the A/C paper, the editor believes there was a moral obligation on A and the new author (B) to acknowledge the earlier paper and/or the collaborative efforts of C.
>
> However, A claims that (1) s/he wrote all of the A/C paper, (2) asked C to identify his/her own material, (3) offered to delete any such material from the final paper with B, (4) received no instructions regarding what to delete and (5) proceeded to use whatever he liked and drop whatever he did not like. There is no way for anyone now to know exactly what A and/or C wrote in the various versions of the A/C paper or what exactly each contributed to the ideas that were presented in the PowerPoint presentation.
>
> The editor felt that there was a clear obligation on the part of A to acknowledge the earlier collaborative work with C, and that there was an equally clear obligation on the part of the journal to inform its readers that this acknowledgement was neglected in the A/B paper. A's obligation resulted from (1) all the collaborative efforts between himself and C, (2) the fact that both A and C were listed as authors of the PowerPoint presentation and the various versions of the unpublished paper, and (3) the fact that A's signature on the Statement of Authorship claiming originality of the entire work was not true.
>
> Author A is contesting the retraction and states that the posting has damaged his personal reputation and career. The case was referred to the publisher's Plagiarism and Piracy Task Force, but this committee could not agree, since some felt the editor had acted correctly, but others felt some sympathy with author A.

Advice

The Forum was unanimous in their opinion that they would not recommend retraction for misattribution of authorship or a missing acknowledgement (which could be resolved by a correction) or as a form of punishment for the authors (as stated in the COPE guidelines). A correction, rather than a retraction, would appear to be more appropriate in this case. An article should be retracted only if the findings are unreliable or in cases of serious misconduct such as plagiarism. Also, COPE does not advocate banning offending authors from publication for any period of time as it may have legal implications. The advice from the Forum was to retract the retraction using carefully agreed wording and publish a correction that acknowledges the original co-authorship of the original complainant. The Forum advised the editor to check the journal's guidelines on retraction and consult COPE's guidelines on retraction.

Resolution

On-going"

Source: http://publicationethics.org/case/lack-acknowledgement-contributor, accessed August 9, 2010.

The Editor and Publisher accepted COPE's suggestion and published a correction.

X & Y Case

The following summary was taken from the material required by editors according to Springer's *Policy on Publishing Integrity.*

"...In accordance with Springer's *Policy on Publishing Integrity,* I (1) studied the charges that Professor X made concerning the paper by Y... published for the *[Journal] Online First,* ... (2) sent a summary of the charges to Professor Y, requesting a response, (3) studied the response and (4) reached a decision regarding the appropriate action to take, all things considered.. ..

[The essence of the charges by X concern several passages in Y's *[Journal]* paper that appear identically or nearly identically in some papers by X without acknowledgement of X's papers. The essence of Y's replies is that the passages in question were not taken from X's papers but from some other papers without acknowledgement. Therefore, Y claimed, X's complaint was unwarranted. There was simply "an honest mistake in our referencing".]

... I do not find such mistakes acceptable and I believe that it would be a serious mistake if I agreed to simply have the correct references inserted and went ahead with publication...

More importantly,... the failure to acknowledge other people's papers ... cannot be accepted as a good reason for claiming freedom from any wrong doing in publishing the [*Journal*] paper.

By failing to appropriately acknowledge those other papers certainly and X's papers probably, the Y paper was not an "original" work as affirmed by Y's signature on the *Copyright Transfer Statement…*

All things considered, my recommendations are to (1) proceed with the retraction and follow-up actions as described in the *Policy* and (2) insert a retraction note…"

My recommendation to Springer was accepted and the retraction was inserted as proposed, but the hard copy version of the article had already gone to press and could not be called back. There is no way now to know what impact, if any, the retraction announcement will have on the future of this article and its authors.

Conclusion

Springer's *Policy on Publishing Integrity* is relatively new and retracting articles from *Online First* proved to be more complicated than any of us expected. In our current electronic age, with many electronic databases, abstracting services and so on that rapidly make our publications and parts of our publications visible in many places, retraction is very complicated and may be incomplete in the sense that things sent off to cyberspace often seem to have a life of their own. Besides being new, the *Policy on Publishing Integrity* is a work in progress in the sense that it will probably evolve and become more sophisticated as more editors of the company's some 2500 scholarly journals make use of it.

References

Aesop. (1998). *The complete fables* (O. Temple & R. Temple Trans.). London: Penguin Books.

Cline, A. (2010). *Synoptic gospel problem.* Retrieved May 2, 2010, from About.com Agnosticism/Atheism.

McGovern, U. (Ed.). (1997). *Chambers biographical dictionary.* Edinburgh: Chambers Harrap Publishers Ltd.

McInerney, J. (1998). *Ancient Greek civilization. Chantilly: Parts I and II.* Chantilly, Virginia: The Teaching Company.

Chapter 16
Building the Encyclopedia of Quality of Life and Well-Being Research

Alex C. Michalos

When I began thinking about writing this introduction, about what readers might want to know concerning the history, aims, scope and structure of the first ever *Encyclopedia of Quality of Life and Well-Being Research* (EQOLWR), it occurred to me almost immediately that I had never read the introduction of any encyclopedia. Like most other scholars, throughout my career (over 50 years now) I had read many entries from many different encyclopedias but never looked at any introductions or prefaces. Although such things are written for general, average or imagined readers, my guess is that practically nobody reads them except potential and/or actual encyclopedia editors, and occasionally editorial board members and authors. So, while this introduction is written from the point of view of what an average reader might want to know, the average reader I have in mind is an average editor, or maybe a board member or author.

Before I wrote this introduction, I read several others with considerable enthusiasm, interest and benefit. Indeed, before I decided to undertake building this encyclopedia, I read the introductions to several others. Without naming all the editors and their volumes, I would like to begin by thanking them. I owe a special thanks to a friend of many years, Carl Mitcham, the Editor in Chief of the *Encyclopedia of Science, Technology, and Ethics*. He generously shared his experiences producing that treatise and provided a fine example of an encyclopedia introduction. In the first sentence of the conclusion of his introduction, Mitcham wrote "In the world of high-intensity science and technology, how does one lead the good life?" The EQOLWR may be regarded as a comprehensive summary of ways to define, measure and achieve a good life for individuals and societies.

Michalos, A.C.: 2013. Building the Encyclopedia of Quality of Life and Well-Being Research.

A.C. Michalos (✉)
University of Northern British Columbia, Prince George, BC, Canada
e-mail: michalos@brandonu.ca

A.C. Michalos, *Connecting the Quality of Life Theory to Health, Well-Being and Education*, DOI 10.1007/978-3-319-51161-0_16

While the quantity of our lives is notoriously limited to one per person, its quality is as varied as the perspectives from which it is viewed. Viewed from one perspective, a person may be well-off, but from another not at all well-off (a fact noticed by Heraclitus in the fifth century BCE). Granting this, the whole research field of quality of life studies might be more accurately called 'qualities of life studies'. From this perspective, it is more accurate to speak of "a" rather than "the" good life.

History

Since I gave little thought to ever writing a historical overview or detailed discussion of the development of the encyclopedia, the story told here will be the best reconstruction I can make given the records I can find. Fortunately, my machine keeps email records better than I do. Unfortunately, it has no idea of what is or is not important. So, what we gain in abundance is not always helpful. In any case, like a good gardener, I will try to remove the weeds so the flowering plants can flourish.

The earliest summary I could find of the idea of an encyclopedia of social indicators and quality of life (QOL) research comes from a book proposal form submitted to Kluwer Academic Publishers dated February 2003. In broad strokes I proposed a treatise of 10 volumes, about 1000 pages per volume, with about 3000 articles covering 46 topic areas, with 4000 tables and 1000 figures. I suggested a very ambitious production time of about 5 years. This was a guess based on my review of the 8 volume (500 pages per volume, 1500 articles) *Encyclopedia of Psychology* and the 10 volume *Routledge Encyclopedia of Philosophy* (850 ppv, 2054 articles), both of which took 8 years to complete.

Following that proposal, I have a memo dated 30 June 2003 that I sent to what I called an Editorial Steering Committee (ESC). It is clear from the book proposal and memo that there had been previous discussions among members of the International Society for Quality of Life Studies (ISQOLS) and with representatives from Kluwer who had expressed interest in the idea. The previous discussions probably started in emails sometime before 2001 leading to face to face discussions that year at the ISQOLS conference in Washington, DC and the memo was prepared to facilitate further discussions at the 2003 conference in Frankfurt. In particular, the aim of the memo was to try to identify some scholars to serve on the ESC and to begin sketching a strategic plan of development. In that memo I suggested a set of about 15 Field Committees based on 46 topical fields that were mentioned in earlier discussions. The fields included topics related to quality of life measurement either as constituents, determinants or both, e.g., a person's health could be regarded as a constituent or a determinant of a good life, or both (as Aristotle noticed in the fifth century BCE). Each Field would have 2–4 coordinators and 20–30 editorial board members. The estimated number of articles had escalated from the 3000 in the book proposal to about 4600 (roughly 100 for each topical field) with article lengths ranging from a half page to five pages.

The 46 topical fields that I hoped to aggregate into 15 broader topic areas are listed here. In most cases one could add 'quality of life' before or after the topic name, since that is a basic assumption. Topics included historical antecedents (a) philosophic/religious views of the good life; historical antecedents (b) early views about its assessment/measurement; social indicators and social reporting in the relatively objective indicator tradition; subjective well-being/happiness tradition; QOL, a mix of traditions; data collection for single cases, focus groups, sample surveys; scales and scale construction; index construction; secondary analysis; forecasting; QOL of the elderly, of children and adolescents; disabilities; poverty; communities; income, consumption; gender; quality of work life and job satisfaction; work; marriage and family quality; community; religion/spirituality; leisure activities; health and health-related QOL; mental health; sex; housing and neighborhood quality; travel/tourism; sports; education; business; politics, government; science, technology; literature, performance and visual arts (music, dance, theatre, architecture); QOL in diverse countries; cities; states and provinces; environmental quality; urban development; planning; regional development; national development; globalization; sustainable development; process of welfare production. Besides these topics, it was assumed that there would be some short biographies mostly of recent scholars who had passed away, but also of some ancient writers whose works display the antiquity of many of our research questions and some answers.

If we could get 15 aggregated fields out of those 46 and 20–30 board members for each of the 15, we would have a large board with from 300 to 450 members. To identify potential article topics, my plan was to circulate a long list among field coordinators and have some sort of ranking procedure to obtain a final short list. Since my five volume *North American Social Report: A Comparative Study of the Quality of Life in Canada and the USA from 1964 to 1974* had a total set of indexes with about 1350 subject topics, the 4600 topics proposed for the ISQOLS project seemed unproblematic. Beginning with that list, I prepared a list of 4300 potential article topics working from indexes of research studies on social indicators, quality of life, sustainable development, statistics, health-related quality of life, economic accounts, back issues of the journal *Social Indicators Research* and *SINET: Social Indicators Network News*, and a variety of web sites. I imagined that given a team of workers, a longer list could be generated fairly easily, although I had not imagined exactly how.

Alas, after making some calculations about what it might cost (in time, energy and money) to deliver the 10 volume treatise, it rapidly became clear that Kluwer could not afford it. The company might have funded something smaller, but nothing smaller seemed very interesting to me. Once we reached that point in our discussions, I lost interest and withdrew from further discussions.

From 2003 to 2008, I pretty much had given up on the idea of an encyclopedia altogether. I had the suspicion that with its search engines, the internet replaced any need we might have had for encyclopedias. Unfortunately, I don't have any good records indicating further discussions about it, although I suppose there must have been some. Sometime in that period, Kluwer had been bought out by Springer, and my friend and main contact with Kluwer, Myriam Poort, began representing Springer. In an email letter dated 23 December 2008, Myriam wrote to me summarizing issues we discussed at the World Business Ethics Forum sponsored by Hong Kong Baptist University a couple weeks earlier. Here is the paragraph of interest to our history.

> We will both look for a possible Editor to develop the Encyclopedia of Social Indicators as originally proposed by you. I have given this some more thought. What do you think about the following construction? You would be the Editor and would define the set up and have general overview. We would appoint a young and upcoming co-editor who is responsible for managing the projects, contacts with authors and reviewers and the day to day business. This way the project would not burden your workload but it would have your name connected to it, which, I believe, is essential for its success given your presence and authority in the field of Social Indicators. A young and upcoming Editor may be eager to take on the job to establish his or her name in the field.

Here is my reply the next day.

> Maybe this would work if we could find such a person. Let's think and look and see what we come up with. I was thinking about the encyclopedia this morning and it occurred to me that it would be an even more impressive project if we included a full account of the health-related quality of life research tradition in it. I do have stuff from that tradition in my proposal, but I am thinking of giving it more attention just because it is a very big field now. Have you ever tried interesting any of those people in an encyclopedia of health-related qol? They are generally pretty narrowly focused on medical practice and health issues, but all that stuff is relevant to qol studies. Still, they may want to go their own way.

On 5 January 2009 I wrote,

> I reread all the material I had on the encyclopedia…We should talk some more, especially so you can give me an idea of what size project you have in mind (number of volumes, investment dollars, possible fees to authors, to me, etc. what timelines for delivery, that sort of thing). I am still thinking that health-related quality of life research should be included fairly substantially and I also think the project might go more smoothly if it were not an ISQOLS or an ISOQOL [International Society for Quality of Life Research] project. Then I would be freer to develop it using the best ideas and talent we can find.

She replied 13 January,

> …I agree completely that health-related qol should be a substantial part of the encyclopedia and that it will take multiple years to complete such work. Also, I see the advantages of keeping the work separate from any Society.

On 12 February she wrote,

> …I am very enthusiastic about publishing an encyclopedia that covers the entire field of quality of life/well-being, including health-related quality of life. I have written already to our Reference Editorial Office that you may be visiting Germany early in April and asked if someone can join our meeting. I look forward to exploring this idea in further detail with you and look forward to your notes.

While we were both committed to including health-related quality of life research in the encyclopedia, in the fall of that year (2009) Springer published a *Handbook of Disease Burdens and Quality of Life Measures.* On Springer's website that book is described as "a state-of-the-art book on the measures of disease" containing about 200 contributions. More precisely, it is about the "impact of disease" on everything "from the financial costs of treatment to the effects of a particular condition on the quality of life". It is therefore more narrowly targeted than this encyclopedia, but provides a natural and welcome complementary treatise.

In response to some material I sent to her which I cannot find, on 26 February she sent me a relatively long email sketching her views about what Springer would provide and how things would work. Among other things, she said the encyclopedia would have

> ...a dedicated Editor available...for as much time as needed...it is generally the Section Editors...who send out informal invitations. Naturally, the Editor-in-Chief will also make invitations. Springer can take care of all invitations should you not wish to contact authors ahead informally...[Encyclopedia of Quality of Life Research]...sounds like a good working title...Perhaps at a later stage we can think of a number of titles...Aim/Focus: To provide a comprehensive reference work emphasizing the past 50 years or so of scientific research on the quality of life, including health-related quality of life...Editorial Structure: I agree a flat structure will probably work best [i.e., no committees between the EiC, board members and authors]...Size:...Our MRW's [Major Reference Work] usually count about 800 pages per volume which would make it a 7 to 8 volume work...We should probably find a balance between an acceptable price and size...Workload:...something we should also discuss...Time Frame: I would prefer to initially plan for a total of 4 years... Compensation:...I would like to get feedback from our Sales Staff....

In the following weeks after this letter, further exchanges occurred leading to signing a contract on 23 June 2009. The contract committed me to delivering and the publisher to publishing a manuscript with a "maximum of 8000 and no less than 6400 printed pages" (i.e., roughly 8–10 volumes). The estimated publication date was August 2012.

Aims

Having sketched the history of how this encyclopedia came to be, it is worthwhile to consider why. Without claiming any particular order of importance, the following aims are most salient.

One important aim is to display in one place the vast scope and complexity of scientific and other scholarly research on quality of life mainly over the last 50 years. This is something that search engines of the internet do not do very well. They are good at finding everything remotely relevant to a topic, but not very good at finding quite specific things significantly related to a topic. When I became interested in this field of research in the late 1960s, there was no central resource bank of relevant exploration and knowledge. Researchers published in their own disciplines, e.g., sociologists wrote for sociologists in journals devoted to the discipline, sharing the same sorts of education, assumptions, language, practices and goals. A sociologist could write and publish papers dealing with quality of life or well-being issues, but such papers often enough would not find an interested audience outside of the discipline. I recall reading well-written grant proposals well into the 1980s and 1990s in which, for example, the relevant literature from economics would be taken into account, without any notice of the vast literature in sociology, psychology and political science dealing with the same subject matter. My assessments would include something like 'If this proposal were aimed only at enlightening economists about the topic, it might be worth funding. However, the proposal is aimed to break new ground in the field of quality of life research and that it cannot do because the field is much greater than the economic literature reveals'.

When I started the journal *Social Indicators Research* in 1973, it had the subtitle "An International and Interdisciplinary Journal for Quality of Life Measurement". The most important aim in creating the journal was to attract research papers to a single site, relieving me as well as other interested scholars of some of the burden of looking for them all over the place. To some extent, that venture paid off exactly as I hoped it would. Over the years, the journal not only attracted relevant papers but it helped create a network of authors and readers from diverse disciplines, inside and outside the academy. An encyclopedia is a good instrument for building the same sort of central repository only, in this case at least, its focus is to assemble a comprehensive review over a particular period of time.

A second aim of the encyclopedia follows from the first. The diverse network of scholars that is loosely assembled by contributing to and drawing from a common source is likely to stimulate cross-disciplinary research leading to a greater progressive, comprehensive and coherent vision of the field. By assembling a greater variety of building blocks, a greater variety of buildings will emerge.

An improved vision of the field provides a rough road map giving some direction to the next 10–20 years of research, a third aim of the encyclopedia. One of the marks of an established field of research is researchers' sense of its current boundaries, the frontiers representing limits of our knowledge and inviting future explorations. Readers of an encyclopedia can get an overview of the density of research in different areas, where the focus has been and where it might go next. For example, in this encyclopedia, with some searching, one can see that the impacts on the quality of life are profoundly under-studied regarding arts-related activities, natural and human-crafted environments, sports, religion, sex, sustainability and good governance.

Because the possession of a good measure of the quality of life is a necessary condition for possessing a good measure of its sustainability, I hoped to include more essays dealing with issues of sustainable development. The relationship between these two measures was made quite clear as long ago as 1987 in the Brundtland Commission on Environment and Development Report when they wrote, "Sustainable development is development that meets the needs of the present without compromising the ability of future generations to meet their own needs… beyond their basic needs these people have legitimate aspirations for an improved quality of life". In short, we have to measure what we want to sustain, what resources are required to sustain it and the rates of change of each relative to the other.

Fourth, the encyclopedia should provide an authoritative, well-informed resource serving the needs not only of scholars and students, but of ordinary citizens, elected and un-elected government officials, non-governmental organizations (NGOs) and socially responsible corporations. This is a huge challenge for authors and readers with very different kinds of education, life experiences, needs, wants and goals. While all of those who helped build this encyclopedia hope that most of it will be accessible and useful to most interested readers, one cannot expect that every essay will serve the purposes, interests and education of every reader.

Notwithstanding the limitations just mentioned, the encyclopedia has been built with an aim (the fifth) to improving private and public policy analyses and discussions leading to better decisions and policy making concerning the quality of life of individuals and societies. At a minimum, I hope that the treatise will contribute to the development and spread of evidence-based and value-based decision and policy making. In particular, it is hoped that a contribution will be made to democratic practices and democracy in general.

Sixth, I aimed to have an international and multi-disciplinary Editorial Board of distinguished scholars and a collection of essays by equally distinguished authors. That would ensure that readers directed to this encyclopedia would find a comprehensive collection of relevant, reliable and valid research reports.

Seventh, I aimed to make maximum use of the latest technology to link encyclopedia essays to other works available in electronic form. The strategy of the encyclopedia is to have relatively short essays with many links to other relevant essays so readers will be helped to build a package of information that most precisely fits their needs. Links made in this encyclopedia will be picked up in Springer's approximately 200 other reference works. Besides publication in hard copy and ebook versions, the encyclopedia will be open-ended and online allowing authors to update essays and editors to insert additional essays. If and when the next edition of the encyclopedia is produced, all updated and brand new essays will be integrated into it.

Finally, while the focus is on the last 50 years of research, my aim was to build a treatise worthy of its illustrious scholarly predecessors extending at least to the fifth century BCE. I would like to think that this is the sort of work Plato or Aristotle might have appreciated and even produced if they had access to resources available today.

Besides pursuing these seven relatively professional aims, there were a couple of more personal motives for undertaking the work. One was simply the attraction of the challenge of building such a large treatise. It has been more of a challenge and required considerably more work than I imagined. Originally, I estimated about 10 h per week over 4 years. For the last 2 years it has been about 30 h per week and we will complete 5 years by the time the volumes and ebook come out. In fact, since signing the contract in 2009, I am sure I have averaged much more than 10 h per week.

A second motive proceeded from asking myself ‘Now that I am in my 70s, of the things I am able to do, what is it that I most love doing?’. The answer came quickly and unequivocally. I most enjoy learning and building. It seemed to me that building an encyclopedia would keep me as close to my first loves as I could get at this stage of my life. I think building an encyclopedia requires more organizational than creative skills, though I suppose I would be hard pressed to distinguish creating a good organization and work plan from creating anything else. An Editor in Chief has to have a fairly clear product in mind, design a strategic plan of action, build a team willing and able to implement the plan and then keep the team moving along until the goal is achieved. Of course, patience is certainly a virtue with this sort of activity, though not, I think, one that I have in great measure.

It is worth mentioning here that I have not aimed to produce a treatise free of bias. On the contrary, I have a bias toward free discussion from diverse perspectives. The encyclopedia is not intended to be free of controversial assessments or of some repetition of discussions of various topics. In a work of this sort and size, coming from authors with diverse backgrounds, interests and perspectives, writing on topics that usually do not have established boundaries, one should not expect universal agreement. Like a great university or a great scholarly journal, a great encyclopedia should provide a shared public space for the exploration of what is true, beautiful and morally good.

Structure and Scope

So far, I have described how and why the encyclopedia came to be. In this section I will provide an overview of the procedural structure on which the treatise has been built and upon which its contents rest. The place to begin is with the question ‘What procedure was used to determine which topics should appear in the encyclopedia?’. The procedure adopted was largely a consequence of the assumption made that a scientific field of research is whatever its key researchers say and/or show it is. Beginning with that assumption, it is obvious that an empirical or inductive procedure of selection is required.

It would be foolish to deny that any a priori criterion of relevance to quality of life or well-being research was used. It has already been shown that a group of ISQOLS scholars agreed that 46 broad-based areas of concern were appropriate, although no criterion was suggested for deciding what is appropriate. That list was never abandoned. However, what was specifically excluded a priori was an attempt to create a conceptual structure or theory that would provide a neat place for all and only those topics belonging to the field. No such theory exists and it is my view that our current understanding of what belongs in the field is still so unclear, diverse and complex that any a priori designed theory would be a mythological procrustean bed that would mislead and constrain future research.

Our procedure began in July 2009 with a key word search undertaken by Springer’s Daniel Quinones of 16 Springer journals with some focus directly or indirectly on quality of life and well-being research. The journals included the five central ones, *Social Indicators Research*, Quality *of Life Research; Journal of Happiness Studies; Applied Research on Quality of Life; Child Indicators Research*; plus *American Journal of Community Psychology; American Sociologist; Asia Europe Journal; Gender Issues; Journal of Housing and Built Environment; Cross-Cultural Gerontology; International Journal of Politics, Culture and Society; Ecohealth; and Sex Roles.* This produced about 13,500 candidate topics for the encyclopedia. I added these to the 4300 gathered earlier and began reading through the lot deleting duplicates and likely outliers, and combining near synonyms.

It rapidly became clear that I would need additional help to continue all the sorting and culling that would be required over the next few months. So I invited my friend and colleague, Maurine Kahlke, with whom I had collaborated in several projects over the past 8 years or so, to join the Editorial Board and work with me. By January 2010 it was clear that her contribution was more like that of an Associate Editor than a standard Board member. So she was invited to and became the Associate Editor. By November 2009 we had reduced the roughly 17,800 topics to 10,000. From this number, we intended to get down to about 3000. For this, we estimated that we needed the help of about 200 Board members.

Prospective Board Members were invited from the boards of the five central journals and a variety of other sources including scholars who had published particularly relevant and good papers and/or books, who had been particularly good reviewers of manuscripts for the central journals, and members of the two central professional societies, ISQOLS and ISOQOL. The earliest formal invitation letter to prospective Board members seems to have been mailed out to 232 people in October 2009. By March 2011, our prospective list became an actual list of 177 members. By May 2012 the list had decreased to 156 as Board members withdrew or were dropped for one reason or another. Although Board members have continued to come and go over the life of the project, that number has been fairly steady to the end. Their names and brief bios are listed in the encyclopedia.

On 3 November 2009, a letter was sent to 172 Board members describing the voting procedures that would be used to obtain a working list of topics. The letter follows.

Voting Procedures for Encyclopedia Entries

When all returns are in we will have about 200 editorial board members and 260 pages of candidate entries. In order to share the burden of selecting entries, reducing about 10,000 candidate-entries to 3000 entries, the following procedures will be used.

The 10,000 candidate-entries were obtained from key word searches in 16 journals central to quality of life research. Many candidate entries have numbers in parentheses following them (e.g., child wellbeing (6)) indicating the number of times that key word appeared in diverse articles.

The board members will be divided into 10 equal-sized groups based on our alphabetical list, e.g., Board Group 1 = BG1 = members Aaronson to Cerin, BG2 = Chamberlain to Eckermann, etc. to BG10.

The 260 pages of candidate entries will also be divided into 10 groups of about 26 pages each based on our alphabetical list, e.g., Entry Group 1 = EG1 = Abdominal pain to Cancer care, EG2 = Cancer patients to Cultural health index, etc. to EG10. On average, in 26 pages there are about 935 candidate-entries.

Each Entry Group will be randomly assigned to each Board Group.

Each Board Group member will receive a complete list of all candidate-entries, about 260 pages, 10,000 items in an EXCEL file.

Then each Board Member will be asked to read only the 26 pages of entries in the Entry Group assigned to him or her and provide the following information:

1. In the EXCEL file: Enter an X in the column in front of each candidate-entry that in your opinion should be included in the encyclopedia, keeping in mind our approximate limit of 3000 entries. Simply ignore entries that do not appear important to you.
2. In addition to the first task and also in the EXCEL file, feel free to browse the entire 260 pages entering Ys in the column in front of candidate-entries that you believe should also be included.
3. The expertise of our board members varies across a huge research territory and we need each member to try to make sure vital topics are not neglected. Therefore, in addition to returning the updated EXCEL file via email, in your covering letter to me, please list any candidate-entries that you believe should be but are not yet included in the email message.

We are allowing about 3 weeks for all members to vote on all candidate-entries.

At the end of the voting period, we will count Xs and Ys in support of every candidate entry. Extra listed candidate-entries will also be counted, with numbers of times an item is emailed in substituting for Xs.

A selection will be made by the Editor-in-Chief with the advice of some editorial board members of a final list of entries based partly on (1) numerical support for each candidate-entry, (2) original number of times the candidate-entry appeared as a key word in some journal article and (3) a qualitative assessment of the importance of the candidate-entry to the total set of entries from the point of view of covering the broad scope of the encyclopedia.

After a selection of entries has been made, Board Members will receive another set of procedures for assigning on average about 15 entries to each Member (some will no doubt do less and some probably more) who then has the responsibility of identifying authors to be invited to write short, medium or long articles. Springer's Reference Works Department will look after the contacts, follow-ups and so on.

By 26 December 2009 about 90 (52%) of the Board members had produced a list of about 7650 candidate topics with one or more supporters. We took about the top ranked 3500 of those topics for the next step in our procedures. For the next step, Board members were asked to select around 15 topics for which they would be willing to try to find authors, obtain essays, have two peer reviews of each, get any required revisions and finally approve them. The completion of these tasks required quite a commitment in time from our members but we managed to get about 1838 topics selected by April 2010. In that month, we sent out another letter headed “Completing Assignments of Board Members’ Responsibilities for EQOLR Entries” [Encyclopedia of Quality of Life Research was our working title] which, among other things, provided more and asked for more information. Here are the most important passages concerning entry/topic selection.

> To complete our matching of topic entries to Board Members, you will find an EXCEL file also attached to this letter. This file has 2 parts.
>
> First, it begins with a list of all entries organized alphabetically according to Board Members’ last names. You can read this part of the file to get a quick overview of your current assignments and everyone else’s. You will see that assignments run from 1 (which is too few) to 76 (which is too many). You will also see that, not counting the dozen or so new Board Members on this list who will be making selections for the first time this round, nearly 40 of our original Board Members have not made any selections. It is, unfortunately, likely that we will have to find replacements for most of these 40 people in order to complete our ambitious plan for the EQOLR. This letter is our last *Cri du Coeur* for a response.
>
> Second, following the list of entries organized according to Board Members’ last names, there is a list of all unclaimed/unassigned entries organized alphabetically.
>
> Each of us now has 5 questions to answer about entries in the EXCEL file.
>
> 1. Do you want to drop any entries for which you are currently assigned responsibility to find authors? If so, which?
> 2. Would you be willing and able to add any entries to your list from the list of currently unclaimed/unassigned entries? If so, which? To add any, simply put an x in the column in front of those entries and return the EXCEL file, or just write the entry names in a return letter to me.
> 3. Are there still important entries of any sort that you think we should add, whether you can look after them or not? For examples, there are hundreds of standardized tests, several hundred places (cities, counties, countries, regions) and perhaps a few dozen departed pioneers, all of which might merit an entry. If so, please write in the names in a return letter to me.
> 4. In the column immediately following each of your entries, can you recommend the length of the article probably needed from one of these 3 types: Short = 100 to 600 words, Medium = 600 to 1800 words or Long = 1800 to 3000 words? Encyclopedia pages have roughly 600 words per page. Where you are able to do so, simply write in S, M or L in that column for each entry. (There are sample entries and templates for entries on the Encyclopedia website: http://refworks.springer.com/QURE/.)
> 5. Can you recommend any good scholars who might be willing and able to join the Editorial Board to take responsibility for some of the remaining unclaimed/unassigned entries? If so, please write in the name(s) and email address(es) if you have it(them).

…The Associate Editor, Maurine Kahlke, and I will create a final list of Board Member names matched to entries, and this list will be distributed to all Members at the end of the exercise. Hopefully, the list will be in your hands by June 1, 2010. We will allow ourselves the month of June to sort out problems of any sort.

Finally, as indicated in our earlier correspondence, in order to have most of the writing and reviewing of entries going on during the 10 months from July 2010

> to April 2011, we ask Board Members to not begin contacting prospective authors until July 1, 2010. Until we have the final list, we cannot say exactly who will be responsible for what. As much as possible, we would like to have the bulk of the entries written and reviewed in that 10 month period, so most of them are contemporaries and authors do not suffer delays in publication of the whole EQOLR waiting for others. Our work plan allows about 4 months for an author to write an entry.

As it turned out, by September 2010 we still had 27 Board members who had not made any selections and they were dropped from the Board. However, by January 2011 we had increased the Board numbers to 196 and decreased the number of topics to 3308 with 2444 (74%) selected by some member. Out of the 2444 selected topics, Board members had identified authors for 582 (24%). We had made progress, but there was still much to be done. From roughly the beginning of 2011 to the middle of 2012 I undertook a more detailed examination of abstracts in about 50 journals covering the years from 2009 to 2012 identifying additional topics and authors where we seemed to have fewer essays that I thought we should have.

The January report to all Board members became the first of reports released about every two months for the remaining months of the project. In the January report, we said "our deadline for the press to receive final versions of all articles should be January 1, 2012". A year later at the end of January we sent out a report to all Board members and authors indicating that no more essays would be accepted for the first edition hard copy and ebook versions of the encyclopedia after 28 February 2013. Essays coming in after that date would be considered for the next edition and for the online open-ended version of circulation with Digital Object Identifiers (DOIs).

The hard copy and ebook versions were released in March 2014.

On behalf of Maurine and myself, we would like to thank the Springer Reference Works staff for making contacts, reminding editors and authors to meet deadlines, copy-editing material written in different styles, working with unfamiliar software and essay templates, and a set of guidelines for authors that appears to provide more information than anyone would want.

Chapter 17
Milestones of Quality of Life Research in Canada, 1960s to 2014

Alex C. Michalos

Introduction

While the quantity of our lives is notoriously limited to one per person, the quality is as varied as the perspectives from which it is viewed. So, it would be more accurate to discuss the qualities of life or aspects of human well-being, although the historical fact is that the terms most often used are 'quality of life' and 'well-being' as if they designated one thing. These terms, like 'justice', 'love' and 'democracy', are generally open-textured and not closed by general agreement on a single thing.

Social Indicators Research 1973

The journal *Social Indicators Research* had the subtitle "An international and interdisciplinary journal for quality of life measurement". It was founded in 1973 and published its first issue in 1974. The founder was Alex C. Michalos who was then at the University of Guelph. At this writing the journal has generated 113 volumes. Michalos served as editor for 40 years and was replaced by Filomena Maggino beginning January 2014. The journal was the first and remains the most comprehensive journal devoted to quality of life studies. It is a deep mine of research from all over the world, about topics and issues coming from authors all over the world, peer reviewed by scholars from all over the world. Celebrating the first 30 years of the journal, a collection of citation classics was published in Michalos

---

Michalos, A.C.: 2016. Milestones of quality of life research in Canada, 1960s to 2014.

A.C. Michalos (✉)
University of Northern British Columbia, Prince George, BC, Canada
e-mail: michalos@brandonu.ca

A.C. Michalos, *Connecting the Quality of Life Theory to Health, Well-Being and Education*, DOI 10.1007/978-3-319-51161-0_17

(2005) which contains an article written in 1978 providing a detailed account of the origins and nature of the journal. A collection of articles written between 1985 and 2003 mostly covering issues in Canada was published in Michalos (2003). In particular, there are articles on quality of life measurement connected to aggregating indicators to measure sustainable human well-being, militarism, migration, job and marital satisfaction, optimism, health of adults, health of older people, leisure activities, public services, criminal victimization, policing services, feminism, ethnicity and modern prejudice, trust and multiple discrepancies theory.

Table 17.1 lists the 10 most frequently cited articles in *Social Indicators Research* in its first 40 years of publication. Five (with *) were in the top 10 in the first 30 years too (Michalos 2005, p. 32).

Table 17.1 Top 10 cited articles from *Social Indicators Research* 1974–2014

Cites	Article
519	Diener, E.* Assessing subject well-being: progress and opportunities 1994, v. 31, n. 2, 103–157
478	Lyubomirsky, S. and H.S. Lepper A measure of subjective happiness: Preliminary reliability and construct 1999, v. 46, n. 2, 137–155
372	Diener, E. and E. Suh Measuring quality of life: economic, social and subjective indicators 1997, v. 40, ns. 1–3, 189–216
349	Michalos, A.C.* Multiple discrepancies theory (MDT) 1985, v. 16, n. 4, 347–413
333	Diener, E. and R. Biswas-Diener Will money increase subjective well-being? 2002, v. 57, n. 2, 119–169
302	Veenhoven, R.* Is happiness relative? 1991, v. 24, n. 1, 1–34
288	Diener, E., E. Sandvik, L. Seidlitz and M. Diener The relationship between income and subjective well-being 1993, v. 28, n. 3, 195–223
266	Cummins, R.A. The domains of life satisfaction: an attempt to order chaos 1996, v. 38, n. 3, 303–328
230	Shin, D.C. and D.M. Johnson* Avowed happiness as an overall assessment of the quality of life 1978, v. 5, n. 4, 475–492
199	Andrews, F.M. and S.B. Withey* Developing measures of perceived life quality: results from several national surveys 1974, v. 1, n. 1, 1–26

Perspectives Canada 1974, 1977 and 1980

In 1974 Statistics Canada launched a collection of statistical time series beginning with the title *Perspective Canada I.* Because so many readers had noted that the first two volumes were really about "a set of perspectives rather than a single integrated view", beginning with the third volume, the series was re-titled *Perspectives Canada*, with an 's' (*Perspectives Canada III* 1980). Unfortunately, the third volume turned out to be the last in the series.

A short time after the appearance of the first volume, Michalos was told by the Chief Statistician (Sylvia Ostry) that the volume represented something like an "entry fee" for Statistics Canada. The characterization was appropriate in two senses insofar as the volume was the first investment in a new line of research and publication, and a demonstration that Canada's official statistical agency had joined the group of other nations (e.g., the United States, Germany, United Kingdom, Sweden, the Netherlands) building national social reports of one sort or another. Good overviews of country activities in the early years of the field's development may be found in Berger-Schmitt and Jankowitsch (1999) and Hass et al. (2002).

In the introductory chapter of the third volume, readers are told that the

> ...book is more than a collection of statistics. It is rather a set of descriptive essays which rely primarily on statistics to provide a variety of perspectives on the social and economic future of Canadian life...the volume contains selected social statistics brought together within some covering theme. The ultimate intention of the series is to complement this approach by publishing, in addition, indicators of social well-being – what have traditionally been called 'social indicators'...Economic indicators are measures of our country's economic well-being...Social indicators will issue from theories about sub-components of the social system such as health and education and the elements of well-being that these bring to individuals...Thus the role of *Perspectives Canada* will be to describe our social and economic well-being both in terms of indicators that should allow us to assess our position, and in terms of discussions of the social changes that interplay to effect that well-being (*Perspectives Canada III* 1980).

The perspectives of the third volume were organized around 15 themes described in 15 chapters, namely, population, family, health, education, work, income and consumption, social security, leisure, crime and justice, Indians and Métis, urban profiles, environment, use of energy, general perceptions on the quality of life, vignettes of Canada and the United States. Each chapter is stocked with charts and tables, but no precise list of statistical time series or candidate-social indicators used. So there is also no complete list for the whole volume and no clear, comprehensive assessment of Canadian society, its progress or regress. (An interesting assessment of *Perspective Canada II* and the U.S. *Social Indicators 1976* can be found in Brusegard 1979.)

Quality of Canadian Life: Social Change in Canada 1977, 1979 and 1981

This was a pioneering set of national surveys undertaken by Tom Atkinson, Bernard R. Blishen, Michael D. Ornstein, H. Michael Stevenson and Bryn Greer-Wotton at the Institute for Behavioral Research (IBR), York University. While several publications appeared following the 1977 survey, I have found only one publication based on the joint use of the 1977 and 1979 surveys, and nothing seems to have been published about the quality of life items from the 1981 survey. Atkinson (1979) used national survey data from Meisel (1973) and LeDuc et al. (1974) to craft a trend line from 1968 to 1977 for three roughly comparable general life satisfaction questions.

The text of each of the questions was:

- 1968 Would you say that in general you are very satisfied, fairly satisfied, a little dissatisfied, or quite dissatisfied with your life so far?
- 1974 Let's think about your life as a whole. Would you say that you are very satisfied, fairly satisfied, a little dissatisfied or very dissatisfied with your life as a whole right now?
- 1977 All things considered, how satisfied or dissatisfied are you with your life as a whole? Which number comes the closest to how you feel?

1	2	3	4	5	6	7	8	9	10	11
Completely Dissatisfied					Neutral					Completely Satisfied

(Atkinson 1979, Appendix)

In an earlier study, Atkinson (1977) had shown that the two highest responses in the 1977 scale were comparable to the 'very satisfied' responses in the 1968 and 1974 scales. Using this alteration of the 1977 scale, the percentages of each sample responding 'very satisfied' were 39% in 1968 (N = 2734), 34% in 1974 (N = 1234) and 35% in 1977(N = 3289), a modestly downward trend over the decade (Atkinson 1979). Canada's 1977 percent of 'very satisfied' respondents ranked fourth among eight European countries surveyed in 1975, with Denmark first at 54%, then Republic of Ireland (50%) and Belgium (36%) (Atkinson 1979, Table 17.2).

Atkinson (1980) summarized more findings from the 1977 survey, including a rank ordering of Canadian respondents' satisfaction with 13 domains of life plus life as a whole, city and province of residence and country. Summing scores for the top two response categories (i.e., 11 and 10), percentages of respondents 'very satisfied' were as follows: marriage 60%, children 59%, neighborhood 44%, friends 41%, job 32%, housing and leisure activities each 31%, housework 29%, romantic life (of unmarried persons) 28%, health and amount of leisure time each 25%, financial situation 20%. Domain rankings with marriage, children and/or living partner at the top and financial situation at the bottom are quite usual for quality of life surveys (Michalos 2003, 2005). The rank orders for political jurisdictions were respondents' cities 44%, provinces 39% and Canada as a whole 22%. Governments getting higher satisfaction ratings as they get closer to respondents is also a fairly typical finding.

Blishen and Atkinson (1980, p. 25) used the 1977 survey results to assess the degree to which Anglophone and Francophone Canadians had different perceptions of the quality of life that might have helped "to inform the participants in the national debate about one element in their desire to continue or discontinue the present conferation". Overall quality of life was measured by the satisfaction with life as a whole question and responses were compared to a question about satisfaction with life in Canada. Briefly, what they found was that

> Francophones are more satisfied than Anglophones with life in general and with their current financial situation, but Anglophones are more satisfied than Francophones with life in Canada. In both language groups, life satisfaction tends to increase with age and income...However, these data do not provide support for the assumption that the Francophone discontent now evident in Canada, particularly in the Province of Quebec, is related to satisfaction with life in general or with financial situation. We would conclude that support for independence in Quebec draws very little on economic discontent and frustration...Although both sides in the political debate over Quebec's future often use economic arguments, it would seem that they are not likely to be the reasons that carry the issue (Blishen and Atkinson 1980, pp. 38–39).

Mckennell et al. (1980, p. 112) used data from national surveys in Britain, Canada and the USA in the 1976–1977 period to show that "Around 50 to 60 percent of the variance in feelings about life-as-a-whole can be accounted for by a linear additive combination of the evaluations made in some dozen separate domains. Moreover, the greater part of the explained variance is accounted for by just the first half dozen from the set of domains". This so-called Bottom-Up approach to explaining satisfaction and/or happiness with life as a whole on the basis of satisfaction with particular domains was the most frequently used model throughout the 1970s. From the 1980s on, so-called Top-Down models and Bi-Directional models have also been used (Michalos 2005; Mallard et al. 1997).

In the final important piece of research coming from the IBR surveys, Atkinson (1982) used a panel format in which a representative sample of 2,162 Canadians were interviewed in 1977 and again in 1979. According to Michalos and Kahlke (2010, p. 404) "Apart from some results dealing with a subset (N = 285) of the national sample used in Campbell et al. (1976), this was the first published report 'on the stability of QOL measures over time'". It also became a citation classic from *Social Indicators Research* (Michalos 2005). Respondents in 1979 were asked if their lives in general and for specific domains were essentially the same as in 1977, better or worse. As well they were asked which of 16 significant life events they had experienced in that period, e.g., divorce/separation, serious injury, new job or house. Comparing responses to satisfaction questions and these life change assessments, he reported that

> The hypothesis that the No Change group would have more stable QOL scores than those reporting change is supported when the perceptual indicator of change is used as the independent variable but not when the event measures are involved...[As well] Relationships between self-reported change and satisfaction levels are always higher than between events and changes in satisfaction (Atkinson 1982, pp. 122, 126).

Michalos and Kahlke (2010, p. 431) replicated some of Atkinson's results using 27 of the most frequently used quality of life measures on a panel of 462 residents of British Columbia distributed across 3 different points in time in 2005, 06 and 07. Among other things, they found that 46% of their respondents reported changes in their life circumstances using each of Atkinson's two different measures of change. They also found that the quality of life indicators "behaved more often than not (61.7%) as expected using the 'perceptual indicator of change' but less often than not (37.3%) as expected using 'event measures'". (The author owes special thanks to Michael Ornstein and Bryn Greer-Wootten for information on the IBR surveys.)

North American Social Report 1980–1982

The first and most comprehensive attempt to assess the overall quality of life in Canada was undertaken as part of a larger project comparing the quality of life in Canada with that in the United States in the period from 1964 to 1974 (Michalos 1980a, b, 1981a, b, 1982). He began by constructing a classificatory scheme from which questions could be generated and into the conceptual slots of which data could be sorted. After a few years (of 12 required) collecting reasonably comparable statistics on Canada and the United States and placing these pairs neatly into appropriate conceptual pigeonholes, the exercise appeared to be a waste of time. The indicators tended to aggregate themselves in the sense that some of them seemed to fit together as one episode of a story while others belonged to a somewhat different episode. There was virtually no indicator that could not be integrated into a different episode or a different part of the total picture. There was no indicator that absolutely had to go here rather than there on pain of talking nonsense or radically distorting the "true" picture—whatever that might be. Accordingly, the sets of paired indicators considered in each of the resulting chapters of the treatise were there because they were available, seemed to provide important information about the quality of life in the two countries and seemed to belong next to the other indicators in the chapter. (The procedure was pragmatic as defined in Michalos et al. 2011.)

The 13 areas of concern are: population; death, disease and health care; housing; crime and justice; recreation; transportation and communication; education; science and technology; government and organizations; natural environment and resources; economics; religion; morality and social customs. Indicators used were objective (e.g., crime rates) and subjective (e.g., satisfaction with personal future), negative (e.g., crime rates) and positive (e.g., educational achievement). Negative indicators are such that as their indicator numerical values increase, some aspect of the quality

Table 17.2 Comparative quality of life scores, 1964–1974

Social indicators	Canada	USA
Population density	2	1
Illegitimate live births	15	4
Crude death rate	11	0
Abortion rate	1	0
Percent Canadian/American immigrants	13	6
Canadians/Americans changing citizenship	9	13
Population subtotal	*51*	*23*
Infant mortality	15	4
Percent of smokers	0	1
Believers in connection between smoking and cancer	0	1
Suicide	9	10
Tobacco and alcohol expenditures	8	11
Selected reportable diseases	17	2
Blindness	10	0
Hospital occupancy	6	10
Mean stay in hospitals	0	9
Surgical operations	2	14
Patients in public mental hospitals	13	4
Patients in public institutions for mentally retarded	11	3
Food energy available	3	12
Supplies of nutrients	5	9
Food expenditures	14	5
Physicians	6	11
Registered nurses	9	0
Hospital beds	9	0
Combined personal/gov. health care expenditure	10	7
Health subtotal	*147*	*113*
Violent crime	14	5
Favouring death penalty	0	3
Property crime	16	3
Violent crime clearance	0	10
Property crime clearance	10	0
Violent crime convictions	0	5
Property crime convictions	5	0
End-of-year prisoners	8	8
Practicing lawyers	0	8
Criminal justice expenditures	2	15
Criminal justice subtotal	*55*	*57*
Voter turnout	4	1
Favouring voter franchise extension	0	2

(continued)

Table 17.2 (continued)

Social indicators	Canada	USA
People have no say	1	1
Voting is only way to influence	0	2
Government rating	1	1
Head of state approval	5	5
Foreign aid	10	9
Favouring admission of Red China to UN	1	0
Military expenditures	14	4
West and USSR can live peacefully	1	0
Arab-Israel sympathies	3	0
Satisfied with nation's world position	1	0
Perceived national achievement	0	1
Unionized labour force	18	0
Female share of unionized labour force	7	2
Working days lost	2	8
Politics subtotal	*67*	*36*
R&D personnel	0	11
Immigrant professionals	13	8
R&D expenditures	13	4
Cost per patent	3	7
Patents per 1000 R&D personnel	3	7
Automatic dishwashers	7	12
Science/technology subtotal	*39*	*49*
Foreign student enrolment	18	3
Pupil-teacher ratios	10	9
Expenditures per student	2	19
Female percent of degrees	9	11
Degrees per 1000 20–34 year olds	7	14
Female percent of M.D.s	18	3
Satisfaction with education	0	2
Education subtotal	*64*	*61*
Households with TV	5	10
Objectionable TV	1	0
Hunting licences	11	6
Horseracing attendance	17	4
Pro football attendance	6	13
Boating	1	0
Bicycling	1	0
Snowmobiling	1	0
Camping	1	0
Water skiing	1	0

(continued)

Table 17.2 (continued)

Social indicators	Canada	USA
Theatre expenditures	13	8
National park lands	14	7
Park visits	4	17
Copyrights to residents	8	9
Recreation subtotal	*84*	*74*
Energy consumption per capita	13	8
Energy production/consumption	17	4
Selected metals production/consumption	14	5
Total chemicals export/import	5	12
Lumber production/consumption	16	5
Forest area burned	11	10
Air pollution	12	13
Resources subtotal	*88*	*57*
Households with cars	3	15
Motor vehicle accident deaths	6	13
Motor vehicle accident injuries	10	5
Overseas travel	18	3
Canadian/American travel	3	14
Households with telephones	13	7
Telephone conversations	4	17
First class mail	5	14
Newspaper circulation	0	11
Transportation/communication personal expenditures	15	6
Transportation and communication subtotal	*77*	*105*
Crowded housing	1	2
Adequate plumbing	0	3
Home ownership	1	2
Housing expenditures	15	6
New single family dwellings	5	16
Achieved housing requirements	10	9
Building fire losses	11	10
Housing subtotal	*43*	*48*
GNP per capita	10	11
Manufacturing output per hour	9	2
Shared decision-making on family spending	0	1
Personal saving per capita	5	16
Female to male income ratios	13	9
Gini coefficient	3	12
Inflation rate	5	5
Taxes as percent of GNP	5	14

(continued)

Table 17.2 (continued)

Social indicators	Canada	USA
Unemployment rate	8	12
Female/male unemployment difference	15	6
Percent of poor people	0	4
Bankruptcy rate	14	7
Balance of payments	13	8
Net public debt	20	1
Economics subtotal	*120*	*108*
Belief in the devil	1	0
Belief in life after death	1	0
Belief in heaven	1	0
Belief in hell	1	0
Religion subtotal	*4*	*0*
Marriage rate	6	15
Average family size	4	15
One-parent families	3	0
Divorce rate	15	6
Median duration of marriages ending in divorce	8	5
Satisfaction with personal future	1	2
Expect a better year	0	1
Disapprove of racial intermarriage	1	0
Move from coloured neighborhood	1	0
Vote for female President/Prime Minister	1	0
Morals deteriorating	1	0
Honesty deteriorating	1	0
Happiness deteriorating	1	0
Peace of mind deteriorating	1	0
Find life exciting	1	0
Morality and social customs subtotal	*45*	*44*
Combined total all indicators	*884*	*775*

Source Michalos (1980a, b, 1981a, b, 1982)

of life is getting worse and positive indicators are such that as their indicator numerical values increase, some aspect of the quality of life is getting better.

The percent change upward or downward of an indicator value is called its 'flow value' and its value at any point in time is called its 'stock value', e.g., an annual infant mortality rate (stock value) might be something like 20 deaths per 1000 live births and it might have an annual decrease or increase of 5% from some year to the next, which would be good or bad, respectively. The comparative quality of life for Canada and the USA was crudely measured by (1) scoring one point per year for every year to the country whose stock value was preferable, (2) one point per year for every year to the country whose flow value was preferable, (3) summing the points to obtain a final score for each country for all usable indicators, and (4) using the final scores as measures of the comparative quality of life in each country, and assessing the country with the highest score as having the highest quality of life. Combining points for stock and flow values, the results of the investigation are summarized in Table 17.2. Precise definitions of the indicators may be found in the original work.

The conclusion reached from this crude assessment was that on the basis of over 135 indicators and over 1659 indicator values, it seemed fair to say that the quality of life in the 1964–74 period was comparatively or relatively higher (i.e., better) in Canada than in the United States. If one looks at the first and last recorded stock values for the usable indicators for each country independently of the other country, one may get a sense of the direction in which the two countries moved in that period. Interestingly, both countries looked worse on 44 indicators, while Canada looked better on 49 and the United States looked better on 48. So, on the basis of the broadest set of indicators available, it appears that both countries made progress over the period. (Selections from this treatise plus some new material appeared in *Perspectives Canada* III 1980.)

General Social Survey 1985

Initiated in 1985, Statistics Canada's General Social Survey (GSS) was intended "to monitor changes in the living conditions and well-being of Canadians" and it "has served as evidence behind key government programs to improve the well-being of Canadians" (Statistics Canada 2013b, p. 4). The GSS is based on cross-sectional random samples of residents aged 15 years and older, in the ten provinces, conducted over a 6–12 month period, with sample sizes of around 10,000 until 1999 when they were increased to about 25,000. The larger sample sizes allows significant estimates of conditions at the national, provincial and some census metropolitan areas, as well as of "sub-population groups such as single-parent families, visible minorities and seniors". The program began using Random Digit Dialing and currently uses internet and telephone technology. Each survey obtains standard demographic information (e.g., age, sex, education, ethnicity) and is roughly related to six themes, namely, caregiving, families, time use, social identity, volunteering and victimization. Table 17.3 lists the core content, new content and response rates for the 26 cycles that have appeared in the 1985–2012 period.

Using seven cycles of the GSS and three of the Canadian Community Health Survey (CCHS), Bonikowska et al. (2014) published a review of answers to questions concerning respondents' feelings about their "life as a whole right now". The questions had ten- or eleven-point response categories running from very dissatisfied to very satisfied. The usable sample sizes for the GSS surveys ranged from 15,390 to 24,951, and those for the CCHS were much larger, ranging from 61,673 to 63,542. While the average scores on these life satisfaction questions

Table 17.3 GSS cycle numbers, collection dates and response rates

Cycle	Collection date	Core content	New content	Response rate
26	2012	Caregiving and care receiving	Consequences of caregiving	65.7
25	2011	Family	Family transitions	65.8
24	2010	Time use/stress and well-being	Simultaneous activities, work-life balance	55.2
23	2009	Victimization	Internet victimization	61.6
22	2008	Social networks	Coping with change	57.3
21	2007	Family, social support, retirement	Work/family history, retirement experiences and plans	57.7
20	2006	Family history	Family transitions	67.4
19	2005	Time use	Social networks, trust and transportation	58.6
18	2004	Victimization	Use of restraining orders, stalking and social disorder	74.5
17	2003	Social engagement	Social/civic participation, trust and values	78.0
16	2002	Social support and aging	Retirement planning and experience	74.5
15	2001	Family history	Education history, mobility	80.9
14	2000	Technology-computer, internet	Use of computers, impact of technology on privacy, access to information	80.8
13	1999	Victimization	Spousal, senior abuse/perceptions	81.3
12	1998	Time use	Sports participation/culture	77.6
11	1996	Social support	Tobacco use	85.3
10	1995	Family	Effects of tobacco smoke	81.4
9	1994	Education, work and retirement	Transition into retirement	81.2
8	1993	Personal risk	Alcohol and drug use	81.6
7	1992	Time use	Culture, sport and unpaid-work activities	76.8
6	1991	Health	Various health topics	80.2
5	1990	Family and friends	Relationships and interactions with family and friends	75.8
4	1989	Education and work	New technologies and human resources	80.7
3	1988	Personal risk	Victim services	82.4
2	1986	Time use, social mobility	Language	78.9
1	1085	Health	Social support	83.4

Source Statistics Canada (2013b, p. 11)

ranged from 7.6 to 8.3, the scores were strikingly similar and rounded to the nearest whole number they were exactly the same, 8. The GSS scores rounded to the first decimal point for 2003 = 7.9, 2005 = 7.7, 2006 = 8.0, 2008 = 7.9, 2009 = 8.3, 2010 = 7.6, 2011 = 8.1 and the CCHS scores for 2009 = 8.0, 2010 = 8.0, 2011 = 8.0.

Using 13 fairly standard demographic predictors, Ordinary Least Squares regressions showed that from 16 to 22% of the variation in life satisfaction scores could be explained, i.e., roughly 80% of the variation required some other predictors. The 13 predictors used were sex, age group, marital status, number of children, educational attainment, immigration status, labour force activity, household income, household size, homeownership, self-assessed health status, region of residence, and urban/rural residence. Such low explanatory power for such predictors is a well-known fact of social indicators research. The missing 80% of work to be done can be provided by introducing some human agency predictors (e.g., discrepancies between what respondents have and want, or have and relevant others have, or have and had expected to have) and some domain satisfaction predictors (e.g., satisfaction with one's family, friendships, leisure activities) (Michalos 2003).

Canadian Social Trends 1986

A few years after publishing *Perspectives Canada III,* around 1983–84 a decision was made at Statistics Canada to discontinue that series and create an annual compendium of social indicators. The first issue was released in the summer of 1986, edited by David Brusegard. The Editor's Note said that

> This introductory issue of *Canadian Social Trends* begins a quarterly discussion of social trends and conditions in Canada. This continuing series is based on the recognition by Statistics Canada that a large number of Canadians…require factual information about the direction and scope of social change so characteristic of Canadian society…[the series] will also serve as a vehicle to inform its readers of other information sources and services available from Statistics Canada and how these can be obtained…[it] will be topical… comprehensive…selective…analytical…[and] presented in non-technical language (Brusegard 1986, p. 2).

It was exactly the sort of publication that many social indicators researchers hoped to see. As noted above, there was good evidence that most people, including most of the presumed target audience, were not interested in a biannual, very dense volume of statistics like the *Perspectives Canada* series. We thought that a magazine-like production with "graphic and tabular exhibits" that were "attractive and easy to understand" would be a more appropriate vehicle to serve the needs of most people.

Although the focus was described as being on "social trends", more often than not the time series discussed were social indicators in the standard sense of statistics with some significance for measuring the quality of life or well-being. The magazine also became an excellent vehicle for publishing articles based on General

Social Survey results which, as we have just seen, were focused on the well-being and living conditions of Canadians. From the first issue to the Winter issue of 2006, each issue ended with a summary list called "Social Indicators". Table 17.4 gives the list of social indicators from the first issue. Figures were provided for every year from 1978 to 1985.

From the Autumn 1986 issue through 1991 Craig McKie was editor and four issues per year came out. The last issue containing Social Indicators came out in Winter 2006. There were 9 pages of figures, covering the period from 1971 to 2005. The number of issues per year was reduced to two in the 2007–11 period. In 2012 there was only one issue (Summer), which was the last one ever to appear. An attached letter to subscribers said that "The cancellation is the result of a thorough review of the Agency's activities to manage its resources and priorities in the

Table 17.4 Social indicators from Canadian social trends

Population	*Health*
Canada (000s)	Suicide rate per 100,000, men/women
Annual growth rate	% of population 15 + who are regular
Immigration	Cigarette smokers, men/women
Emigration	Gov. expenditure on health
Family	(1982 $000,000)
Birth rate (per 1,000)	*Justice*
Marriage rate (per 1,000)	Crime rates per 100,000
Divorce rate (per 1,000)	Violent, property, homide
Families experiencing unemployment	*Government*
Labour force	Expenditures on social programs
Total employment (000s)	(1982 $000,000)
Goods sector (000s)	As a % of total expenditures
Services sector (000s)	As a % of GNP
Total unemployment (000s)	UI beneficiaries (000s)
Unemployment rate	OAS/GIS beneficiaries (000s)
Part-time employment rate	Can. Assistance Plan beneficiaries (000s)
Women's participation rate	*Economic indicators*
Unionization rate—% of paid workers	GNP annual change
Income	Annual inflation rate
Average family income—1982$	Urban housing starts
% of families with low income	
Women's full-time earnings as a % of men's	
Education	
Elem. and sec. enrolment (000s)	
Full-time postsec. enrolment	
Doctoral degrees awarded	
Gov. expenditures on education	
(1982 $000,000)	

Source Canadian Social Trends, 1986

current fiscal environment while maintaining a balanced national statistical program that accurately measures the economy and society". (The author owes special thanks to Craig McKie and David Brusegard for information on *Canadian Social Trends*.)

Comparative Charting of Social Change 1991

In 1991, the first volume of this book series appeared under the general editorship of Simon Langlois of the University of Laval. By 2013, the series had 12 volumes. Two have a purely Canadian focus, *Recent Social Trends in Canada, 1960–2000* (Roberts et al. 2005) and *Recent Social Trends in Quebec, 1960–1990* (Langlois et al. 1992). The introductory chapter of the Canadian study describes the work as "an exercise in social cartography". The aim was

> …to map out various domains of the social landscape of Canada and identify how they have changed in recent decades. This has been principally a descriptive exercise, not an explanatory one…Describing recent social trends in Canada is an interesting and worthwhile exercise. Interpreting these trends, however, is a larger project. Interpretation requires placing particular events in a larger context: it requires answering the 'compared to what?' question. It is at this point that this social trends volume fits into the larger project of the Comparative Charting of Social Change (CCSC) group (Roberts et al. 2005, pp. 6–7).

Other volumes in the series cover Bulgaria, France, Germany, Greece, Italy, Russia, Spain and the United States. Each volume is organized using a "78-trend classification scheme". So interested readers can pick any of these countries to compare to their own. Such comparisons are not undertaken in this volume, but there is a modest evaluation offered at the end of the first chapter.

> The social trends evident in the volume suggest that Canada has made considerable progress toward finding an appropriate balance between encouraging the cultivation of rights and freedoms, while remembering that members of our society are interdependent and share a common fate…these same trends can also be interpreted to indicate that Canadian society is a civil place (Roberts et al. 2005, p. 16).

The areas of concern and 78 indicators are summarized in Table 17.5. Precise definitions of the indicators can be found in the book.

Global Report on Student Well-Being 1991–1993

If one thinks of a scientific theory as an organized (at best, axiomatic) set of propositions leading to testable predictions, then the field of quality of life or well-being studies has always been short on theories. Multiple Discrepancies Theory (MDT) was described and tested in Michalos (1985). An international exploration of the strength of the theory was undertaken with convenience samples

Table 17.5 Recent social trends indicators

Context	*Mobilizing institutions*
Demographic trends	Labour unions
Macro-economic trends	Religious institutions
Macro-technological trends	Military forces
Age groups	Political parties
Youth	Mass media
Elders	*Institutionalization of social forces*
Microsocial	Dispute settlement
Self-identification	Institutionalization of labour unions
Kinship networks	Social movements
Community and neighbourhood types	Interest groups
Local autonomy	*Ideologies*
Voluntary associations	Political differentiation
Sociability networks	Confidence in institutions
Women	Economic orientations
Female roles	Radicalism
Childbearing	Religious beliefs
Matrimonial models	*Household resources*
Women's employment	Personal and family income
Reproductive technologies	Informal economy
Labour market	Personal and family wealth
Unemployment	*Life style*
Skills and occupational levels	Market goods and services
Types of employment	Mass information
Sectors of the labour force	Personal health and beauty practices
Computerization of work	Time use
Labour and management	Daily mobility
Work organization	Household production
Personnel administration	Forms of erotic expression
Size and types of enterprises	Mood-altering substances
Social stratification	*Leisure*
Occupational status	Amount and use of free time
Social mobility	Vacation patterns
Economic inequality	Athletics and sports
Social inequality	Cultural activities
Social relations	*Educational attainment*
Conflict	General education
Negotiation	Vocational education
Norms of conduct	Continuing education
Authority	*Integration and marginalization*
Public opinion	Immigrants and ethnic minorities

(continued)

Table 17.5 (continued)

State and service institutions	Crime and punishment
Educational system	Emotional disorders and self-destruction
Health system	Poverty
Welfare system	*Attitudes and values*
The state	Satisfaction
	Perception of social problems
	Orientations toward the future
	Values
	National identity

Source Roberts et al. (2005)

of surveys of 18,032 undergraduates in 39 countries in the period from 1984 to 1986. The English questionnaire was translated into 19 other languages: German, Arabic, Bengali, French, Portuguese, Spanish, Finnish, Greek, Hungarian, Hebrew, Japanese, Korean, Dutch, Norwegian, Swedish, Chinese, Thai, Turkish and Croation. Results of the study were published in four volumes (Michalos 1991a, b, 1993a, b). Explanations were provided for life satisfaction and happiness, and for satisfaction with family, friends, living partner, self-esteem, employment, finances, housing, transportation, religion, education, recreation and health.

Briefly, the postulates of MDT are as follows.

- H1: Reported net satisfaction (happiness or subjective wellbeing) is a function of perceived discrepancies between what one has and wants, relevant others have, the best one has had in the past, expected to have 3 years ago, expects to have after 5 years, deserves and needs.
- H2: All perceived discrepancies, except that between what one has and wants, are functions of objectively measurable discrepancies, which also have direct effects on satisfaction and actions.
- H3: The perceived discrepancy between what one has and wants is a mediating variable between all other perceived discrepancies and reported net satisfaction.
- H4: The pursuit and maintenance of net satisfaction motivates human action in direct proportion to the perceived expected levels of net satisfaction.
- H5: All discrepancies, satisfaction and actions are directly and indirectly affected by age, sex, education, ethnicity, income, self-esteem, social support, temperament, current mood, community, natural environment, life events/issues.
- H6: Objectively measurable discrepancies are functions of human action and conditioners.

The central hypotheses of the most successful single discrepancy theories in the literature are built into H1, on the basis of their supporting evidence (Michalos 1985) and the assumption that each hypothesis could add some explanatory power to MDT. These successful single discrepancy theories include aspiration theory, social comparison theory, equity theory, need theory, person-environment fit theory and cognitive dissonance theory. H3 affirms the model from Campbell et al. (1976)

while H2 adds direct effects to that model and objectively measurable discrepancies, with the latter affirming the existence of an external world beyond perceptions. H4 is similar to an expected utility hypothesis insofar as it posits expected net satisfaction as a motivator for action. H5 includes a set of features known to have some influence on discrepancies, satisfaction and action, and H6 provides a loop from actions back to the world from which the actions emerged.

Because there were big differences in the numbers of students in samples from different countries, to avoid having results biased by the countries with the biggest samples, an attempt was made to systematically select samples of 250 students from each country, 125 males and 125 females. This was possible for 80% of the total sample, giving us a balanced working sample of 9092. The total world sample (N = 18,032) and balanced sample (N = 9092) were probably not representative of the world's university undergraduate population in any statistically important sense, but they were the most extensive samples of that population that had ever been collected. Forty percent of the balanced sample was female, 80% aged from 17 to 15, 90% single, never married, and 63% unemployed.

Table 17.6 lists the participating countries' mean and standard deviation scores for satisfaction and happiness with life as a whole, and the zero order correlations between these scores. The individual country means are based on the total samples from each country. The last row of the table gives the figures for the balanced world sample (N = 9092), while the row labeled 'Total Mean' gives the figures for the total world sample (N = 18,032). Scores for 6 Less Developed Countries and for 33 Developed Countries are given in the second and third last rows, respectively.

The average percent of variance explained by MDT in life satisfaction and happiness scores for 38 countries (Switzerland omitted) was 42% and 40%, respectively. Life satisfaction scores' percents of variance explained ranged from a high of 67% for Finland to a low of 30% for Korea, while happiness figures ranged from a high of 74% for Tanzania to a low of 13% for Portugal (Michalos 1991a, pp. 125–127). The mean total effect (MTE) values for the various predictors in applications of MDT to life satisfaction and happiness showed that the self-wants discrepancy was the strongest predictor of the lot, with 40% for life satisfaction and 26% for happiness. In second place, was the self-others discrepancy, with 29% for life satisfaction and 24% for happiness. Third place self-needs dropped to 12% and 10% for life satisfaction and happiness, respectively. The demographic variables (sex, age, working status, level of education and ethnic background) accounted for one (mostly) to 2% (Michalos 1991a, pp. 127–129).

The data set for this global survey was used in Diener et al. (1995) and in Mallard et al. (1997). In the latter study it was shown that the relationship of domain satisfaction scores to scores for life satisfaction vary by type of domain and country. For some domains in some countries, domain satisfaction scores predict life satisfaction scores but not *vice versa* (a so-called Bottom-Up relationship). For some domains and countries, life satisfaction scores predict domain satisfaction scores but not *vice versa* (a Top-Down relationship), and for some domains and countries, the causal arrows run in both directions between domain scores and life satisfaction scores (a Bi-Directional relationship). For example, for Canada, the relationships

Table 17.6 Participating countries' mean and standard deviation scores for satisfaction and happiness with life as whole, and Pearson correlations

Country	Satisfaction		Happiness		Pearson correlation between satisfaction and happiness*
	Mean	SD	Mean	SD	
Austria	4.92	1.01	4.48	1.12	0.65
Bahrain	4.96	1.22	4.86	1.30	0.55
Bangladesh+	4.31	1.10	5.00	1.16	0.68
Belgium	5.21	0.80	4.99	1.07	0.62
Brazil	4.94	1.02	5.04	1.11	0.59
Cameroon	4.12	0.90	4.02	0.96	0.34
Canada	5.11	0.94	5.06	1.20	0.67
Chile	4.97	0.84	4.70	1.03	0.49
Colombia	5.12	0.86	5.02	1.10	0.60
Egypt+	4.55	1.06	4.44	1.12	0.52
Finland	5.44	0.99	5.01	1.16	0.67
Germany	4.84	0.96	4.97	1.11	0.61
Greece	4.83	0.90	4.42	0.92	0.53
Hungary	4.77	0.72	4.52	0.96	0.63
India+	4.72	1.09	4.82	1.43	0.48
Israel	4.98	0.85	4.58	1.39	0.50
Japan	4.09	1.05	4.49	1.11	0.49
Jordan	4.49	1.12	4.53	1.19	0.52
Kenya+	4.46	1.01	4.46	1.11	0.58
Korea	4.21	1.50	4.38	1.17	0.57
Mexico	5.12	0.79	5.17	1.09	0.52
Netherlands	5.17	1.02	5.23	1.08	0.72
New Zealand	5.06	0.96	5.07	1.22	0.69
Norway	5.14	0.89	4.96	1.02	0.53
Philippines	5.02	0.92	4.90	1.11	0.55
Portugal	3.26	1.52	2.25	1.66	NA
Puerto Rico	5.18	0.94	5.02	1.17	0.56
Singapore	4.76	0.95	4.73	1.00	0.65
S. Africa	4.53	1.14	4.37	1.17	0.49
Spain	4.55	0.89	4.52	0.94	0.48
Sweden	4.96	1.09	5.19	1.21	0.67
Switzerland	5.08	0.83	4.95	1.06	0.67
Taiwan	4.35	0.95	4.56	1.21	0.50
Tanzania+	4.97	1.23	4.95	1.22	0.65
Thailand	4.61	0.94	4.07	1.05	NA
Turkey+	4.21	1.02	4.61	1.09	0.63
UK	5.20	0.87	5.22	1.11	0.65
USA	5.28	1.00	5.27	1.20	0.67

(continued)

Table 17.6 (continued)

Country	Satisfaction		Happiness		Pearson correlation between satisfaction and happiness*
	Mean	SD	Mean	SD	
Yugoslavia	4.70	1.14	4.54	1.22	0.62
Total Mean	4.77	1.00	4.70	1.14	0.58
Dev.C.Mean	4.82	0.99	4.70	1.13	0.58
L.D.C.Mean	4.54	1.09	4.71	1.19	0.59
World	4.76	1.11	4.71	1.27	0.59

+ Below 142-country median on per capita GNP and literacy rate
*$p < 0.001$
Source Michalos (1991a)

between life satisfaction and satisfaction with health, finances, family relations, friendships, living partner, recreation and education are Bi-Directional, but for the United States, the relationship between life satisfaction and these domain variables is Bi-Directional for all but health and education. The relationship between life satisfaction and satisfaction with paid employment is Top-Down for the United States but Bottom-Up for Canada. The relationship between life satisfaction and satisfaction with religion is Top-Down in both countries.

Aboriginal Peoples Surveys 1991–2012

The first national Aboriginal Peoples Survey was conducted by Statistics Canada in 1991 and it was found so useful to researchers for the Royal Commission on Aboriginal Peoples (1996) that requests were made for further studies. A second survey was undertaken in 2001 and a third after the 2006 Census, after which the survey became a quinquennial study. Here we will review the fourth survey, undertaken in 2012.

The aim of all these surveys is to provide "key statistics to inform policy and programming activities aimed at improving the well-being of Aboriginal Peoples". In particular, the purpose "is to identify the needs of Aboriginal people and focus on issues such as education, employment, health, language, income, housing and mobility" (Statistics Canada 2012a, p. 1).

The target population of the 2012 APS was

> …the Aboriginal identity population of Canada, 6 years of age and over as of February 1, 2012, living in private dwellings excluding people living on Indian reserves and settlements and in certain First Nations communities in Yukon and the Northwest Territories (NWT). The concept of 'Aboriginal identity' refers to those persons who reported identifying with at least one Aboriginal group, namely, First Nations (North American Indian), Métis or Inuit, those who reported being a Status Indian (Registered Indian or Treaty Indian, as defined by the Indian Act of Canada), or those who reported being a member of a First Nation or Indian Band (Statistics Canada 2012a, p. 2).

This target population is narrower than those used in earlier surveys and the sample was drawn not from a Census long form but from respondents to the 2011 National Household Survey. So comparisons to earlier surveys are not recommended. The total number of Aboriginal respondents was "about 28,410" (Statistics Canada 2012a, pp. 2–5). The 11 general themes in the survey covered by over 150 indicators are Aboriginal Identity, Household Composition, Mobility, Education, Aboriginal Language, Residential School, Labour Market Activities, Traditional Activities, Income, Health and Housing (Statistics Canada 2012b, p. 1). Here we review selections from one published report from the 2012 survey, on education and employment (Statistics Canada 2013c). We also consider results from a published report combining data from four cycles of the Canadian Community Health Surveys (CCHS) 2007 to 2010 (Statistics Canada 2013a). Responses to similar questions taken from both surveys "yielded similar results".

Because there are significant differences in the living conditions and culture of the three kinds of Aboriginal groups, in these reports results are given for each group independently. Occasionally comparisons with the non-Aboriginal populations are made with each group. In the 2006 census 1,172,790 (about 4% of the total population of Canada) "identified themselves as an Aboriginal person", 60% were First Nations people, 33% Métis and 4% Inuit. About 3% had other Aboriginal identities. On average, the Aboriginal population was and still is younger than the non-Aboriginal population. Forty-three percent of First Nations people lived on reserve. (Statistics Canada 2013a, p. 4).

From the CCHS (Statistics Canada 2013a) samples of Aboriginal people 12 years of age and older, not living on reserves, we learned that in the 2007–2010 period all three groups self-reported poorer health than the non-Aboriginal population, with First Nations people 50%, Métis 54% and Inuit 55% claiming 'very good' or 'excellent health', compared to 63% of the non-Aboriginal population. Fifty-six percent of First Nations people and 48% of the non-Aboriginal population "reported being diagnosed with one or more chronic conditions". "All three groups had higher rates of asthma", 13–14% compared to 9% for the non-Aboriginal population. All three groups had "higher rates of daily smoking", with First Nations people 32%, Métis 30% and Inuit 39%, compared to 15% for the non-Aboriginal population. All three groups had higher rates of heavy drinking, with First Nations people 26%, Métis 27%, Inuit 26%, compared to 19% for the non-Aboriginal population. All three groups had higher obesity rates, First Nations people 25%, Métis 22% and Inuit 26%, compared to 16% for the non-Aboriginal population. For First Nations people 45 years and older, the diabetes rate was 19%, compared to 11% for the non-Aboriginal population. Notwithstanding their relatively much poorer health, 92% of Inuit, 89% of First Nations people and 90% of Métis reported that they were satisfied with life as a whole, compared to 93% for the non-Aboriginal population.

From the APS 2012, for each of the three groups, we can create a rough profile of the educational and employment experiences of sampled Aboriginal people. Here we limit our review to a selection of indicators for First Nations people living off reserve.

Seventy-two percent of First Nations people living off reserve, 42% of Inuit and 77% of Métis aged 18 to 44 had “a high school diploma or equivalent (‘completers’)”, compared to 89% for the non-Aboriginal population. Twenty-eight percent of First Nations people, 58% of Inuit and 23% of Métis in this age group “were not attending high school and had not met the requirements for a high school diploma (‘leavers’)”, compared to 11% for the non-Aboriginal population. Forty-three percent of First Nations people in this age group, 26% of Inuit and 47% of Métis had “a post-secondary qualification; that is, a certificate, diploma or degree above the high school level”, compared to 64% for the non-Aboriginal population (Statistics Canada 2013c, p. 6).

Table 17.7 lists some statistics from APS 2012 indicating the different life experiences and life chances of off reserve First Nations people 18–44 in the high school completers versus the leavers groups.

Reviewing the numbers in this table, it seems as if the completers and leavers lived in different worlds with different experiences and life chances. Clearly, the quality of life of the completers was better than that of the leavers.

Cooke et al. (2004) claimed that “there has not been a systematic attempt to describe the changes in the relative well-being of Aboriginal people and other Canadians in a single, easily understood set of indicators”. Following up an earlier study by Beavon and Cooke (2003), they applied a version of the UN Human Development Index (UNDP 1996) to address this problem for the five census years 1981 to 2001. The comparison groups used were the Registered Indian population according to the Canadian Indian Act of 1976 versus all Canadians who were not registered. The division is rough because many First Nations peoples, Inuit and Métis are not registered and therefore they are included in the general population numbers.

The HDI is built on the assumption that human development means “the enlargement of choices made possible by education and literacy, a decent material standard of living, and a long and healthy life” (Cooke et al. (2007, p. 3). Indicators used for education and literacy were “the proportion of the population fifteen years and older that had attained Grade 9 or better…and the proportion of the population nineteen years and older that had attained a high school diploma/technical/post-secondary education with or without a high school diploma” (Cooke et al. 2004, p. 52). Estimates of average individual income were made from Census average incomes “adjusted to include the entire population with and without income in the denominator” (Cooke et al. 2004, pp. 52–53). Overall HDI scores are calculated by taking the average of index scores made for each of the three domains. The authors summarized their results as follows.

> The gap in HDI scores between Registered Indian and other Canadians was reduced from 0.18 in 1981 to 0.12 in 2001. While both populations improved in terms of human development between 1981 and 2001, gains have been greater for the Registered Indian population…Although there have been substantial gains made by Registered Indians in life expectancy and education, the 1981–2001 period saw much less progress in terms of average annual income…The average annual income for Registered Indians did improve over the entire 1981–2001 period, from $6,840 to $10,094, but remained well below the level experienced by other Canadians (Cooke et al. 2004, pp. 53–55).

Table 17.7 Selected indicators of life experiences and life chances for First Nations high school completers and leavers 18–44, percents*

Life experiences and chances	Completers	Leavers
Mainly A and B grades in last year of school (LYS)	80	51
Often skipped classes LYS	18	42
Often arrived late LYS	17	31
Participated in sport activity at least once a week LYS	50	40
in art/drama/music at least once a week	26	20
in school group/club at least once a week	21	9
Volunteered at least once a week LYS	29	23
Read books four or more times a week LYS	51	43
Most or all closest friends LYS skipped classes once a week or more	23	33
Had reputation for causing trouble	8	18
Thought completing high school very important	77	51
Planned further education	61	34
Dropped out	10	26
Parents spoke or visited your teacher LYS	51	42
Attended school event in which you participated	55	32
Participated in other school activities	31	21
Siblings dropped out	43	68
Mother graduated from high school	74	55
Father graduated from high school	64	50
Felt safe at school in LYS	94	85
I was happy	87	72
Most students enjoyed being at this school	85	77
Racism was a problem	33	40
Bullying was a problem	46	54
Presence of drugs was a problem	46	53*
Violence was a problem	30	43*
Post-secondary graduate	54	16*
Never attended post-secondary school	22	70*
Employed	72	47*
Unemployed	9	15*
Not in labour force	20	37*

Source Statistics Canada (2013c)
*All statistics significantly different from completers' percentage ($p < 0.05$)

The rising tide did not raise all ships equally. Within the class of Registered Indians, the overall HDI scores for women increased a bit more than the scores for men, driven mainly by the stronger educational performance of women. The period-long gap between the life expectancy scores of Registered Indian men and women is unclear, but the gender gap in earnings for men and women was reduced, though the men still had higher incomes than the women throughout the period.

Comparing the development of on- and off-reserve Registered Indians, they found that the latter had better scores than the former throughout the 1981–2001 period, although the gap between the two groups decreased from the beginning to the end of the period.

Cooke et al. (2007) took their application of the HDI again in a somewhat altered form to Aboriginal peoples in Australia, Canada, New Zealand and the United States for the period of 1990–2000. To nobody's surprise, they immediately found that in all four countries "minority Indigenous populations" had "much poorer health and social conditions than their non-indigenous compatriots". Comparisons of the overall HDI scores showed that in that decade, the gap decreased the most for United States Non-Aboriginals versus American Indian and Alaska Native scores. Australia had the worst performance, with the gap between Aboriginal and Torres Strait Islander scores versus Australia Non-Aboriginal scores increasing. The gaps for Canada Non-Aboriginal versus Canadian Aboriginal, and for New Zealand Non-Aboriginal and Māori decreased practically the same amount.

Social Indicators Research Book Series 1997

Under the general editorship of Michalos, the first volume of this book series was published in 1997. By 2014, 53 volumes appeared in the series. (By the end of 2015, 60 volumes.) None are focused on Canada although books in the series contain several essays by Canadian authors about various aspects of the quality of life in Canada.

Centre for the Study of Living Standards Index of Economic Well-Being 1998–2009

Building on Osberg (1985), Osberg and Sharpe (1998) created the Index of Economic Well-Being (IEWB). The IEWB is built on four components and 14 sub-components briefly described in Osberg and Sharpe (2011). The "basic hypothesis" of the index is that "a society's economic well-being depends on total consumption and accumulation, and on the individual inequality and insecurity that surrounds the distribution of macroeconomic aggregates". More precisely,

1. *Effective per capita consumption flows* is measured by per-capita market consumption adjusted for household size and life expectancy, government spending per capita, changes in the value of leisure time (all 3 in constant $).
2. *Net societal accumulation of stocks of productive resources* measured by capital stock per capita, R&D per capita, human capital, net international investment position per capita, less: social cost of environmental degradation per capita (all 5 in constant $).

3. *Income distribution* measured by income inequality, poverty rate and gap (poverty intensity).
4. *Economic security from job loss and unemployment, illness, family breakup and poverty in old age* measured by risk from unemployment, financial risk from illness, risk from single parent poverty, risk from poverty in old age.

In the standard procedure used by Osberg, Sharpe and their collaborators, each of the four components is given the same weight and each of the weights, of each sub-component is distributed equally within its component. For example, each of the components accounts for 25% of the index score and each of the 3 sub-components in the first component has a weight of 1/3 of 25%, each of the 5 sub-components in the second component has a weight of 1/5 of 25%, and so on. Thus, for example again, in the standard procedure, each of the two sub-components of the third component are worth twice as much as each of the four sub-components of the fourth component.

Considerable efforts have been made by the researchers to test the sensitivity of various alternative weighting schemes. Sharpe and Andrews (2012) concluded that "Among explicit weights, the original weights of the IEWB were best. Although the original weights are supported, they were controversial – a shift to equal weights mitigated this controversy – it appears equal weights remain least objectionable". This conclusion is consistent with analyses in Hagerty and Land (2007, 2012). In the latter article, they wrote that

> We recommend that the weights used be proportional to surveys of citizen's own weights for various indicators…This procedure maximizes agreement between citizens and the index, and has the further advantage of protecting the index from political manipulation of the weights and indicators. If surveys of citizen's weights are not available, then equal weighting minimizes the worst disagreements (Hagerty and Land 2012, p. 198).

The results of applying IEWB to Canada and the United States for the period of 1980–2009 show that, considering both stock and flow values, the former performed better than the latter. The index values for Canada in 1980 and 2009 were 0.412 and 0.575, respectively. For the United States the values were 0.355 and 0.482, respectively. For Canada over the whole period there was an improvement of 39.8% and for the United States there was an improvement of 35.7%.

How Canada Performs: A Report Card on Canada 1999–2013

The Conference Board of Canada (CBC) is a not-for-profit, applied research organization affiliated with but independent from the Conference Board, Inc. of New York. Its *Report Card on Canada* is supposed to measure "how well Canada is meeting its fundamental goal of creating a high and sustainable quality of life for all Canadians". Because for many indicators we do not have measures of the levels of reserves, recycling, reclamation, renewability, resilience and rates of change and no idea of the causal connections among them, these *Report Cards* cannot tell us how sustainable the reported quality of life might be, although they provide quite a bit of information about the quality of life.

According to the current Project Director, Brenda Lafleur, The *Report Cards* were initiated in 1999 and have evolved over time. In 1999 there were 40 indicators and 7 peer review countries. By 2013 the *Report Cards* had increased in size, with 6 domains with indicators distributed as follows: economy = 8, innovation = 21, environment = 14, education and skills = 20, health = 11 and society = 16. Indicators are selected on the basis of the information they provide on the performance value of some domain, their reliability and timely availability, their relevance and capacity for being altered by policy, and general agreement about the desired direction of movement of indicator values (i.e., about negative and positive indicators). Precise definitions of all indicators are not provided in the published documents. Indicator values are selected from the most recent figures available and about 80% of the data are drawn from the Organization for Economic Co-operation and Development (OECD) (CBC 2013, p. 2, methodology, p. 1). Since comprehensive tables are not provided for all years and data values, it is impossible to guess the level of precision attained.

Grades are assigned to indicator values by means of benchmarking scores from 38 "peer countries". The countries are regarded as "high income" by the World Bank, excluding those with populations less than one million people, geographic areas less than 10,000 km^2, or 5-year averages of gross domestic product ranked below the mean score of the 38. Using these filters 17 peer countries remained: Australia, Austria, Belgium, Canada, Denmark, Finland, France, Germany, Ireland, Italy, Japan, Netherlands, Norway, Sweden, Switzerland, United Kingdom and United States.

For each indicator, country scores are rank ordered from best to worst, after which data points are normalized by the formula: indicator value minus minimum value, divided by maximum value minus minimum value, multiplied by 100. The indicator value for the best-performing country then has a score of 100 and the worst of zero, and composite indexes for domains individually and collectively are created for each country based on the averages for all the indicators. For each domain rank ordered composite normalized score, the difference between the best and worst performance score is calculated and divided by four. A country's *Report Card* rating for a domain is A if its score is in the top quartile, then B, C or D if the score is in the second, third or fourth quartile, respectively. When grades for all domains and countries are determined, a similar procedure is used to obtain overall country grades. Assigning 4 points for A-grades, 3 for Bs, 2 for Cs and 1 for Ds, it is possible (neglecting the fact that strictly speaking ordinal values cannot be manipulated using standard arithmetic rules) to obtain overall numerical values for each country which can then be averaged to assign grades. CBC does not do this,

Table 17.8 Composite overall, domain and indicator values, Canada and USA, 2013

Composite overall, domain and indicator values	Canada	USA
Economy	*3*	*3*
Income per capita	2	3
GDP growth	3	3
Labour productivity growth	3	2
Inflation	4	4
Unemployment rate	3	3
Employment growth	3	4
Inward foreign direct investment performance index	1	1
Outward foreign direct investment performance index	2	1
Innovation	*1*	*4*
Scientific articles	3	2
Patents by population	1	2
Patents index	1	1
High and medium-high technology manufacturing	1	1
Knowledge intensive services	2	4
Export market share: aerospace	2	3
Export market share: electronics	1	3
Export market share: office machinery and computers	1	3
Export market share: pharmaceuticals	1	1
Export market share: instruments	1	2
Trademarks	1	1
ICT investment	1	4
New firm density	3	NA
Venture capital	1	4
Public R&D spending	3	2
Business R&D spending	1	3
Top-cited papers index	3	4
Patenting firms less than 5 years old	1	2
Ease of entrepreneurship index	3	2
Connectivity	1	3
Government online services index	3	4
Environment	*2*	*1*
Nitrogen oxides emissions	1	2
Sulphur oxides emissions	3	4
VOC emissions	1	2
PH10 concentration	3	3
Municipal waste generation	1	1
Water quality index	4	2
Water withdrawals	2	1
Threatened species	4	2

(continued)

Table 17.8 (continued)

Composite overall, domain and indicator values	Canada	USA
Forest cover change	3	4
Use of forest resources	4	3
Marine trophic index	1	1
Greenhouse gas emissions	1	1
Low emitting electricity production	4	2
Energy intensity	1	2
Education and skills	*4*	*2*
High school completion	4	4
College completion	4	2
University completion	3	4
Ph.D. graduates	1	1
Science, math, computer science and engineering grads.	2	1
Students with reading skills: low-level	4	2
Students with reading skills: high-level	4	2
Students with math skills: low-level	4	1
Students with math skills: high-level	3	1
Students with science skills: low-level	4	1
Students with science skills: high-level	2	1
Adult literacy rate: low-level	2	1
Adult literacy rate: high-level	2	1
Performance of disadvantaged schools	4	2
Participation in non-formal, job-related education	2	2
Equity in outcomes	4	3
Foreign student index	3	1
Gender gap in tertiary attainment	3	4
Returns to post-secondary education: men	2	4
Returns to post-secondary education: women	3	4
Health	*3*	*1*
Life expectancy	3	1
Self-reported health status	4	4
Premature mortality	4	1
Mortality due to cancer	2	3
Mortality due to circulatory diseases	4	2
Mortality due to respiratory diseases	3	2
Mortality due to diabetes	2	2
Mortality due to musculo-skeletal system diseases	2	2
Mortality due to mental disorders	3	2
Infant mortality	2	1
Mortality due to medical mis-adventures	3	2
Society	*3*	*1*

(continued)

Table 17.8 (continued)

Composite overall, domain and indicator values	Canada	USA
Self-sufficiency: Jobless youth	3	2
Self-sufficiency: Disabled income	4	1
Equity: elderly poverty	4	2
Equity: child poverty	2	1
Equity: working age poverty	1	1
Equity: income inequality	2	1
Equity: income mobility	4	1
Equity: gender income gap	2	2
Social cohesion: voter turnout	2	1
Social cohesion: confidence in parliament (congress)	2	1
Social cohesion: homicides	4	1
Social cohesion: burglaries	3	3
Social cohesion: life satisfaction	4	3
Social cohesion: acceptance of diversity	4	4
Social cohesion: social network support	3	1
Social cohesion: suicides	3	3
Average of 6 domain composite scores	*3*	2

but Table 17.8 lists the composite overall, domain and indicator values for Canada and the United States for 2013. The composite overall score for Canada is 3 = B and for the United States 2 = C.

Federation of Canadian Municipalities Quality of Life Reporting System 1999

In 1999 the Federation of Canadian Municipalities (FCM) initiated its Quality of Life Reporting System (QOLRS). The FCM was organized in 1901 as "the national voice of municipal governments…dedicated to improving the quality of life in all communities by promoting strong, effective, and accountable municipal government". Currently the federation includes over 1,775 municipal governments, covering Canada's "largest cities and regional municipalities, small towns, rural municipalities, and the 18 provincial and territorial municipal associations" (FCM 2013, p. 1).

Twenty-four communities, representing over 17 million people, 54% of the Canadian population, located in seven provinces, participate in the QOLRS. According to the FCM, the

…quality of life is enhanced and reinforced in municipalities that do the following:

- Develop and maintain a vibrant local economy;
- Protect and enhance the natural and built environment;
- Offer opportunities for the attainment of personal goals, hopes and aspirations;
- Promote a fair and equitable sharing of common resources;
- Enable residents to meet their basic needs; and
- Support rich social interactions and the inclusion of all residents in community life (FCM 2013, p. 1).

Generally speaking, the QOLRS is designed "to monitor quality of life at the local level", help "formulating public policy" and "serve as a planning tool for municipalities" (FCM 2013, p. 1). Because the system does not have a single index summarizing results from each indicator in some kind of common metric, different assessments of progress or regress may be made based on the same set of indicators. In FCM (2013, p. 55), there are ten areas of concern and 87 indicators as follows. (Precise definitions of indicators can be found in the report.)

1. *Demographic and Background Information*: Population growth, household size, family composition, average income, renters and owners, population mobility, immigration, language spoken at home, visible minorities, Aboriginal population.
2. *Affordable, Appropriate Housing*: Rental housing affordability, homeowner affordability, core housing need, substandard units, changing face of homelessness, vacancy rates, rental housing starts, monthly rent, cost of housing, overcrowding.
3. *Civic Engagement*: voter turnout, women in municipal government, volunteering, charitable donations.
4. *Community and Social Infrastructure*: Social housing waiting lists, rent-geared-to-income housing, subsidized child care, community and social services occupations, recreation facilities, cultural facilities, long-term care facilities, recreation programs, libraries, access to health care professionals.
5. *Education*: education levels, literacy levels, classroom size, composite learning index, education occupations.
6. *Employment and Local Economy*: Business bankruptcies, consumer bankruptcies, hourly wages, change in family income, building permits, unemployment, immigrant unemployment, quality of employment, labour force replacement.
7. *Natural Environment*: air quality, commuting distance, mode of transportation, density, water consumption, wastewater treatment, waste diversion, recreational water quality, drinking water quality, ecological footprint.
8. *Personal and Community Health*: low birth weight babies, teen birth rate, premature mortality, infant mortality, body mass index, smoking status, life expectancy, physical activity, prevalence of asthma, mental health.
9. *Personal Financial Security*: families receiving social assistance, families receiving Employment Insurance, incidence of low-income families, children living in poverty, income gap, social assistance rates, working poor, community affordability, transit affordability, food insecurity.

10. *Personal Safety*: Young offenders, violent crimes, property crimes, criminal code offences, police per capita, weapons violations, drug violations, traffic incidents, emergency services occupations.

The most interesting feature of this set of indicators is the total absence of any measures of how people perceive, feel and evaluate their lives, or the lives of other people in their communities or anywhere else. Assuming that the quality of life in a community is a function of the actual conditions of residents' lives and what they make of those conditions, this set of indicators has significant omissions. While the authors tell us that research has shown that community investments "contribute to inclusion, trust, cohesion and enhanced levels of social engagement" (FCM 2013, p. 5), suggesting that these are important aspects of a good life or a life of a good quality, there is no indication that the QOLRS uses such data, although we have seen that Statistics Canada has plenty to share. Hopefully, some use of such data will be made in the future.

Status of Women in Canada 2000

On the recommendation of the Prime Minister, Lester Pearson, on February 16, 1967 the Privy Council appointed five women and three men to form the Royal Commission on the Status of Women. They were given the mandate to

> ...inquire into and report upon the status of women in Canada, and to recommend what steps might be taken by the Federal Government to ensure for women equal opportunities with men in all aspects of Canadian Society, having regard for the distribution of legislative powers under the constitution of Canada, particularly with reference to federal statutes, regulations and policies that concern or affect the rights and activities of women and, without restricting the generality of the foregoing, to inquire and report on:
>
> 1. Laws and practices under federal jurisdiction concerning political rights of women;
> 2. The present and potential role of women in the Canadian Labour force, including the special problems of married women in employment and measures that might be taken under federal jurisdiction to help in meeting them;
> 3. Measures that might be taken under federal jurisdiction to permit the better use of the skills and education of women, including the special re-training requirements of married women who wish to re-enter professional or skilled employment;
> 4. Federal Labour laws and regulations in the application to women;
> 5. Laws, practices and policies concerning the employment and promotion of women in the Federal Civil Service, by Federal Crown Corporations and by Federal Agencies;
> 6. Federal taxation pertaining to women;
> 7. Marriage and divorce;
> 8. The position of women under the criminal law;
> 9. Immigration and citizenship laws, policies and practices with respect to women; and such other matters in relation to the status of women in Canada as may appear to the Commissioners to be relevant (Royal Commission on the Status of Women 1970, pp. vii–viii).

The 488 page *Report of the Royal Commission on the Status of Women in Canada* (hereafter *Report*) was submitted on September 28, 1970 and tabled in the House of Commons on December 7, 1970. The rich body of information assembled in the *Report* and its 167 recommendations created the foundation upon which most policies related to gender equality have been initiated. In particular, that information formed the foundation over the next 25 years until the next comprehensive report given by the Status of Women Canada (1995) in the *1995 Beijing Platform for Action* for the United Nations Fourth World Conference on Women in Beijing (hereafter *Platform*).

While it is practically impossible to demonstrate that a particular policy, program or change in the status of women in those years was the effect of something in the *Report*, it does seem reasonable to use information in the *Report* as a starting point for an evaluation of progress made in the 1970–96 period. In fact, because the *Report* drew upon statistics gathered as far back as 1930, in some cases it was possible to evaluate progress over nearly 70 years.

The *Report* was divided into ten chapters, covering the most salient areas of concern in the late 1960s. Although the aims of the two documents are not exactly the same, one way to illustrate the difference in the range of issues between then and 1996 is to compare the 10 areas of the *Report* with the 12 areas of concern identified in the Platform. The two lists are in Table 17.9.

Inspection of the two lists reveals that there were six roughly identical broad areas of concern in the *Report* and *Platform*, four areas in the *Report* that were not

Table 17.9 Report and platform concerns

Areas of concern in the report	Areas of concern in the platform
Women in the Canadian economy	Women and the economy
Education	Education and training of women
Women and the family	x
Health	Women and health
Taxation and child care allowances	x
Poverty	Women and poverty
Participation of women in public life	Women in power and decision-making
Immigration and citizenship	x
Criminal law and women offenders	x
x	Violence against women
x	Women and armed conflict
A plan for action	Institutional mechanisms for the advancement of women
x	Human rights for women
x	Women and the media
x	Women and the environment
x	The girl child

Source Michalos (2000)

emphasized in the *Platform* and seven areas emphasized in the *Platform* that were not emphasized in the *Report*. Thus, altogether seventeen distinct broad areas of concern were identified in the two lists. Using 14 social indicators, roughly six broad areas may be compared here to measure progress or deterioration toward gender equality in Canada over the 1970–95 period: women and the economy, education and training, poverty, violence against women, women and the family. Each indicator in the list below is followed by a plus sign (+) to signify that over the period in question there was progress or a minus sign (−) to signify that over the period there was deterioration. The ratio of indicators where progress was made to the total set of indicators will be used as a general measure of progress.

1. Real average annual wages by gender −
2. Gender equality index for total earnings +
3. Percentage of women and men employed +
4. Gender equality workload indexes +
5. Percentages of men and women attending school +
6. Women as percentage of full-time university enrolment +
7. Percentages of university degrees granted to women +
8. Gender equality indexes for training −
9. Ratio of female to male poverty rates +
10. Total sexual assault rates −
11. Average ages at first marriage +
12. Custody of children involved in divorces +
13. Proportion of births to unmarried women +
14. Ratio of supply to demand for childcare spaces −

Since ten of the 14 indicators show some progress, we may conclude that all things considered, there is more evidence of improvement than of deterioration toward gender equality in the 1970–95 period. (The material in this section was drawn from Michalos (2000) with some modification.)

The Well-Being of Nations 2001

Using data from a variety of sources drawn from the 1996–1999 period, Prescott-Allen (2001) produced Canada's most complex set of indexes representing human and ecological well-being for roughly 180 countries. Allowing that "no method can provide a definitive assessment", he claimed that his "Wellbeing Assessment" method

> ...provides a framework for reflection and debate about the relationships between people and the ecosystem, the factors that are crucial for ecosystem wellbeing and human well-being, the indicators that best represent these factors, and performance criteria for each indicator...[his book] is offered as both a contribution to the debate and a first approximation of national conditions (Prescott-Allen 2001, pp. 10–11).

There are four equally weighted main indexes with unequally weighted sub-indexes and indicators. The Human Wellbeing Index (HWI) has five dimensions and 36 indicators and the Ecosystem Wellbeing Index (EWI) has five dimensions and 51 indicators. The Wellbeing Index (WI) is a graphic index representing the "intersection" of the HWI and EWI, and the Wellbeing/Stress Index (WSI) "measures the ratio of human wellbeing to ecosystem stress". More precisely, by substracting EWI from 100, the author obtains an Ecosystem Stress Index (ESI) and dividing HWI by ESI he obtains WSI.

"The underlying hypothesis of Wellbeing Assessment", we are told, "is that sustainable development is a combination of human wellbeing and ecosystem wellbeing" (Prescott-Allen 2001, p. 4). While this is uncontroversial, the particular kind of "combination" offered is problematic. Graphically tracing measures of performance for HWI on the vertical axis and for EWI on the horizontal axis, the author believes that the intersection of lines representing the two performance measures provides a "Barometer of Sustainability" which is equivalent to a Wellbeing Index (WI) (Prescott-Allen 2001, pp. 8–9). However, because we have no idea of the levels of reserves, recycling, reclamation, renewability, resilience and rates of change for the two performance measures and no idea of the causal connections between them (or among all the indicators represented by them), we have no idea of how sustainable the relationships may be and, therefore, how sustainable any wellbeing might be. Apart from these structural problems, the author recognizes the great difficulties shared by all researchers in selecting "performance criteria", e.g. the use of international targets, generally accepted thresholds, diverse expert opinion.

"Performance measures" provide the author's solution to the problem of reducing the multidimensional space of diverse raw data scores to a unidimensional scale. Essentially, the procedure is similar to that used by school teachers when they assign grades to students based on their performance, or rather the relationship between desired and actual performance. There are five categories of performance mapped onto a scale running from 100 to 0 thus: good = scores from 100 to 81, fair = 80–61, medium = 60–41, poor = 40–21 and bad = 20–1. The base of the scale is 0. Overall index scores are produced by averaging and summing scores, much like a teacher determines final grades and grade point averages based on several courses. While these performance measure procedures strictly speaking produce ordinal numbers, the latter are manipulated using the basic operations of arithmetic as if they were cardinal numbers. In this respect, the procedures are no better or worse than those usually used by teachers and administrators.

The five dimensions and indicators of the HWI and EWI are as follows.

Human Wellbeing Index

- *Health and Population*

  Life expectancy at birth
  Healthy life expectancy at birth
  Total fertility rate

Population with insufficient food
Prevalence of stunting (low height for age) in children under 5
Prevalence of underweight (low weight for age) in children under 5
Population with safe water and basic sanitation

- *Wealth*

Gross domestic product per person
Annual inflation rate
Annual unemployment rate
Present value of debt service as a percentage of exports of goods and services
Present value of debt service as a percentage of gross national product
Ratio of short-term debt to international reserves
Gross public debt as a percentage of gross domestic product
Annual central government deficit/surplus as a percentage of gross domestic product

- *Knowledge and Culture*

Net primary school enrollment
Net secondary school enrollment
Tertiary school enrollment
Main telephone lines and cellular phones per 100 persons
Faults per 100 main telephone lines
Internet users

- *Community*

Political rights rating
Civil liberties
Press freedom
Corruption perceptions index
Deaths from armed conflicts
Military expenditure as a percentage of gross domestic product
Homicides
Rapes
Robberies
Assaults

- *Equity*

Ratio of richest 20%'s income share to poorest 20%'s
Ratio of male income to female income
Average difference between male and female school enrollment rates
Women's share of seats in parliament

Ecosystem Wellbeing Index

- *Land*

  Converted land as a percentage of total land
  Natural land as a percentage of total land
  Annual change in native forest area
  Protected land (+ inland waters) as a percentage of total land (+ inland waters)
  Degraded land as a percentage of cultivated modified land

- *Water*

  Dam capacity as a percentage of total water supply
  Flow dammed for hydropower as a percentage of dimmable flow
  Dissolved oxygen in inland waters
  Biochemical oxygen demand (BOD)
  Chemical oxygen demand (COD)
  Nitrogen in inland waters
  Phosphorus in inland waters
  Alkalinity of inland waters
  Acidity of inland waters
  Total suspended solids in inland waters
  Fecal coliforms in inland waters
  Arsenic in inland waters
  Cadmium in inland waters
  Chromium in inland waters
  Copper in inland waters
  Lead in inland waters
  Mercury in inland waters
  Nickel in inland waters
  Zinc in inland waters
  Water withdrawal as a percentage of internal renewable supply

- *Air*

  Carbon dioxide emissions per person
  Use of ozone depleting substances (ODSs)
  Annual mean ambient air concentration of sulfur dioxide
  Days ambient air concentration of sulfur dioxide exceeds WHO guideline
  Annual mean ambient air concentration of nitrogen dioxide
  Days ambient air concentration of nitrogen dioxide exceeds WHO guideline
  Days ambient air concentration of ozone exceeds WHO guideline
  Days ambient air concentration of carbon monoxide exceeds WHO guidelines
  Annual mean ambient air concentration of suspended particulate matter (SPM)
  Annual mean ambient air concentration of fine particulates 10 micrometers or less in diameter (PM10)
  Annual mean ambient air concentration of lead

- *Species and genes*

  Threatened species in a group as a percentage of total species in that group: plants
  Threatened species in a group as a percentage of total species in that group: animals
  Number of not-at-risk breeds per million head of a species
  Ratio of threatened to not-at-risk breeds of a species

- *Resource use*

  Energy consumption per hectare of total area
  Energy consumption per person
  Food produced per harvested hectare
  Fertilizer consumed per 1,000 harvested hectares
  Food production as a percentage of supply
  Depleted + overexploited fishery species as a percentage of assessed species
  Tons of fishing fleet capacity per km^2 of continental shelf and/or inland water area
  Tons of catch per ton of fishing fleet capacity
  Fish production as a percentage of supply
  Timber feelings + imports as a percentage of net annual increment (NAI)
  Timber production + imports as a percentage of volume (Prescott-Allen 2001, pp. 300–306)

Applying his performance measure approach to figures for 180 countries in the 1996–1999 period, Prescott-Allen (2001, pp. 267–268) found that for his overall Wellbeing Index, Canada ranked seventh with a score of 60.5 (just barely fair) and the United States ranked twenty-seventh with a score of 52.0 (medium) out of a possible 100. On the Human Wellbeing Index, Canada and the United States scored 78 and 73, respectively, and on the Ecosystem Wellbeing Index, Canada and the United States scored 43 and 31, respectively. On the Ecosystem Stress Index, Canada and the United States scored 57 and 69, respectively, while on the Wellbeing/Stress Index, Canada and the United States scored 1.37 and 1.06, respectively. Collectively these figures indicate that the quality of life or wellbeing of Canadians was superior to that of Americans in the period examined.

Vital Signs 2001

In 2001 the Toronto Community Foundation initiated "a new way to engage their community in understanding and monitoring the health and vitality of Toronto on an ongoing basis". Annual reports have been produced each year that provide "a snapshot of quality of life and community vitality". In 2006, the initiative became a national program which by 2013 included over 30 communities all across the country from Wolfville, Nova Scotia to Victoria, British Columbia (http://www.vitalsignscanada.ca/en/about).

There is considerable variation in the kinds of settlement areas designated as "Vital Signs communities". The term may be applied to Canada as a whole, to provinces (e.g., Nova Scotia), CMAs (e.g., Hamilton), cities (e.g., Hamilton), particular regions (e.g., Lower Mainland British Columbia) or sets of cities (Lethbridge-Medicine Hat, Alberta).

While there was a core set of indicators recommended for all participating communities, for a variety of reasons, not all communities had the same indicators. In time, the idea of a central core for all communities was abandoned. As well, different communities occasionally had data for different years. Given these limitations, it was not possible to construct a single comprehensive index including all indicators for all communities. However, it was and is possible to craft a profile of several communities over different periods of time that would at least provide some sense of trends in different areas of concern.

Below is a list of the 44 indicators used in *Canada's Vital Signs 2011.*

Youth unemployment rate as a proportion of the overall unemployment rate, Canada, 1976–2010, per cent
Youth versus total unemployment rates in Canada, 1976–2010
Unemployment rates for youth (15–24 years), Vital Signs communities, 2010.
Seasonally unadjusted unemployment rates for youth (15–24 years), Major CMAs [Census Metropolitan Areas], 2010 and 2011, per cent
Self-reported obesity rates (age 18 and over) in Canada, 2003, 2005, and 2007–2010
Obesity rates (age 18 and over) in Major CMAs, 2010
Obesity rates (age 18 and over) in Vital Signs communities, 2010
Obesity rates (age 18 and over) by province, 2010, per cent
Business and consumer bankruptcies in Canada, 2000 and 2010
Business and consumer bankruptcies in Canada, 2000–2010
Business and consumer bankruptcies, Major CMAs, 2009
Business bankruptcies per 1,000 businesses, Vital Signs communities, 2009
Consumer bankruptcies per 1000 persons, Vital Signs communities, 2009
Child poverty rate in Canada, after-tax, 2000, 2008 and 2009
Incidence of child poverty in Canada, 2000–2009, per cent
Incidence of child poverty in Vital Signs communities, pre-tax, LIM, 2009
Incidence of child poverty in Major CMAs, 2009, per cent
Households that composted kitchen or yard waste, Canada, 2006, per cent
Per cent of households that composted kitchen waste, selected Vital Signs communities, 2009
Per cent of households that composted yard waste, Vital Signs communities, 2009
Per cent of households that composted kitchen waste, Major CMAs, 2009
Per cent of households that composted yard waste, Major CMAs, 2009

Proportion of population (15 years and older) that have not completed high school, Canada, 1990–2010
Proportion of population (15 years and older) that has not completed high school, Vital Signs communities, April 2010
Proportion of population (15 years and older) that have not completed high school, Major CMAs, 2010
Proportion of population (age 25–64) that have not completed high school, Vital Signs communities, 2006
Rental vacancy rates for rental row and apartment 2 bedroom units in Vital Signs communities, April 2011, per cent
Rental vacancy rates for rental row and apartment 2 bedroom units in Vital Signs communities, April 2010, per cent
Rental vacancy rates for rental row and apartment 2 bedroom units in Major CMAs, April 2010 and April 2011, per cent
Employment levels in Canada, January 2008–July 2011, seasonally adjusted, monthly, thousands of workers
Employment levels in Canada, 1976–2010, thousands of workers
Employment growth, Canada and Vital Signs communities, 2010, per cent
Employment growth, Major CMAs, 2010, per cent
Percentage voter turnout for federal elections, Canada, 2000, 2004, 2006, 2008 and 2011
Percentage voter turnout for the federal election, Vital Signs communities, 2011
Percentage voter turnout for the federal election, Major CMAs, 2011
Total Criminal Code traffic violations per 100,000 in Canada, 1998–2010
Criminal Code traffic violations by type, rate per 100,000 persons Canada, 1998–2010
Total Criminal Code traffic violations per 100,000 in Vital Signs communities, 2010
Total Criminal Code traffic violations per 100,000 in Major CMAs, 2010
Attendance at classical or symphonic music performances in selected Vital Signs CMAs (population age 15+), 2010, per cent
Attendance at popular music concerts in selected Vital Signs CMAs (population age 15+), 2010, per cent
Attendance at theatrical performances in selected Vital Signs CMAs (population age 15+), 2010, per cent
Attendance at cultural or artistic festivals in selected Vital Signs CMAs (population age 15+), 2010, per cent

Issue-specific national reports began being released in 2012. The first was focused on youth issues and the second on food. The general presentation format in these reports tended to have relatively descriptive narratives with some statistics, but no tables or figures.

Canadian Policy Research Networks (CPRN)

CPRN was established in 1994, "following a commitment by six federal agencies to contribute annual funding for the next five years" (CPRN 2009, p. 6). Funding continued until 2006 when the new Conservative government cancelled the grant. From 2006 to 2009 CPRN carried on with ad hoc contributions and project funding. Then beginning in 2010, Carleton University accepted all of the CPRN publications and administrative documents for its archives and also "agreed to host and maintain the CPRN website for seven years" until 2017. From its beginning in 1994 until 2009, CPRN produced over 700 policy research publications covering such topics as social innovation, civic engagement, Canadian values, environmentally sustainable communities, health and ageing, labour markets, education, job quality and affordable housing. Broadly speaking, the aim of the organization was to create knowledge and lead public dialogue on social and economic issues that are important to the well-being of Canadians" (CPRN 2009, p. 6).

In the fall of 2000, CPRN initiated a set of forty focus groups across the country involving about 350 Canadians who spent 3 hours discussing "what is important for quality of life" and what "information they need to assess progress". According to Michalski (2002), the report of results of these discussions "offers the first attempt to develop a Canadian quality of life report card based on the preferences and values expressed by Canadians…". Nine thematic groups and 40 indicators emerged from the discussions. In the CPRN (2002) *Report Card*, for each indicator a baseline value was selected as near to 1990 as possible and then compared to the most recent value, as near to 2000 as possible. For each indicator, "CPRN assigned a score indicating progress (or not) over the 1990s", with three options, Better, Mixed/No Changed or Worse. Table 17.10 is a summary of their results, with a plus (+) sign attached to an indicator if the trend showed that something had become better, a minus (−) sign if something had become worse, and a zero (0) if there was no change or mixed results.

Together, there were 11 cases in which things got better, 12 cases in which things got worse, 13 cases with mixed or unchanged results, and 4 cases without indicator values. "In summation then," Michalski (2002, p. 78) concluded, "Canada has earned a mixed review in assessing the quality of life during the 1990s. While the majority of Canadians arguably enjoyed an overall better quality of life at the end of the 1990s, any number of specific indicators could cast a more negative light on that generalization". The hope was expressed that the exercise would be "repeated every five years", but there has been no follow-up.

Table 17.10 CPRN themes and indicators

Democratic rights and participation
Exercising democratic rights: voter turnout −
Tolerance of diversity –
Health
Quality of the health care system 0
Physical health status 0
Mental health status +
Lifestyle +
Education/learning
Access to universal primary/secondary education system 0
Educational attainment +
Access to post-secondary education: tuition costs as percent of family income 0
Participation rates and enrolment NA
Access to lifelong learning −
Adult literacy rates 0
Child/youth literacy rates 0
Environment
Air quality –
Water quality +
Waste management +
Resources devoted to developing renewable energy sources 0
Access to clean, healthy public outdoor green spaces NA
Social programs and conditions
Low income rates −
Adequacy of income supports in meeting basic needs −
Availability and affordability of child care +
Living wages –
Food bank usage 0
Affordability of housing −
Community
Satisfaction with police, courts, prison and parole systems 0
Sense of personal safety and changes in crime rates +
Level of civic involvement 0
Availability of programs and services NA
Personal well-being
Personal time stress or control over time −
Degree of social interaction, intimate connections and social isolation 0
Sense of personal financial security 0
Economy and employment
Unemployment and labour force participation rates +

(continued)

Table 17.10 (continued)

Percentage of involuntary part-time workers +
Job security, satisfaction and working conditions 0
Bankruptcies (personal and business) +
Income/wealth distribution –
Consumer debt levels –
Government
Level of public trust +
Accountability/stewardship of public values and funds –
Public governance NA

Canadian Index of Well-Being 2011

The Canadian Index of Well-Being (CIW) was initiated by the Atkinson Charitable Foundation of Toronto in 1999. Between that year and 2011 when the first version of the index appeared, the foundation supported a variety of necessary organizational steps. A good history can be found on the website of the CIW. Here it is enough to say that such steps included meetings with experts and practitioners, nation-wide focus groups and round-tables, creation of a Canadian Research Advisory Group and a smaller management team, and commissioning background studies in key areas of concern that were scrupulously peer reviewed and published on the website.

The logo for the CIW includes a subtitle saying "measuring what matters", which suggests a broad understanding of well-being. It is assumed that 'overall well-being' is roughly synonymous with 'overall quality of life'. While the quantity of our lives is notoriously limited to one per person, its quality is as varied as the perspectives from which it is viewed. Viewed from one perspective, a person or society may be well off, whereas from another perspective, not at all well off. After some negotiation in the Canadian Research Advisory Group, it was decided that most of the phenomena relevant to the well-being of Canadians at the present time could be conceptualized in eight domains. The eight domains and references to commissioned reports on each domain are as follows: living standards (Sharpe and Arsenault 2010), healthy populations (Labonte et al. 2010), community vitality (Scott 2010), democratic engagement (Moore et al. 2010), leisure and culture (Smale et al. 2010), time use (Brooker and Hyman 2010), education (Guhn et al. 2010) and the environment (Morgan 2011). After reviewing a large number of available indicators, eight headline indicators (headliners) were selected for each domain. Headliners are indicators that collectively provide a comprehensive sample of all those available in a domain. All indicators are weighted equally and all domains are weighted equally.

The technical problem of constructing a unidimensional scale to reasonably represent a multidimensional construct of human well-being was solved by creating a mean percentage change rate ratios scale (percentage change scale, for short). Because percentage change scales allow trade-offs between deteriorations on some indicators to be compensated by improvements in others, they may be regarded as compensatory scales.

To create comparable index values from raw data values, the baseline value of each of the 64 headliners was set at 100 for the year 1994. Percent change increases from 100 indicate some improvement in some aspect of the quality of life and decreases indicate some deterioration. For negative indicators like crime rates, inverses of raw scores were created before percent changes were calculated. The aggregation function used for the index values for the eight headliners within each domain as well as for the composite index of the eight domains is a simple average or mean score.

Table 17.11 gives an overview of the final average scores for each of the eight domains, the 64 indicators, and the CIW itself. From this table, one can see that there were 39 headline indicators showing improvements or positive changes over the 15 year period from 1994 to 2008, and 25 showing deterioration or negative change. Over the whole period, Canadians enjoyed an 11.0% improvement in their over all wellbeing.

The CIW is now housed at the University of Waterloo and annual reports are made using most of the original headliners with some changes made to replace discontinued time series or to employ finer measures than those originally available.

Table 17.11 CIW list of indicators for all domains, with percent gains and losses 1994–2008

Domain and indicator names	Percent gains and losses
Living standards	
Ratio of top to bottom quintile of economic families, after tax	−13.9
After tax median income of economic families, 2007$	24.0
Percent of economic families in poverty	48.9
Scaled value of economic security	−8.7
Percent labour force with long-term unemployment	160.4
Percent of labour force employed	8.8
CIBC index of employment quality, 1994 QI = 100	−0.8
RBC housing affordability index	−7.7
Domain average	*26.4*
Healthy population	
Percent self-rated health as excellent or very good	−6.7
Percent claiming to have diabetes	−49.2
Life expectancy at birth, years	3.3
Percent of daily or occasional smokers among teens aged 12–19	83.3
Percent with probable depression	−11.7
Percent rating patient health services as excellent or good	2.8
Percent aged 65 years or more getting influenza immunization	34.2
Average number of remaining years expected to be lived in good health (Average HALE 15+)	−3.9

(continued)

Table 17.11 (continued)

Domain and indicator names	Percent gains and losses
Domain average	*6.6*
Community vitality	
Percent reporting participation in activities	27.3
Percent with 6 or more close friends	10.1
Property crime rate per 100,000 population	34.0
Violent crime rate per 100,000 population	1.1
Percent who feel safe walking alone after dark	10.3
Percent disagreeing that they worry less about the needs of others	55.6
Percent who provide unpaid help to others on their own	15.1
Percent reporting unpaid volunteer work in the past 12 months	12.3
Domain average	*20.7*
Democratic engagement	
Percent of voter turnout at federal elections	−11.8
Percent that are not interested in politics at all	36.6
Percent strongly agree it is every citizen's duty to vote in federal Elections	14.7
Percent reporting that they are very or fairly satisfied with the way democracy works in Canada	3.1
Percent reporting that policies of the federal government have made them better off	106.6
Ratio of registered to eligible voters	6.7
Percent of women in parliament	24.4
Net Official Development Aid as a percent of Gross National Income	−25.6
Domain average	*19.3*
Leisure and culture	
Average percent of time spent on the previous day in social leisure activities	−18.5
Average percent of time spent on the previous day in arts and culture activities	−5.4
Average number of hours in the past year volunteering for culture and recreation orgs.	−19.5
Average monthly frequency of participation in physical activity lasting over 15 min	24.5
Average attendance per performance in past year at all performing arts performances	0.5
Average visitation per site in past year to all National Parks and National Historic Sites	−21.4
Average number of nights away per trip in the past year on vacation trips to destinations over 80 km from home	11.3
Expenditures in past year on all aspects of culture and recreation as a percent of total household expenditures	4.2

(continued)

Table 17.11 (continued)

Domain and indicator names	Percent gains and losses
Domain average	*−3.0*
Time use	
Percent of 20–64 years old working ≥ 50 h per week	21.5
Percent of 20–64 years old reporting high levels of time pressure	−16.3
Percent of 20–64 years old giving unpaid care to seniors	−10.8
Percent ≥ 65 reporting daily active leisure activities	−4.5
Percent ≥ 65 reporting annual formal volunteering activities	9.2
Percent of 12–17 years old spending ≥ 2 h per day on TV or video games	−14.2
Percent 6–9 years old having $\geq$ weekly structured activities	9.0
Percent 3–5 years old read to daily by parents	1.5
Domain average	*−0.6*
Education	
Ratio of childcare spaces to children aged 0–5 years	66.7
Percent of children doing well on 5 developmental domains	3.6
Ratio of students to educators in public schools	8.2
Average of 5 social and emotional competence scores for 12–13 years old	−3.7
Basic knowledge and skills index for 13–15 years old	−0.2
Percent of PISA scores explained by socio-economic background	22.2
Percent of 20–24 population completing high school	5.8
Percent of 25–64 population with a university degree	47.4
Domain average	*18.7*
Environment	
Ground Level Ozone (population weighted in parts per billion)	−3.5
Absolute GHG Emissions (megatons of CO_2 per year)	−15.0
Primary Energy Production (petajoules)	17.7
Water Yield in Southern Canada (km^3)	3.9
Viable Non-Renewable Energy Reserves Index	60.7
Viable Metal Reserves Index	−37.3
Canadian Living Planet Index	−23.8
Marine Trophic Index	−5.3
Domain average	*−0.3*
Composite Canadian Index of Well-Being	*11.0*

Source Michalos et al. (2011)

Encyclopedia of Quality of Life and Well-Being Research 2014

The final contribution to quality of life research in Canada meriting some attention is the 12 volume *Encyclopedia of Quality of Life and Well-Being Research* (Michalos 2014). The encyclopedia had an editorial board of about 155 members from 32 countries, 1300 authors from 58 countries and 2200 articles. It had several aims. The first aim was to display in one place the vast scope and complexity of scientific and other scholarly research on the quality of life over the last 50 years, i.e., to serve as a central repository of all relevant exploration and knowledge accumulated over this period. Second, it was intended to stimulate cross-disciplinary and cross-national or cross-cultural research, leading to a greater progressive, comprehensive and coherent vision of the field. Such a vision would provide a rough road map giving some direction to the next 10–20 years of research, a third aim. Fourth, it was aimed at providing an authoritative, well-informed resource serving the needs not only of scholars and students, but of ordinary citizens, elected and unelected government officials, nongovernmental organizations (NGOs), and socially responsible corporations. Fifth, it was supposed to improve private and public policy analyses and discussions leading to better decisions and policy making concerning the quality of life of individuals and societies. Sixth, it was intended to contribute to the development and spread of evidence-based and value-based decision and policy making. Lastly, the encyclopedia was to use the latest technology to link its articles to other works available in electronic form. The strategy was to have relatively short articles linked to relevant articles across Springer's approximately 200 other reference works, so readers could build a package of information that most precisely fits their needs. (Adapted from Michalos 2014).

References

Atkinson, T. H. (1977). *Is satisfaction a good measure of the perceived quality of life?* Paper read at the Annual Meeting of the American Statistical Association, August.

Atkinson, T. H. (1979). *Trends in life satisfaction among Canadians, 1968–1977*. Occasional Paper #8 (February). Montreal: Institute for Research on Public Policy.

Atkinson, T. H. (1980). Public perceptions on the quality of life. *Perspective Canada III*, Statistics Canada (pp. 275–292).

Atkinson, T. H. (1982). The stability and validity of quality of life measures. *Social Indicators Research, 10*(2), 113–132.

Beavon, D., & Cooke, M. (2003). An application of the united nations human development index to registered Indians in Canada. In J. White, D. Beavon, & P. Maxim (Eds.), *Aboriginal conditions* (pp. 213–230). Vancouver: UBC Press.

Berger-Schmitt, R., & Jankowitsch, B. (1999). *Systems of social indicators and social reporting: The state of the art*. Mannheim: Centre for Survey Research and Methodology (ZUMA).

Blishen, B., & Atkinson, T. H. (1980). Anglophone and Francophone differences in perceptions of the quality of life in Canada. In A. Szalai & F. M. Andrews (Eds.), *The quality of life: Comparative studies* (pp. 25–40). Beverly Hills: SAGE Publications.

Bonikowska, A., Helliwell, J. F., Hou, F., & Schellenberg, G. (2014). An assessment of life satisfaction responses on recent statistics Canada surveys. *Social Indicators Research, 351*, 1–38.

Brooker, A. S., & Hyman, I. (2010). *Time use domain report*. Waterloo, Ontario: Canadian Index of Well-Being and University of Waterloo.

Brusegard, D. (1979). Rethinking national social reports. *Social Indicators Research, 6*, 261–272.

Brusegard, D. (1986). Editor's note. *Canadian Social Trends, 1*, 2.

Campbell, A., Converse, P.E., & Rodgers, W.L. (1976). *The quality of American life*. New York: Russell Sage Foundation.

Conference Board of Canada. (2013). *How Canada performs: A report card on Canada*. Ottawa, Conference Board of Canada.

Cooke, M., Beavon, E., & McHardy, M. (2004). Measuring the well-being of aboriginal people: An application of the united nations human development index to registered Indians in Canada, 1981–2001. In J. P. White, P. Maxim, & D. Beavon (Eds.), *Aboriginal policy research: Setting the agenda for change* (Vol. 1, pp. 47–69). Toronto: University of Toronto Press.

Cooke, M., Mitrou, F., Lawrence, D., Guimond, E., & Beavon, D. (2007). Indigenous well-being in four countries; An application of the UNDP's human development index to indigenous peoples in Australia, Canada, New Zealand and the United States. *BMC International Health and Human Rights, 7*(9), 1–11. doi:10.1186/1472-698X-7-9.

CPRN. (2002). *Quality of life in Canada: A citizen's report card*. Ottawa: Canadian Policy Research Networks Inc. http://relocatecanada.com/pdfdocuments/qualityoflife.pdf.

CPRN. (2009). *Farewell: Annual report*. Ottawa: Canadian Policy Research Networks Inc. http://www.cprn.org.

Diener, E., Diener, M., & Diener, C. (1995). Factors predicting the subjective well-being of nations. *Journal of Personality and Social Psychology, 69*, 851–864.

Federation of Canadian Municipalities. (2013). *Quality of life in Canadian communities: Mending Canada's frayed social safety net*. Ontario, Federation of Canadian Municipalities: The Role of Municipal Governments.

Guhn, M., Gadermann, A. M., & Zumbo, B. D. (2010). *Education domain report*. Waterloo, Ontario: Canadian Index of Well-Being and University of Waterloo.

Hagerty, M. R., & Land, K. C. (2007). Constructing summary indices of quality of life: A model for the effect of heterogeneous importance weights. *Sociological Methods and Research, 35*, 455–496.

Hagerty, M. R., & Land, K. C. (2012). Issues in composite index construction: The measurement of overall quality of life. In K. C. Land, A. C. Michalos, & M. J. Sirgy (Eds.), *Handbook of social indicators and quality of life research* (pp. 181–200). Dordrecht: Springer.

Hass, J. L., Brunvoll, F., & Hoie, H. (2002). *Overview of sustainable development indicators used by national and international agencies*. Oslo: Statistics Norway.

Labonte, R., Muhajarine, N., Winquist, B., & Quail, J. (2010). *Healthy populations domain report*. Waterloo, Ontario: Canadian Index of Well-Being and University of Waterloo.

Langlois, S., Baillargeon, J. P., Caldwell, G., Fréchet, G., Gauthier, M., & Simard, J. P. (1992). *Recent social trends in Quebec, 1960–1990*. Montreal: McGill-Queen's University Press.

LeDuc, L., Clarke, H., Jenson, J., & Pammett, J. (1974). A national sample design. *Canadian Journal of Political Science, 7*, 701–708.

Mallard, A. G. C., Lance, C. E., & Michalos, A. C. (1997). Culture as a moderator of overall life satisfaction—Life facet satisfaction relationships. *Social Indicators Research, 40*, 259–284.

McKennell, A., Atkinson, T. H., & Andrews, F. M. (1980). Structural constancies in surveys of perceived well-being. In A. Szalai & F. M. Andrews (Eds.), *The quality of life: Comparative studies* (pp. 111–128). Beverly Hills: SAGE Publications.

Meisel, J. (1973). Working papers on Canadian politics (2nd ed.). Montreal: McGill-Queen's University Press.

Michalos, A. C. (1980a). *North American social report, Vol. 1: Foundations, population and health*. Dordrecht: D. Reidel.
Michalos, A. C. (1980b). *North American social report, Vol. 2: Crime, justice and politics*. Dordrecht: D. Reidel.
Michalos, A. C. (1981a). *North American social report, Vol. 3: Science, education and recreation*. Dordrecht: D. Reidel.
Michalos, A. C. (1981b). *North American social report, Vol. 4: Environment, transportation and housing*. Dordrecht: D. Reidel.
Michalos, A. C. (1982). *North American social report, Vol. 5: Economics, religion and morality*. Dordrecht: D. Reidel.
Michalos, A. C. (1985). Multiple discrepancies theory (MDT). *Social Indicators Research, 16*, 347–413.
Michalos, A. C. (1991a). *Global report on student well-being, Vol. 1: Life satisfaction and happiness*. New York: Springer.
Michalos, A. C. (1991b). *Global report on student well-being, Vol. 2: Family, friends, living partner and self-esteem*. New York: Springer.
Michalos, A. C. (1993a). *Global report on student well-being, Vol. 3: Employment, finances, housing and transportation*. New York: Springer.
Michalos, A. C. (1993b). *Global report on student well-being, Vol. 4: Religion, education, recreation and health*. New York: Springer.
Michalos, A. C. (2000). Evaluation of equality policies for the status of women in Canada. *Social Indicators Research, 49*, 241–277.
Michalos, A. C. (2003). *Essays on the quality of life*. Dordrecht: Kluwer Academic Publishers.
Michalos, A. C. (Ed.). (2005). *Citation classics from social indicators research*. Dordrecht: Springer.
Michalos, A. C., & Kahlke, P. M. (2010). Stability and sensitivity in perceived quality of life measures: Some panel results. *Social Indicators Research, 98*(3), 403–434.
Michalos, A. C., Smale, B., Labonté, R., Muhajarine, N., Scott, K., Guhn, M., et al. (2011). *The Canadian index of wellbeing: Technical report 1.0*. Canadian Index of Wellbeing and the University of Waterloo, Waterloo, Ontario.
Michalos, A. C. (Ed.). (2014). *Encyclopedia of quality of life and well-being research*. Dordrecht: Springer.
Michalski, J. H. (2002). *Quality of life in Canada: A citizen's report card, background report*. Ottawa: Canadian Policy Research Networks Inc.
Moore, K., Swystun, L., Holden, B., Bernardin, H., Dunning, B., & Graham, P. (2010). *Democratic engagement domain report*. Waterloo, Ontario: Canadian Index of Well-Being and University of Waterloo.
Morgan, A. (2011). *Environment domain report*. Waterloo, Ontario: Canadian Index of Well-Being and University of Waterloo.
Osberg, L. (1985). The measure of Economic Well-Being. In D. Laidler (Ed.), *Approaches to economic well-being, Volume 26 of the Royal commission on the economic union and development prospects for Canada (MacDonald Commission)*. Toronto: University of Toronto Press.
Osberg, L., & Sharpe, A. (1998). *An index of economic well-being for Canada*, Research Report R-99-3E, Human Resources Development Canada, December.
Osberg, L., & Sharpe, A. (2011). *Moving from a GDP-based to a well-being based metric of economic performance and social progress: Results from the index of economic well-being for OECD countries, 1980–2009*. Ottawa: Centre for the Study of Living Standards.
Prescott-Allen, R. (2001). *The wellbeing of nations: A country-by-country index of quality of life and the environment*. Washington: Island Press.
Roberts, L. W., Clifton, R. A., Ferguson, B., Kampen, K., & Langlois, S. (Eds.). (2005). *Recent social trends in Canada, 1960–2000*. Montreal: McGill-Queen's University Press.
Royal Commission on Aboriginal Peoples. (1996). *Report of the royal commission on aboriginal peoples*. Ottawa: Minister of Supply and Services Canada.

Royal Commission on the Status of Women. (1970). *Report of the royal commission on the status of women in Canada*. Ottawa: Information Canada.

Scott, K. (2010). *Community vitality domain report*. Waterloo, Ontario: Canadian Index of Well-Being and University of Waterloo.

Sharpe, A., & Arsenault, J. F. (2010). *Living standards domain report*. Waterloo, Ontario: Canadian Index of Well-Being and University of Waterloo.

Sharpe, A., & Andrews, B. (2012). *An assessment of weighting methodologies for composite indicators: The case of the index of economic well-being*. Centre for the Study of Living Standards: Ottawa.

Smale, B., Donohoe, H., Pelot, C., Croxford, A., & Auger, D. (2010). *Leisure and culture domain report*. Waterloo, Ontario: Canadian Index of Well-Being and University of Waterloo.

Statistics Canada. (1974). *Perspective Canada I*. Ottawa: Minister of Supply and Services.

Statistics Canada. (1977). *Perspective Canada II*. Ottawa: Minister of Supply and Services.

Statistics Canada. (1980). *Perspectives Canada III*. Ottawa: Minister of Supply and Services.

Statistics Canada. (2012a). *Aboriginal peoples survey (APS)*. Ottawa: Ministry of Industry.

Statistics Canada. (2012b). *High level indicators—Aboriginal peoples survey 2012*. Ottawa: Ministry of Industry.

Statistics Canada. (2013a). *Health at a glance: Select health indicators of first nations people living off reserve, Métis and Inuit*. Cat. No. 82-624-X. Ottawa: Minister of Industry.

Statistics Canada. (2013b). *General social survey: An overview, 2013*. Cat. No. 89F0115X. Ottawa: Minister of Industry.

Statistics Canada. (2013c). *The education and employment experiences of first nations people living off reserve, Inuit, and Métis: Selected findings from the 2012 aboriginal peoples survey*. Cat. No. 89-653-X–No. 001. Ottawa: Minister of Industry.

Status of Women Canada. (1995). *Setting the stage for the next century: The federal plan for gender equality*. Ottawa: Status of Women Canada.

United Nations Development Program. (1996). *Human Development Report*. New York: Oxford University Press.

Appendix

History in Photographs

See Figs. A.1, A.2, A.3, A.4, A.5, A.6, A.7, A.8, A.9 and A.10.

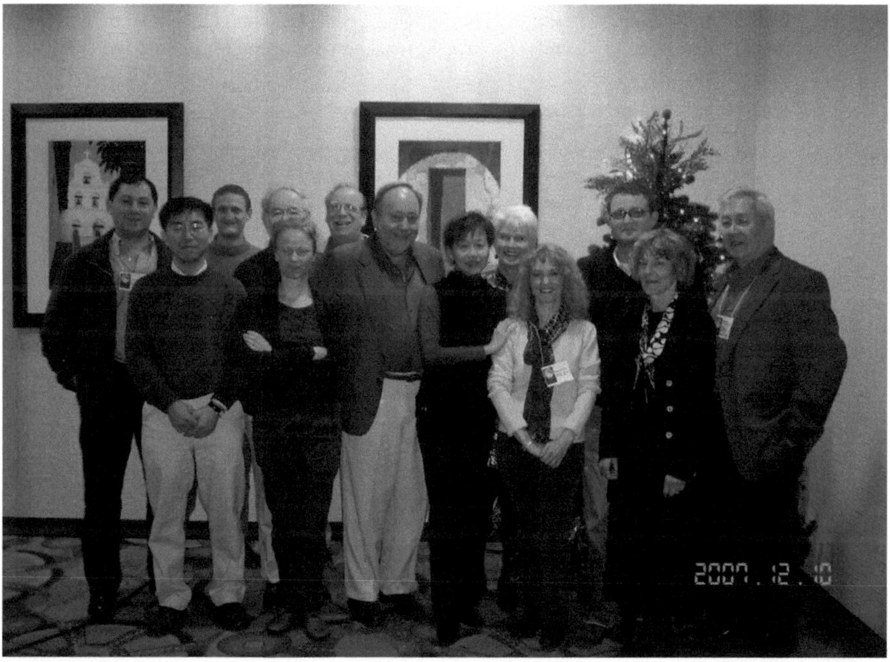

Fig. A.1 Members of ISQOLS meeting at San Diego, California in 2007. From *left* Mariano Rojas, Don Jin, Dave Webb, Richard J. Estes, Peggy Schyns, Richard A. Easterlin, Robert A. Cummins, Anna L. D. Lau, Elizabeth Eckermann, Filomena Maggino, Denis Huschka, Valerie Moller and Mahar Mangahas

A.C. Michalos, *Connecting the Quality of Life Theory to Health, Well-Being and Education*, DOI 10.1007/978-3-319-51161-0

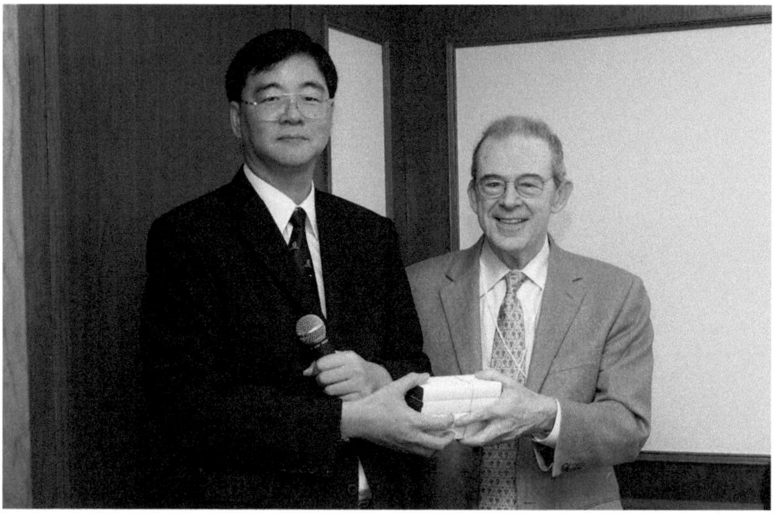

Fig. A.2 Daniel T.L. Shek and Alex at the International Conference on Human Development and the Environment: Advances in Quality of Life Studies, on the Anniversary of the New Asia College in Hong Kong 2008

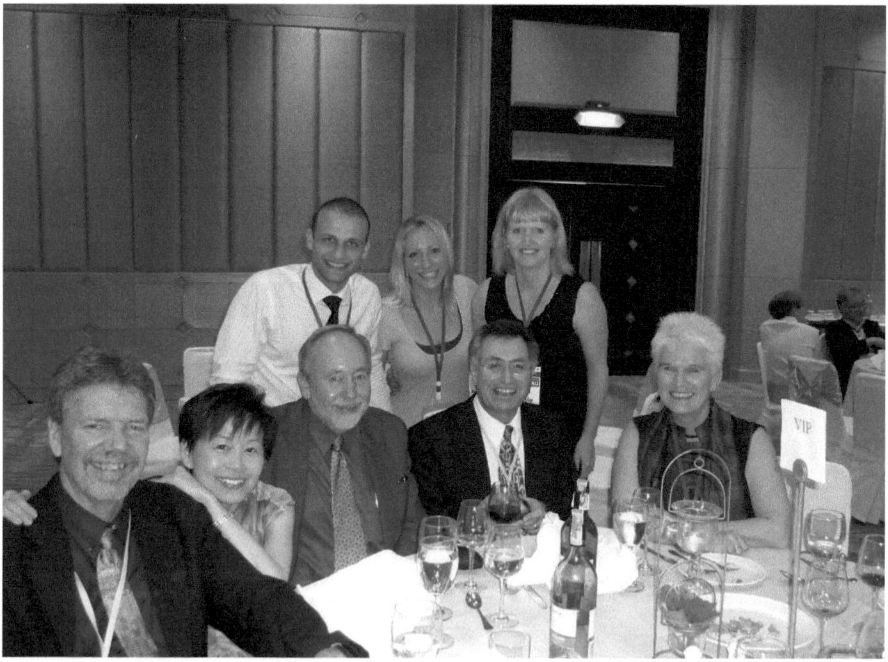

Fig. A.3 Members of ISQOLS meeting at Bangkok, Thailand in 2009. Front row from *left* Don Rahtz, Anna L.D. Lau, Robert A. Cummins, M. Joseph Sirgy, Elizabeth Eckermann. *Back row* Adrian Tomyn, Melissa Weinberg and Melanie Davern

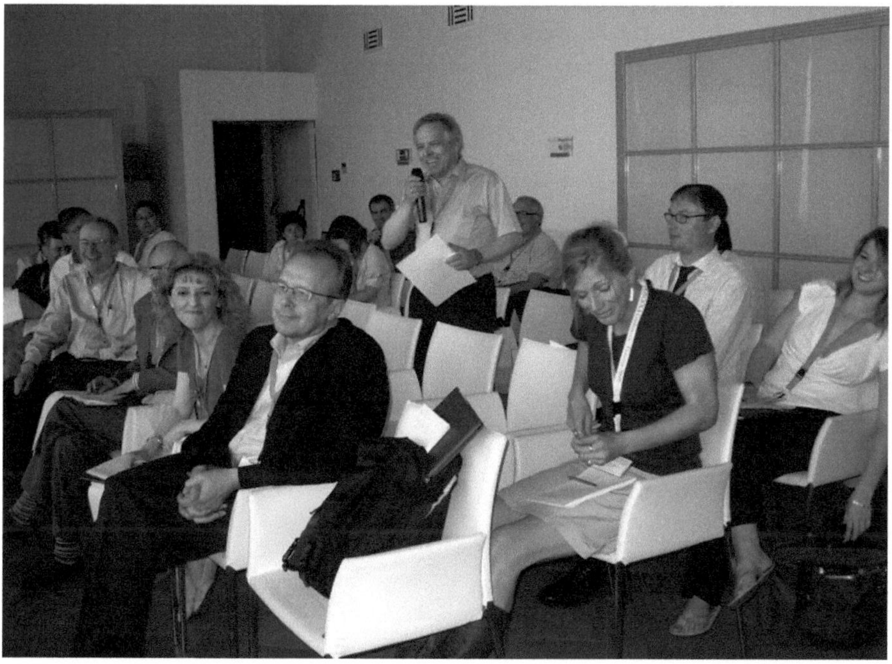

Fig. A.4 Participants in Satellite Conference on Measuring Subjective Well-Being: An Opportunity for National Statistical Offices? at Florence, Italy in 2010. From *left* Alex, Filomena Maggino, Heinz-Herbert Noll, Wolfgang Glatzer

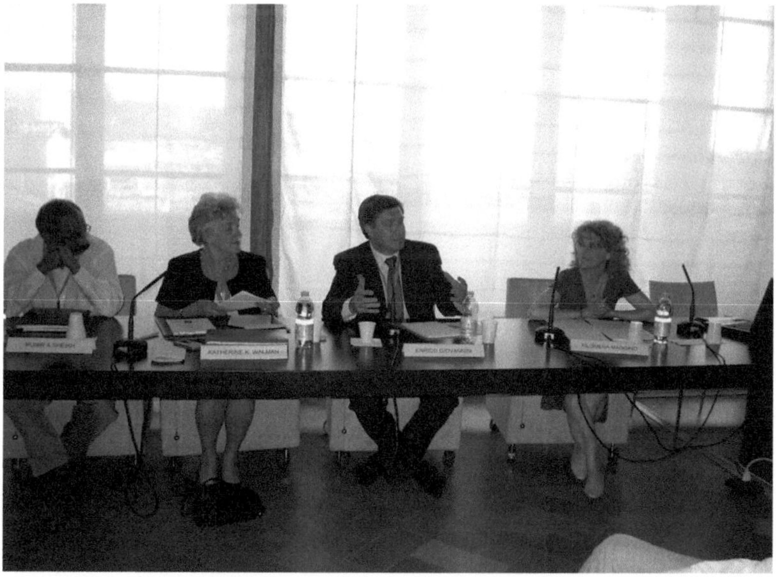

Fig. A.5 Participants in Satellite Conference at Florence in 2010. From *left* Munir Sheik, Katherine K. Wallman, Enrico Giovannini and Filomena Maggino

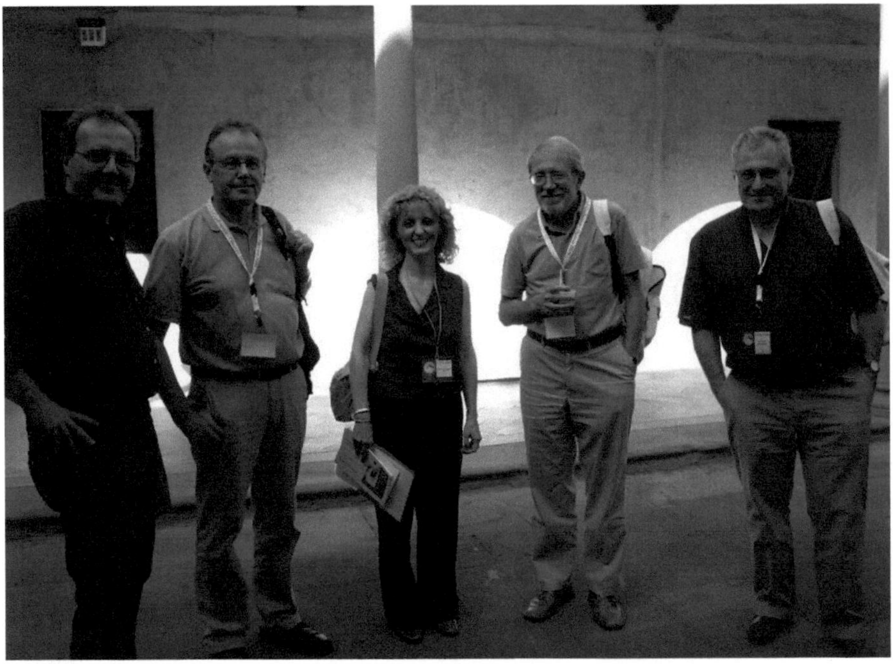

Fig. A.6 Members of ISQOLS meeting at Florence, Italy in 2010. From *left* Giampoalo Nuvolati, Heinz-Herbert Noll, Filomena Maggino, Willem Saris and Daniel Byk

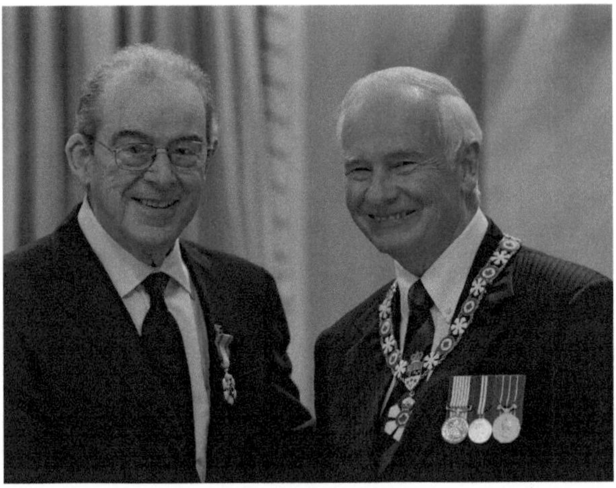

Fig. A.7 Alex becoming a Member of the Order of Canada with the Governor General, David Johnston in 2010

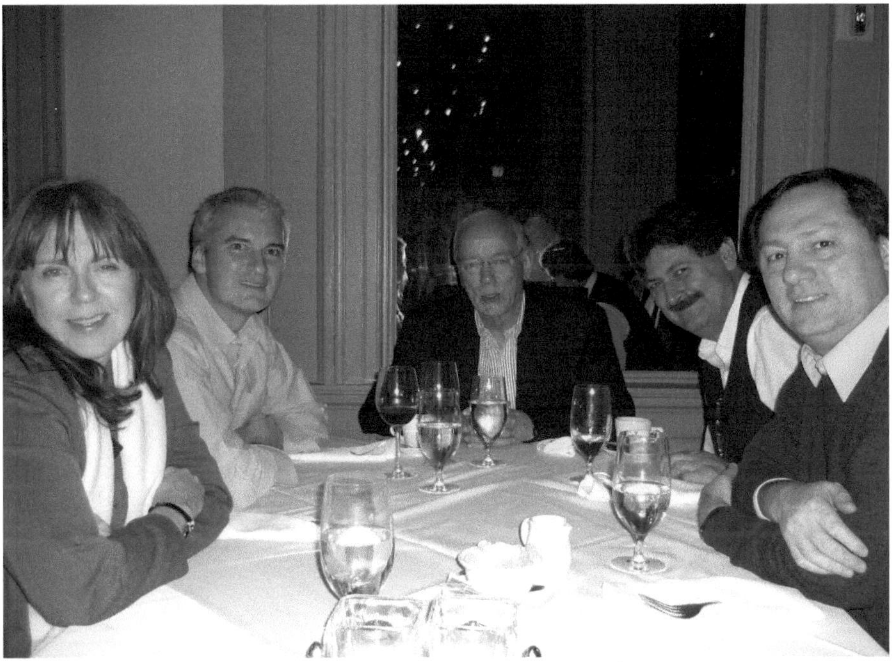

Fig. A.8 Participants in the Halloran Project on the History of Well-Being at Philadelphia, Pennsylvania in 2012. From *left* Rhonda Phillips, Andrew Clark, Kenneth C. Land, Jose Garcia Vega and Mariano Rojas

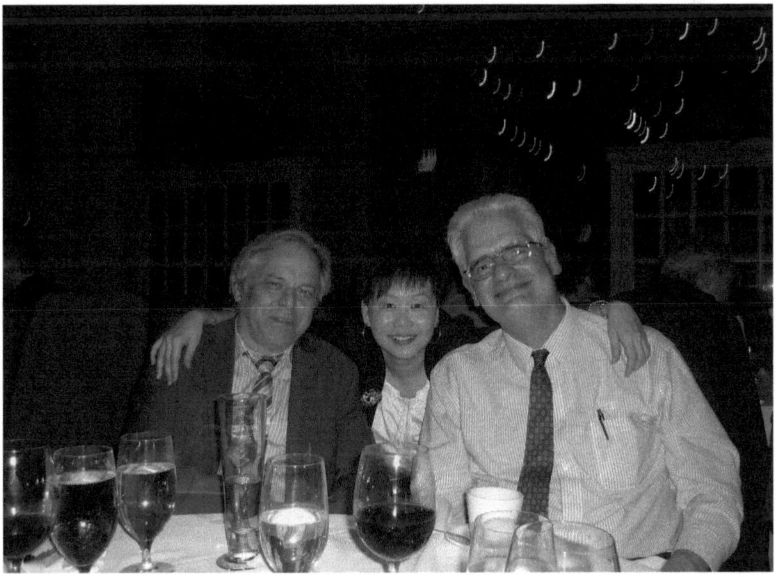

Fig. A.9 Wolfgang Glatzer, Anna L.D. Lau and Michael Frisch at the Halloran meeting in Philadelphia 2012

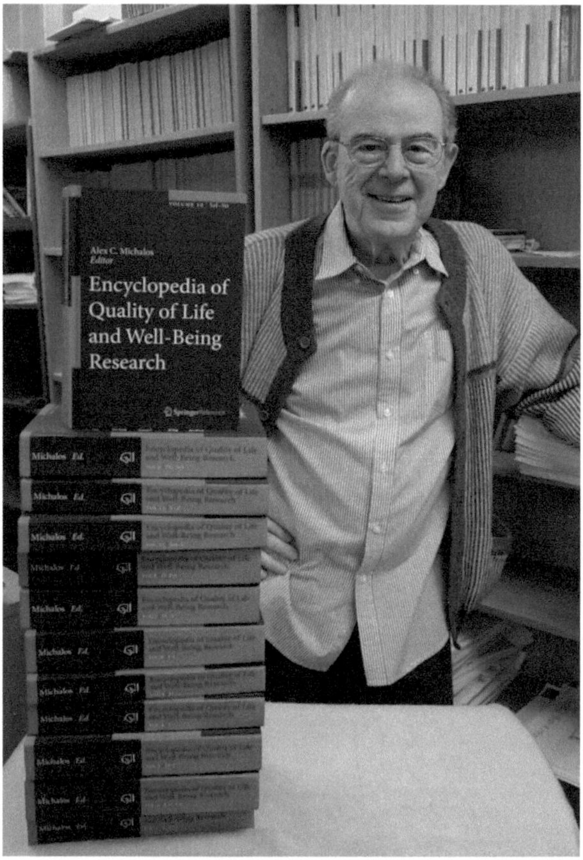

Fig. A.10 Alex with the 12 volumes of the *Encyclopedia of Quality of Life and Well-Being Research* in April 2014

MIX
Papier aus verantwortungsvollen Quellen
Paper from responsible sources
FSC® C105338

If you have any concerns about our products,
you can contact us on
ProductSafety@springernature.com

In case Publisher is established outside the EU,
the EU authorized representative is:
Springer Nature Customer Service Center GmbH
Europaplatz 3, 69115 Heidelberg, Germany

Printed by Libri Plureos GmbH
in Hamburg, Germany